METALS IN MEDICINE

VOLUME 1

Metals for Tissue Engineering and Pharmaceutical Applications

Metals in Medicine, 2-volume set: Volume 1: Metals for Tissue Engineering and Pharmaceutical Applications / Volume 2: Metallic Nanoparticles for Biomedical Applications
ISBN: 978-1-77491-710-7 (hbk)
ISBN: 978-1-77491-713-8 (pbk)

Metals in Medicine, Volume 1: Metals for Tissue Engineering and Pharmaceutical Applications
ISBN: 978-1-77491-711-4 (hbk)
ISBN: 978-1-77491-712-1 (pbk)
ISBN: 978-1-00353-818-9 (ebk)

Metals in Medicine, Volume 2: Metallic Nanoparticles for Biomedical Applications
ISBN: 978-1-77491-714-5 (hbk)
ISBN: 978-1-77491-715-2 (pbk)
ISBN: 978-1-00353-845-5 (ebk)

METALS IN MEDICINE

VOLUME 1

Metals for Tissue Engineering and Pharmaceutical Applications

Sonali Sundram, MPharm

Rishabha Malviya, PhD

GSN Koteswara Rao, PhD

Editors

APPLE ACADEMIC PRESS

First edition published 2025

Apple Academic Press Inc.
1265 Goldenrod Circle, NE,
Palm Bay, FL 32905 USA

760 Laurentian Drive, Unit 19,
Burlington, ON L7N 0A4, CANADA

CRC Press
2385 NW Executive Center Drive,
Suite 320, Boca Raton FL 33431

4 Park Square, Milton Park,
Abingdon, Oxon, OX14 4RN UK

Library and Archives Canada Cataloguing in Publication

Title: Metals in medicine / Sonali Sundram, MPharm, Rishabha Malviya, PhD, GSN Koteswara Rao, PhD, editors.
Names: Sundram, Sonali, editor. | Malviya, Rishabha, editor. | Koteswara Rao, GSN (Gudhanti Siva Nago), editor.
Description: First edition. | Includes bibliographical references and index.
Identifiers: Canadiana (print) 20240466578 | Canadiana (ebook) 20240466594 | ISBN 9781774917107 (set ; hardcover) | ISBN 9781774917138 (set ; softcover) | ISBN 9781774917114 (v. 1 ; hardcover) | ISBN 9781774917121 (v. 1 ; softcover) | ISBN 9781003538189 (v. 1 ; ebook)
Subjects: LCSH: Metals in medicine.
Classification: LCC R857.M37 M48 2025 | DDC 610.28—dc23

Library of Congress Cataloging-in-Publication Data

CIP data on file with US Library of Congress

ISBN: 978-1-77491-711-4 (hbk)
ISBN: 978-1-77491-712-1 (pbk)
ISBN: 978-1-00353-818-9 (ebk)

Dedication

This book is dedicated to

Honorable CEO of Galgotias University

Mr. Dhruv Galgotia

Thank you, sir, for your continuous support and

motivation to undertake this research.

About the Editors

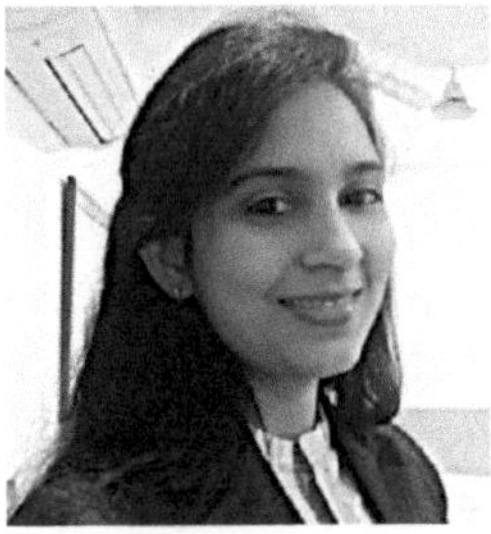

Sonali Sundram,
Assistant Professor, School of Medical and Allied Sciences, Galgotias University, Greater Noida, Uttar Pradesh, India

Sonali Sundram, MPharm, is Assistant Professor in the School of Medical and Allied Sciences at Galgotias University, Greater Noida, Uttar Pradesh, India. Previously, she worked as a research scientist on a project of the Indian Council of Medical Research (ICMR) at King George's Medical University, Lucknow, India. After that, she joined BBDNIIT (Babu Banarasi Das Northern India Institute of Technology), Lucknow. Her PhD (Pharmacy) work was in Neurodegeneration and Nanoformulation. Her areas of interest include neurodegeneration, clinical research, and artificial intelligence. She has authored and edited more than 15 books (published by Wiley, CRC Press/Taylor and Francis, IOP Publishing, Apple Academic Press/Taylor and Francis, Springer Nature and River Publisher) and has organized more than 15 national and international seminars, conferences, and workshops. She has more than eight patents, both national and international, to her credit. She has published six SCI-indexed manuscripts (cumulative impact factor: 20.71) with reputed international publishers. She has delivered oral presentations at international conferences organized in different European countries. She completed both her BPharm and MPharm (Pharmacology) at Dr. A.P.J. Abdul Kalam Technical University, Lucknow, India.

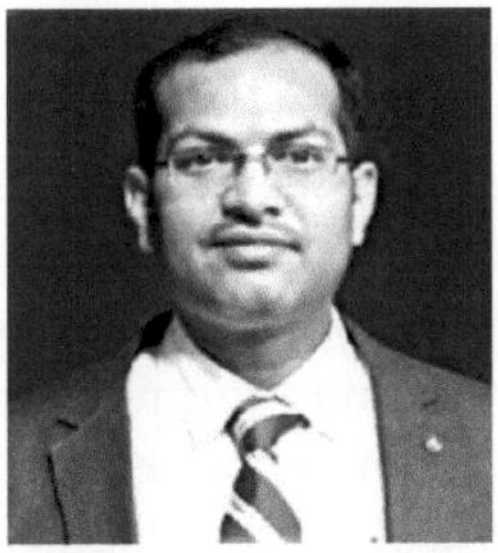

Rishabha Malviya, PhD
Associate Professor, Department of Pharmacy, School of Medical and Allied Sciences, Galgotias University, India

Rishabha Malviya, PhD, has 11 years of research experience and is presently working as Associate Professor in the Department of Pharmacy, School of Medical and Allied Sciences, Galgotias University, India. His areas of interest include formulation optimization, nanoformulation, targeted drug delivery, localized drug delivery, and characterization of natural polymers as pharmaceutical excipients. He has authored more than 150 research/review papers for national/international journals of repute. He has over 50 patents to his name and many publications in reputed national and international journals (with a total of 91 cumulative impact factor). He has also received an Outstanding Reviewer Award from Elsevier. He has edited books (Wiley, Springer Nature, CRC Press/Taylor and Francis, Apple Academic Press, River Publisher, Lambert, etc.) and authored 15 book chapters. His name has been included in the Stanford University's World's Top 2% Scientists, 2020 by Elsevier BV and Stanford University. He is a reviewer, editor, and editorial board member for more than 50 national and international journals. He was an invited author for the magazine *Atlas of Science* as well as a pharma magazine dealing with the B2B industry, *Ingredients South Asia.* He completed his BPharm at Uttar Pradesh Technical University and MPharm (Pharmaceutics) at Gautam Buddha Technical University, Lucknow, Uttar Pradesh, India. His PhD (Pharmacy) work was in novel formulation development techniques.

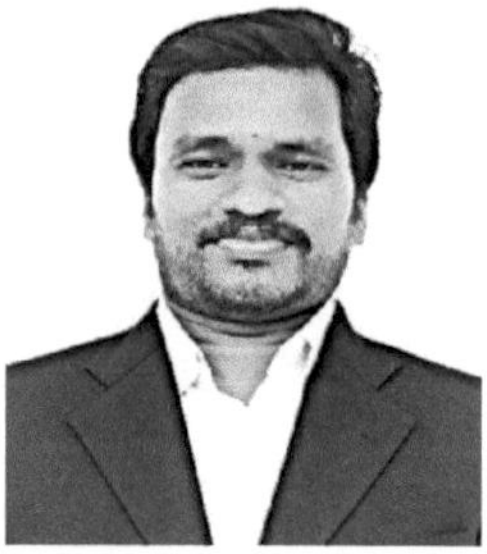

GSN Koteswara Rao, PhD, MPharm, MBA
Professor and Head of the Department of Pharmaceutics, SPPSPTM, SVKM's NMIMS University, Mumbai, India

GSN Koteswara Rao, PhD, MPharm, MBA, is Professor and Head of the Department of Pharmaceutics at SPPSPTM, SVKM's NMIMS University, Mumbai, India. He has 15 years of academic, research, and administrative experience. He has received several awards and is also a recipient of a UGC fellowship. He presented his research outcomes at the American Association of Pharmaceutical Scientists (AAPS) at San Diego, California, USA, in 2017. He has published more than 75 research papers in reputed national and international journals. In addition, he has also published 10 books and book chapters with international publishers such as Elsevier, Springer, and Wiley. He has participated in more than 80 national and international conferences, seminars, symposia, workshops, and faculty development programs. His areas of research interest include formulation design, development of novel drug delivery systems, bioanalytical method development, in vitro and vivo studies, biopharmaceutical evaluation, and pharmacokinetic-pharmacodynamic drug interactions.

Contents

Contributors

R. Abdel-Karim
Metallurgy and Advanced Materials, Faculty of Engineering, Cairo University, Giza, Egypt

Rajasekhar Reddy Alavalaa
Shobhaben Pratapbhai Patel School of Pharmacy & Technology Management, SVKM's NMIMS, V.L. Mehta Road, Vile Parle (W), Mumbai, India

Aparna Badwane
Shobhaben Pratapbhai Patel School of Pharmacy & Technology Management, SVKM's NMIMS, Vile Parle (W), Mumbai, India

Roja Rani Budha
Shobhaben Pratapbhai Patel School of Pharmacy & Technology Management, SVKM's NMIMS, Vile Parle (W), Mumbai, India

Shikha Chaudhary
Department of Pharmacy, School of Medical and Allied Sciences, Galgotias University, Greater Noida, India

Ajaykumar Chittipolu
Vision College of Pharmaceutical Sciences and Research, JNTUH, Hyderabad, India

Uma Sankar Gorla
K L College of Pharmacy, Koneru Lakshmaiah Education Foundation, Guntur, Andhra Pradesh, India

Nachiket Joshi
Shobhaben Pratapbhai Patel School of Pharmacy & Technology Management, SVKM's NMIMS, Vile Parle (W), Mumbai, India

Parth Joshi
Shobhaben Pratapbhai Patel School of Pharmacy & Technology Management, SVKM's NMIMS, Vile Parle (W), Mumbai, India

Mahesh V. Kamble
School of Nanoscience and Biotechnology, Shivaji University, Kolhapur, India

Sathish Kumar Konidala
Department of Pharmaceutical Sciences, School of Biotechnology and Pharmaceutical Sciences, Vignans Foundation for Science, Technology and Research, Vadlamudi, Guntur, Andhra Pradesh, India

Reet Minhasa
Shobhaben Pratapbhai Patel School of Pharmacy & Technology Management, SVKM's NMIMS, Vile Parle (W), Mumbai, India

Sachin V. Otari
School of Nanoscience and Biotechnology, Shivaji University, Kolhapur, Maharashtra, India

Aryan Patel
Shobhaben Pratapbhai Patel School of Pharmacy & Technology Management, SVKM's NMIMS, Vile Parle (W), Mumbai, India

Darshan Patel
Shobhaben Pratapbhai Patel School of Pharmacy & Technology Management, SVKM's NMIMS, Vile Parle (W), Mumbai, India

Mital Patel
Shobhaben Pratapbhai Patel School of Pharmacy & Technology Management, SVKM's NMIMS, Vile Parle (W), Mumbai, India

Kiran D. Pawar
School of Nanoscience and Biotechnology, Shivaji University, Kolhapur, India

Rohit Raj
Shobhaben Pratapbhai Patel School of Pharmacy & Technology Management, SVKM's NMIMS, Vile Parle (W), Mumbai, India

GSN Koteswara Rao
Shobhaben Pratapbhai Patel School of Pharmacy & Technology Management, SVKM's NMIMS, V.L. Mehta Road, Vile Parle (W), Mumbai, India

Naresh Babu Rekha
Nirmala College of Pharmacy, Atmakur, Mangalagiri, Guntur, Andhra Pradesh, India

Komal Sharma
Shobhaben Pratapbhai Patel School of Pharmacy and Technology Management, SVKM's NMIMS, Vile Parle (W), Mumbai, India

Honisha Shah
Shobhaben Pratapbhai Patel School of Pharmacy & Technology Management, SVKM's NMIMS, V.L. Mehta Road, Vile Parle (W), Mumbai, India

Priyal Shah
Shobhaben Pratapbhai Patel School of Pharmacy & Technology Management, SVKM's NMIMS, Vile Parle (W), Mumbai, India

Madhura Tiwari
Shobhaben Pratapbhai Patel School of Pharmacy & Technology Management, SVKM's NMIMS, Vile Parle (W), Mumbai, India

Devdhar Yadav
Department of Pharmacy, School of Medical and Allied Sciences, Galgotias University, Greater Noida, India

Abbreviations

AgNPs	silver nanoparticles
AgO	silver oxide
Al_2O_3	aluminum oxide
ALP	alkaline phosphatase
BMP-2	bone morphogenetic protein 2
CDDP	cis-diamminedichlo-platinum
CeO2	selenium oxide
CLEM	correlative light and electron microscopy
Co	cobalt
CoMOFs	cobalt metal organic frameworks
CP	calcium phosphate
CSNCPs	core-shell nanocomposites
CT	computer tomography
CuO	copper oxide
CuS	copper sulfide
CV	cyclic voltammetry
CVD	chemical vapor deposition
DAB	diaminobenzindine
DNA	deoxyribonucleic acid
DOX	doxorubicin
DPV	differential pulsed voltammetry
ECL	electro-chemilumeinescenc
ECM	extracellular matrix
EIS	electro-chemical impedance spectroscopy
EMWA	electromagnetic wave absorption
FAM	fluorescein amidite
Fe	ferrous
FeONPs	ferrous oxide nanoparticles
FRET	fluorescence resonance energy transfer
GO	graphene oxide
GOx	glucose oxidase
HA	hydroxyapatite
HDPE	high density polyethylene
HRP	horseradish peroxidase

ICG	inert gas condensation
Lox	lactate oxidase
Mg	magnesium
MgO	magnesium Oxide
MOFs	metal organic frameworks
MRI	magnetic resonance imaging
NaOH	sodium hydroxide
Nb	niobium
Ni-IRMOF	nickel-isoreticular metal organic frameworks
NiO	nickel oxide
NIR	near infra-red
NK	natural killer
Nm	nanometer
NMOFs	nanometal-organic frameworks
NOAEL	no observed adverse effect level
NP	nanoparticle
NSAIDS	non-steroidal anti-inflammatory drugs
ORR	oxygen releasing reactions
Pd	palladium
PdNP	palladium nanoparticle
PEC	photoelectron-chemical chemistry
PEG	polyethylene glycol
PET	photoinduced electron transfer
PLGA	poly(l-lactide-co-glycolide acid)
Pt	platinum
PtNP	platinum nanoparticle
QDs	quantum dots
ROS	reactive oxygen species
ssDNA	single-stranded DNA
SWV	square wave voltammetry
Ta	tantalum
TAMRA	trimethylrhodamine
TCP	tricalcium phosphate
TE	tissue engineering
TERM	tissue engineering and regenerative medicines
TGF	transforming growth factor
Ti	titanium
TiO_2	titanium oxide
Zr	zirconium
ZrO_2	zirconium oxide

Foreword

Since metals have unique features that are not found in typical carbon-based drugs, the recent trend in drug discovery can be applied to the development of novel metal-based therapies. This book, edited by Dr. Rishabha Malviya and Dr. Sonali Sundram, is very interesting and represents a distinct field of investigation. One of the most fascinating subjects in the latest report is the use of noble metals in the health sector. The medical field has been most significantly influenced by the widespread use of noble metal nanoparticles, nanocompounds, or nanostructures in many fields of research and technology. This impact influences people's quality of life. Metal nanostructures have the potential for use in biomedicine, which is a brand new and attractive area for research.

The purpose of this work was to consolidate the findings from years of study to present the most exciting applications of metal-based drugs in modern biological and medical research. *Metals in Medicine Volumes 1 and 2* offer an interesting union of disciplines, bringing together the hard science of inorganic chemistry with the complexities and variety of biochemistry and physiology. Those who work in the fields of biological engineering, metallurgical engineering, chemistry, pharmaceutical sciences, and drug development will benefit from both volumes. I believe that this book will be an excellent resource for educators as well as learners with undergraduate, graduate, and postgraduate degrees in the biomedical field.

—**Prof. Roop Krishen Khar**
Director, B. S. Anangpuria Educational Institutes
Ballabgarh Sohna Road, Alampur, Faridabad, India
Director, Formulators Koncept Pvt. Ltd.
Director, Unicure India Ltd.
Former Dean & HOD, Jamia Hamdard, New Delhi, India

Preface

Metals have been used for health and healing for thousands of years. In the last 50 years, there has been significant development in the idea of using modern medicinal chemistry methods to consciously investigate the structure and characteristics of inorganic complexes for medicinal function. In medicine, metal ions are needed for their function as drugs and as diagnostic tools. Potential therapeutic applications of metal complexes is still underexplored, but their study could be beneficial in the development of new therapeutics.

Metals have often attracted the interest of numerous research centers across the world due to their complex biological activity and wide variety of effects on the human organism; for this reason, their usage in medicine is a particular concern. This volume, *Metals in Medicine, Volume 1: Metals for Tissue Engineering and Pharmaceutical Applications,* presents the application of metal-containing compounds that will function as essential tools in medical science for the imaging and diagnosis of disease states in an organism as well as for the treatment of many diseases or for their prevention.

In this book, we present a curated collection of the latest medicinal and inorganic chemical research featuring metals for medicinal applications. This book is published in two volumes, starting with an introduction of metallodrugs and their application in the biomedical fields, including tissue engineering, drug delivery, bioimaging, biosensing, and bone tissue engineering.

Metals in Medicine, Volume 2: Metallic Nanoparticles for Biomedical Applications illustrates the possible applications of different types of metal active drugs in the pharmaceutical and biomedical field. This volume provides valuable therapeutic and diagnostic properties of metallic drugs that will be of significant interest for healthcare readers. This book's concept will connect the fields of inorganic chemistry and medicine. Scientists from a variety of disciplines who are specialized in their fields have contributed to this volume.

Metals in Medicine is intended to serve as a reference for graduate students, postdoctoral researchers, and those working in the fields of materials science, biomedical engineering, and metalloengineering. The contents of these volumes will enable readers to comprehend how metals function as drugs and how they are used in a wide range of fields.

The editors are very thankful to all contributors for helping in this important edition. We also express our warmest gratitude toward Apple Academic Press for their continuous support and guidance.

CHAPTER 1

Recent Advancements in Nanoporous Metal Foams for Biomedical Applications: Processing and Mechanical Properties

R. ABDEL-KARIM

Department of Metallurgy and Advanced Materials, Faculty of Engineering, Cairo University, Giza, Egypt

ABSTRACT

Agricultural, energy, environmental, biosensing, tissue engineering, and biomedical implants are just a few of the applications in which nanoporous (NP) materials may be used. Due to their distinctive chemical and physical characteristics in comparison to other nanoparticles and bulk correspondence well as their configurable porosity and pore geometry (size, shape, and distribution), nanoporous metal foams (NPMFs) are regarded as an essential class of nanoscale materials. They stand out for their reduced weight, great energy absorption, rigidity, and damping capability. Metals such as titanium (Ti) and its alloys, magnesium, and tantalum are porously produced. In this review, the production techniques, properties as well as application techniques of metal foams used as biomaterials, are discussed. The primary constraints and potential future prospects for NPMFs in these fields are also covered.

1.1 INTRODUCTION

Nanoporous (NP) materials also have unique surface and structural properties, a large surface area, customizable pore sizes, tunable pore geometries, and surface topographies with porous architectures. Their applications various

Metals in Medicine, Volume 1: Metals for Tissue Engineering and Pharmaceutical Applications.
Sonali Sundram, Rishabha Malviya, and GSN Koteswara Rao

TABLE 1.1 Surface Morphology and Biomedical Applications of Different NPMFs.[12]

Material type	Material	Pore size and morphology	Biomedical applications
(i) Inorganic	Anodic aluminum oxide (AAO)	5 nm–10 μm, uniform pores, high density	Cell culture, biosensing: drug delivery, molecular sieving, chromatography.
	Si, SiO_2, other semiconductors	2 nm–3 μm, uniform pores, high density	Biosensing, cell culture, drug delivery, biomimicking.
(ii) Organic (pore morphology defined by fabrication process)	Polydimethylsiloxane (PDMS)	800 nm–500 μm	Micropatterning, microfiltration, cell operation, organ on chip, bioassay.
	Polycarbonate (PC)	1 nm–1 mm	Bioassay, separation, filtration, drug delivery, microfiltration, ultrafiltration, micropatterning.
	PE	>20 nm	Organ on chip, microfiltration.
	Polystyrene (PS)	0.7 nm–1 pm	Ultrafiltration, nanopatterning, drug delivery.
	Parylene	5 nm–1 mm	Cell culture, drug delivery, microfiltration.
	PET	100 nm–8 μm	The bioparticle operation, cell culture, and organ chips.
	Polymethyl methacrylate (PMMA)	0.7 nm–5 μm	Drug delivery.
	Polylactic acid (PLA)	300 nm–1 μm	Wound care, bone regeneration, adhesive anchor.
(iii) Polymer composite	Ceramics/polymer Oxide + polymer	nm pore size by pore-filling coating	Micro- and ultrafiltration.

1.2.1 *DEALLOYING APPROACHES*

There are several common dealloying processes, including chemical, electrochemical, liquid metal dealloying (LMD), vapor phase, and solid phase dealloying.[21]

This dealloying method is distinguished by its simplicity of fabrication, ability to manufacture numerous samples concurrently in a batch, ease of tuning the size of the pores and ligaments, suitability for self-supported NP-metal structures, and reduced reliance on extremely corrosive solvents. Drawbacks include the use of caustic solvents, the inclusion of impurities from less-noble metals, the requirement for time-consuming preparation of thicker and more electrodes, and the electrolyte being polluted after dealloying and possibly requiring replacement after each dealloying.[22] The creation of porosity during dealloying is shown in Figure 1.2: (a) The more-noble component (grey) diffuses along the interface to agglomerate,

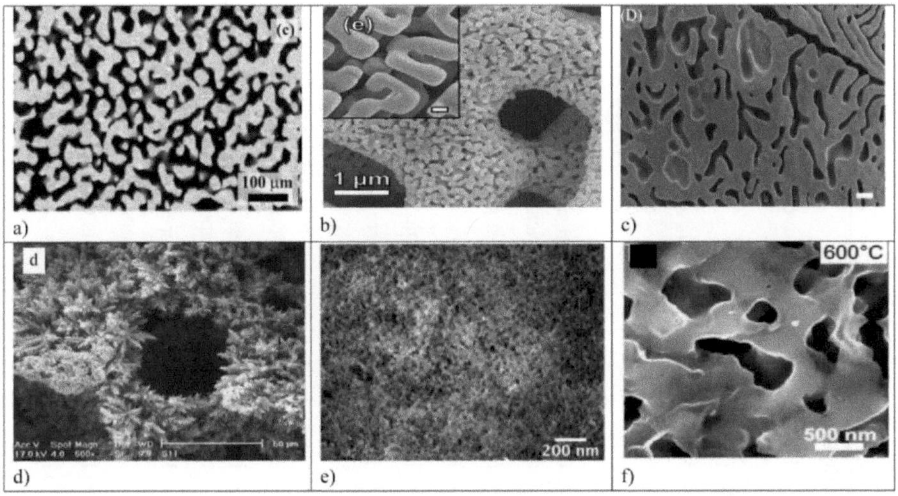

FIGURE 1.1 NP microstructures obtained from different synthesis techniques. (a) Au–foam synthesized through dealloying; (b) Hierarchical Au network prepared by reduction-induced decomposition. Inset shows upper hierarchy level; (c) NP single crystal Au particles prepared by eutectic decomposition of Au–Ge and selective etching of Ge; (d) NP Ag prepared by redox induced replacement of copper foam; (e) Directionally grown Al-ligaments made by galvanic replacement; (f) NP Al with native oxide shell through galvanic replacement reaction.

Source: Reprinted with permission from a) Ref. [15], b) Ref. [16], c) Ref. [17], d) Ref. [18], e) Ref. [19], Ref. [20]

whereas the less noble species' (gray) atoms are dissolved from the alloy. (b) The development of mounds rich in noble materials (yellowish region). (c) The undercutting of the otherwise passivated mounds, which led to the initial formation of the ligament structure.[23]

As the less-noble dissolving element is removed from the surface according to Erlebacher's description of the kinetics of electrochemical dealloying, atoms of the higher noble elements that are still retained condense into groups, exposing patches of unalloyed material to the electrolyte. The construction of a stable porous structure is caused by competition between these two mechanisms' rates—the rate of dissolution and the rate of interface diffusion—and this competition determines the porosity's distinctive length scale. The size of the pores can be modified using experimental variables. For instance, with a greater applied potential, both mechanisms' rates rise, but the dissolution rate increases much more quickly, which shrinks the typical length scale, resulting in a considerably finer porous structure.[24]

TABLE 1.2 Methods for Manufacturing Nanoporous Materials.[1]

Fabrication technique		Advantages	Disadvantages
1. Dealloying	**Electrochemical**	• Better control over porosity and chemical composition than chemical dealloying. • Low-temperature one-step process. • No need to prepare alloy beforehand. • No need for highly concentrated corrosive chemicals. • Low chances of impurity on surface.	• Time-consuming, corrosive solvents, and difficult scalability. • Limited to thin films. • Not suitable for materials of similar electrochemical potentials.
	Chemical	• Control over the size of pores and ligaments. • Used for the fabrication of metal and metal oxides. • Low-temperature and simple process.	• Coarsening (i.e., reduced surface energy/area and degradation of physical properties. • Difficulty in fabricating nonmetallic materials • Use of corrosive solvents. • Impurities from less-noble metals. • Time-consuming and there is no control over the composition of NP structure.
	Vapor phase	• The facile and environmentally friendly fabrication process with no chemical waste. • Recycling metal from precursor alloy.	• Vacuum chamber limits industrial scalability and high-throughput production. • High-temperature process and inapplicable for materials with similar vapor pressure.
	Liquid metal	• More efficient than chemical or • electrochemical dealloying and • more environmentally friendly. • Faster due to operation at higher temperatures.	• Requires high temperatures. • Unavoidable thermal coarsening. • Inapplicable for materials with similar solubility.

TABLE 1.2 *(Continued)*

Fabrication technique	Advantages	Disadvantages
2. Templating Soft	• Good control over geometry, • pore size, and architecture • Simple technique.	• The collapse of NP structures after the removal of soft template. • Low mechanical stability. • Low thermal stability of soft template. • Not scalable approach. • Low yield.
Hard	• Stable NP structures after the removal of the hard template. • Retaining hard geometries.	• Less tunability in the size and structures of nanopores. • Low yield. • High cost and require multiple steps. • Not scalable. • Low mechanical stability of NP materials.
3. Microwave-based fabrication	• High yield, purity, and selectivity; • NP fabrication from metal, metal oxide, polymer, and MOF • Tunability in the size of nanopores and backbone structure via time and microwave power • Rapid process	• Low yield of NP materials. • Low-depth penetration of microwave irradiation limiting the industrial scale production.

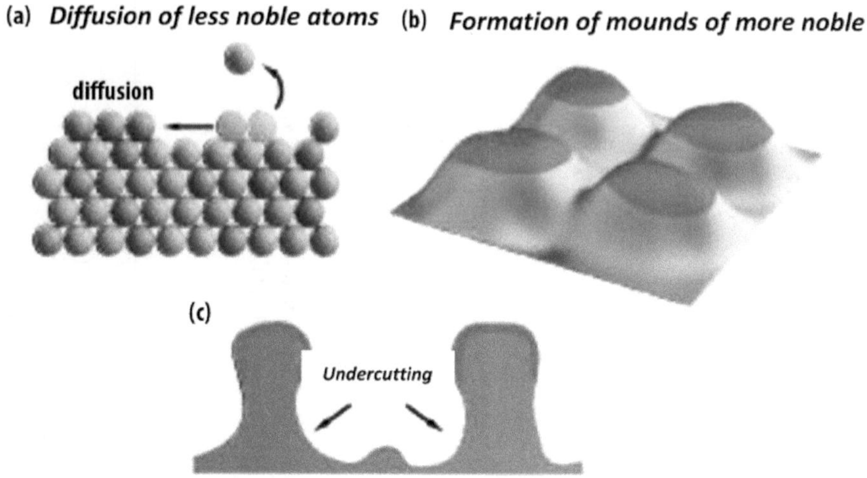

FIGURE 1.2 Evolution in porosity during the dealloying of an Au:Ag alloy. Yellow regions represent Au; uncolored regions represent Ag.

Source: Modified from Ref. [23]

According to diffusion-limited dealloying kinetics, the dealloying rate v may be written as

$$\frac{-dx}{dt} = (D_A - D_N)\frac{\partial x_{\mathrm{A}}}{\partial x} \tag{1.1}$$

where x is dealloying depth, t is dealloying time, x_{A} is the molar fraction of active atoms, and D_{A} and D_{N} are the diffusion coefficients of active atoms and noble atoms, respectively. The integration of eq (1.1) in dealloying depth yields the dealloying rate.

$$v = \frac{(D_{\mathrm{A}} - D_{\mathrm{N}})X_{\mathrm{A}}}{x} \tag{1.2}$$

The relationship between dealloying depth and dealloying duration may be found by integrating eqs (1.1) and (1.2)[24]:

$$x = \{2(D_A - D_N)x_A\}^2 \tag{1.3}$$

One of the early proposals to explain the enrichment of more-noble atoms on the porous skeleton was the volume diffusion hypothesis. It was created by Pickering and Wagner in the latter 1960s. According to this theory, the less-noble component gets depleted close to the surface. The outcome is the formation of a gradient perpendicular to the alloy/electrolyte interface, driving the bulk diffusion of the less valued component to the surface where it may dissolve. Due to the development of surface vacancies brought on by the preferential removal of the less-noble component, this inevitably results in a concentration of the more-noble adatoms on the electrode surface. However, it was discovered that volume diffusion in the unaffected alloy was very sluggish; in fact, when this process was first put forth, even surface diffusion was thought to be too slow. Erlebacher recently added kinetic function to both silver dissolution/diffusion and gold diffusion to further refine the Monte Carlo model. This enabled the simulation of alloy composition and applied potential controlled "real-time" dealloying. The bond-breaking model for the nearest neighbor was used to calculate the rates of diffusion and dissolution. With the dissolution/diffusional probability computed for certain conditions, the surface atoms were selected at random. Equations 1.1 and 1.2, respectively, show the rates of diffusion and dissolution[25]:

$$K_{\text{diss}} = v_E \exp\left(-\frac{aE_{\text{b-}\varnothing}}{k_{\text{B}}T}\right) \tag{1.4}$$

$$K_{\text{diff}} = v_{\text{D}} \exp\left(-\frac{aE_{\text{b}}}{k_{\text{B}}T}\right) \tag{1.5}$$

where stands for the number of closest neighbors, E_{b} is the bond energy, which is first stated as 0.15 eV and is thought to be equivalent for both gold and silver and ϕ is the applied potential (1.75 eV). The Boltzmann constant (k_{B}) and absolute temperature (T) are two terms used interchangeably. the frequency of the order of the Debye frequency, set to 1×10^{13} s^{-1}, was attempted after fitting experimental data of pure silver dissolution ($= 1 \times 10^{4}$ s^{-1}). In the high overpotential Tafel's area, silver dissolution rates were in accordance with the Butler–Volmer equation.[25]

1.2.1.1 *CHEMICAL DEALLOYING*

By carefully choosing the less sensitive species to selectively erode or leach in an acidic or basic media, chemical dealloying has been extensively utilized to create nanostructured metals and metal oxides. Niauzorau et al.[26] claim that cosputtered gold–silver thin films were chemically dealloyed to produce nanostructured gold. Dealloying's porosity properties, including ligament diameter and solid area proportion, were adjusted by regulating temperature and time. Additionally, the relationship between the structural and elemental development of nanoporous gold (NPG) over time and the residual silver concentration was looked at.

1.2.1.2 ELECTROCHEMICAL DEALLOYING

Rahman et al.[27] recently showed how the Ni–Al system ($Ni_{30}Al_{70}$) may be electrochemically dealloyed to create NP nickel. Compared to conventional Au–Ag systems, the dispersion of pore diameters was larger, and the process was very dependent on the parent alloy's composition. Similar to this, NP copper has been created by dealloying a copper-aluminum alloy.

1.2.1.3 LIQUID METAL DEALLOYING "LMD"

Rather than employing an acid environment, this approach uses liquid metal as a channel for the selective dissolving of one element of a multicomponent alloy. The process depends on the positive entropy of mixing the disposable atoms with the liquid metallic "etchant" and the negative entropy of mixing the target metal atoms with the alloy. The synthesis of porous Ti from a binary Cu–Ti alloy in molten magnesium is an analogous case. Upon coming into touch with the Mg liquid, the Cu–Ti binary alloy solid precursor preferentially dissolves into the melt, while the mutual repulsing of the residual Ti atoms and the melt results in a NP structure. A few empirical guidelines for dealloying include (1) For a binary alloy, the two elements must have sufficiently dissimilar equilibrium potentials so that the more-noble (MN) element can remain intact while the less-noble (LN) element, which is electrochemically active, can dissolve away. During dealloying, the nobler element may also undergo a slight disintegration. (2) The MN element's surface diffusivity, D_s, which among other things establishes the rate and duration of the creation of porous structures It is crucial that the surviving nobler atoms have enough mobility to reorganize a stable, self-standing porous structure within the dealloying time. Equation 1.6 can be used to quantitatively determine D_s of adatoms along the solid/solution interface after a coarsening procedure of the ligaments.

$$D_s = [d(t)]\ 4kT\ 32\gamma t\alpha^4 \tag{1.6}$$

where k is the Boltzmann constant (1.38×10^{-23} J.K.$^{-1}$), T is the dealloying temperature, d(t) is the ligament size at time t, and γ is the surface energy of an alloy. Ds was determined in this method to be within the order from 10^{-11} to 1010^{-19} cm^2 s^{-1} for several noble metals.[28]

By dealloying precursor, $(TixZr_{100-x})_y$ Cu_{100-y} alloys in liquid magnesium, a variety of open porous $TixZr_{100-x}$ alloys with various chemical compositions and microstructural features were created. The design of precursor alloys for the LMD is based on both the biocompatibility of the alloying components and the enthalpy of mixture values between Mg and the chosen alloy element [H (Mg-element) mix]. While elements with a positive H (Mg) element mix, such as Ti, Zr, V, or Fe, are immiscible in Mg, those with a negative H (Mg) element mix, such as Al, Si, Cu, or Ni, are miscible and will dissolve in Mg during the dealloying process. Ti, Zr, Nb, Mo, Hf, and Ta are among the elements that can be used in Mg and are both biocompatible and immiscible (see Fig. 1.3).[29]

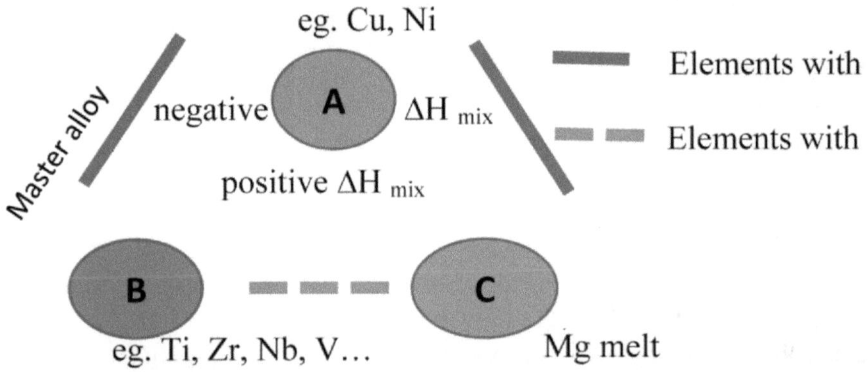

FIGURE 1.3 Enthalpy of elemental mixing during the dealloying of a master alloy AB in a liquid metal C (e.g., Mg melt).

Source: Modified from Ref. [29]

By dealloying Ti (Me) Cu-based alloys (Me = Fe, V, Nb, and Ta) in liquid Mg and then treating them as dealloyed samples with 15 M HF to etch off the non-Mg phases, open NP Mg was created. The creation of a MgF_2-rich layer on the surface of the NP Mg during the last corrosion step passivates the surface, preventing the porous samples from rapidly oxidizing. The precursor alloy's crystalline framework can be tailored using the following techniques: Improving the fabrication constraints and/or alloying; (ii) adjusting the dealloying circumstances, such as time and temperature; and (iii) changing the chemical makeup of the precursor alloy, such as alloying the precursor with elements having a high melting point to refine the NP Mg microstructure.[30]

LMD was effectively employed to create the porous surface layer and, as a result, functionalize the surface of the Ti-6Al-7Nb alloy with a decreased Al content in the surface layer. The Ti-6Al-7Nb alloy samples with functionalized (for instance, porous) surfaces show high cytocompatibility (the property of being safe for cells—an indication of biocompatibility) and improved bone synthesis, which promotes a better Osseo incorporation, especially in biodegradable polymer graft sites. The present results demonstrate the potential uses of LMD for the surface functionalization of biomedical alloys by generating porous surface layers and tailoring their chemical composition. Drug distribution could potentially be accomplished using the LMD-tailored porous surfaces.[31]

1.2.1.4 VAPOR PHASE DEALLOYING

Vapor phase dealloying (VPD) takes advantage of changes in the vapor pressure of elements that are included in the precursor alloy in an effort to selectively vaporize and/or dealloy one constituent.[1]

Pinna et al.[32] have successfully created NP Al beginning from an $Al_{20}Zn_{80}$ nanocomposite generated from ball milling using this method. Under high vacuum, the nanocomposite was annealed at 550°C, and the Zn was selectively removed by VPD due to the difference in vapor pressures. The morphology of the resultant NP material was examined using scanning electron microscopy, which showed pores with sizes ranging from a few to thousands of nm. The NP 3D structure was also studied using serial block face scanning electron microscopy. The majority of base metals' propensity to oxidize makes it difficult to fabricate NP structures from them. Numerous fabrication techniques have been documented to address this issue. For instance, some of them (including Ti, Ta, Si, and Nb) have been produced by substituting a liquid metal for the aqueous solution. VPD has recently been developed in this regard. This method precisely removes one or more alloy elements by taking advantage of variances in the vapor pressures of elemental metals, regardless of how likely it is that the alloy elements may oxidize.

1.2.1.5 SOLID PHASE DEALLOYING

The discrepancy in mixing enthalpies between the components of the precursor alloy and the dealloying medium, which causes selective dissolution, is what drives solid-state dealloying, similar to how LMD works. Wada et al. first introduced this technique in 2016 to create a dealloyed interfacial zone between the two layers of a diffusion pair. They proposed solid-state dealloying as a novel technique to stop coarsening while the porous structure was developing. Lower temperature operation may delay coarsening and provide a finer morphology with a larger surface area. At the interface between the precursor and the solvent, thermally accelerated atomic diffusion mediates coarsening. In further research, solid-state dealloying in thin films has been successfully implemented using a thin precursor film deposited on a solid metal solvent substrate or both the precursor and the dealloying medium in thin film form.[33]

1.3 TEMPLATING APPROACHES

1.3.1 SOFT TEMPLATING APPROACHES

In soft templates, a framework surrounds an organic molecule that serves as the "template." When these organic molecules are taken out, a cavity is left behind that still has its form and structure. The soft template method has a lot of benefits, such as low costs, simple preparation in calm conditions, and accessibility to a wide range of mesoporous structures. On the contrary, it has several drawbacks, such as a basic reliance on challenging sol–gel processes and challenges in managing polymerization and hydrolysis of transition metal ions during preparation. When employing commercial PEO-based copolymers, the soft template method's end products are often susceptible to relative humidity and may have walls that are amorphous or semicrystalline with poor thermal and mechanical stability.[34]

By hydrolyzing tetraethyl orthosilicate in an alkaline solution of water and alcohol, Stöber et al. (1968) produced silica nanoparticles employing the sol–gel process.

$$\mathrm{Si(OEt)_4 + 4H_2O \rightarrow SiO_2 + 2H_2O + 4EtOH} \tag{1.7}$$

The synthesis procedure has now been somewhat altered, entailing the insertion of the template, to prepare other kinds of porous silica nanoparticles using the Stöber method. The soft-templating strategy refers to the simple calcination or solvent-washing method of template removal. Typically, soft templates are made of micelles or supramolecular surfactant aggregates. The substances that generate pores are called porogens or structure-directing agents (SDA) which include nonionic surfactants such as pluronics, triton, tween, and spans as well as anionic surfactants such as sodium lauryl sulfates and sodium dodecyl sulfates; cationic surfactants such as alkyl trimethyl quaternary ammonium surfactants; such as cetyltrimethylammonium bromide (CTAB), gemini, and bolaform; and anionic surfactants.[35]

Polymeric templates that are less stiff are used in soft templating procedures. For instance, two-photon lithography is used to print sacrificial nanoscale polymer frameworks as templates, and metallic lattices are created after an oxidation-resistant metal (such as gold) is sputtered onto the template and removed. Although this technique may manufacture features with 150-nm feature size and good controllability of metal morphology at the nanoscale (10-nm resolution), it is often utilized to create truss structures rather than bicontinuous pore-ligand or gyroid structures. However, research has shown that certain species of polymers have stable nanoscale domains, which makes template-based manufacturing interesting in this context. The most popular method for creating polymeric templates for NP metal manufacturing uses block copolymers' (BCPs) self-organizing properties. Alternate techniques include melt-mixing and foaming. Deposition can be used to metalize polymer templates with different metals (usually nickel is used as an example). After metallization, the template can be removed using polymeric solvents or by thermally degrading sacrifice scaffolds. Because they provide a high degree of structural uniformity and adaptability inappropriate metals, polymeric templating approaches for the manufacture of NP metals are set to revitalize existing efforts in this sector.[36]

1.3.2 HARD TEMPLATING

Self-organizing behavior is most commonly used in the fabrication process. Three processing stages are necessary for the majority of the template-based NP metal production processes (template synthesis, metallization of template, and template removal). Typically, different NP structures are produced using rigid templates comprised of silica, metals, metal oxides, carbon, polystyrene, and calcium carbonate ($CaCO_3$). The shape, size, and quantity of nanoparticles may be controlled by altering the hard templates' pore size, particle size, and morphology. Mesoporous carbon or silica has been used as templates to produce a range of distinctive mesoporous materials, including polymers, fullerenes, biomolecules, carbon nitrides, metal nitrides, boron nitride, and carbon nitride.[35]

The characteristics of the template are historically used to categorize templating procedures for material assembly. Inorganic templates, such as porous carbon compounds, are used in hard templating techniques. Carbon compounds generated from carbides may have homogeneous nanopores with dimensions between 0.65 and 2.1 nm. Additionally, porous carbon has been created using the template approach by first introducing a carbon precursor into the template's pores, which can range in size from 2.532 to 220 nm, carbonizing the material, and then removing the template. For instance, carbonization of zeolite Y is said to have a periodicity of 1.4 nm, whereas mesoporous silica can be used to create porous carbon with high-aspect-ratio pores as small as 400 nm in diameter and as deep as 10 lm. These templates stand out for their depth of porosity, which goes beyond the micrometer range, and their simplicity in removing the template after metallization by burning. Although template removal was not attempted, the electrodeposition of metals into porous silicon (such as Au, Cu, Ni, and Fe) was also demonstrated.[36]

1.3.3 HYDROGEN BUBBLES TEMPLATING TECHNIQUE (DHBT)

Strong adhesion and seamless integration of the catalyst and the substrate are made possible by the direct growth of catalytically influential species on substrates to create self-supporting sensors. This eliminates the need for extra coating or augmented adhesion, exposing more catalytically active surface sites and preventing catalyst subluxation more effectively. Additionally, self-supporting materials' composition and shape can be changed to efficiently tune their electrocatalytic characteristics. There are four different types of self-supporting substrates: metal substrates (foils, meshes, and fabric); carbon-based substrates (clothes, carbon papers, and graphene papers); conductive oxides; and unusual nonconductive substrates (papers, textiles, and sponges). Metal meshes are seen to be the most promising substrates for producing self-supporting catalysts for industrial applications because of their exceptional electrical conductivity and remarkable flexibility. Meshes may also be used as sources of metal for the development of catalyst layers. Currently, solid-phase reactions, vapor deposition, electrodeposition, and wet chemical methods can all be used to build active catalysts on self-supporting substrate surfaces.[37]

During electrodeposition, two different reactions take place:

$$M^{2+} + 2e^{-} = M \tag{1.8}$$

$$d = 0.020\theta(\gamma / g(\rho_l - \rho_g))^{0.5}(1 + 0.2i / (Am^{-2}))^{0.45} \tag{1.11}$$

where θ is the contact angle, g is the gravity of acceleration, γ is surface tension, i is current density, ρ_1 is the liquid density ρ_g is the gas density, γ is the surface wettability.[39]

By affecting how rapidly the HER occurs and the hydrogen bubbles leave the electrode surface with a tiny break-off diameter due to diminished coalescence, the applied current density and process overpotential affect the pace and type of dendrite development. The nucleation rate "w" that occurs during electrodeposition is given in eq 1.12.

$$w = k_{1e^-}\left[\frac{k_2}{\eta_k}\right] \tag{1.12}$$

where η_k is the overpotential and k_1 and k_2 are constants.

According to eq. 1.13, this overpotential in turn influences the nucleation radius (r_c) and grain size.

$$r_c = \frac{\pi h^3 E}{6Z_c\eta_c} \tag{1.13}$$

where Z_e denotes the number of electrons in discharge ions, E denotes the energy of the contact, and h denotes the height created by absorbent atoms.[25]

Impact of current density. Fewer H_2 bubbles develop on the cathode's surface at lower current densities, and this, together with the substrate's plentiful availability of deposition sites, results in the unevenly distributed morphology of NPMFS films. An increase in the deposition current density can lead to improvements in lattice constants, pore size, and grain refinement. A similar relationship holds true when applying a pulsing current, where an increase in the current density amplitude increases the HER and creates smaller H_2 bubbles, resulting in a structure resembling a honeycomb with fewer pores.[39,40]

Impact of the deposition time. The pore diameter grows with longer deposition times at a constant current density. The doubling in pore thickness and size results in a decrease in the number of pores per unit area, or pore density. However, there must be a time restriction since as the structure became more disorganized, the pore wall thickness likewise grew over time. This disordering may cause the porous 3D network in the electrolyte to collapse or for the metal pores to be filled by metal dendrites, which would cause the porous structure to vanish.[39,41]

Temperature's impact: More hydrogen evolution happens as the deposition temperature rises, creating a bigger bubble template. As a result, the space between the bubbles becomes bigger, which expands the pore size of the electrodeposited NPMFMs. The increase in bath temperature, which quickens the electrochemical reaction and ion diffusion rate, decorates the coarser crystal structure with defects that reduce the crystallinity of the deposited foam.[39]

Additions: The reduction of the branches is aided by the alkaline sulfates, chlorides, and bromides. Similar to additives, acetic acid and CTAB operate as bubble stabilizers by lessening the bubbles' hydrophobic force and preventing their coalescence. As a result, the foams' dendritic branches and pore size are reduced. Due to its ability to adsorb on the cathode surface and so raise the cathodic overpotential, NH_4^+ is the most potent suppressant of the deposition of metal foams and hydrogen evolution among all additions. As a result, stronger layers are formed together with a bigger pore width of the metal foam and less dense branching. Even though NH_4 was present, the addition of Cl^-, PEG, and MPSA led to the formation of a highly dense porous structure with smaller pores and thinner walls, which allowed for the reversal of surface porosity. The combination of benzotriazole (BTA, which is a suppressant in and of itself) and $(NH_4)_2SO_4$ led to the development of grape-like foams with great ductility but low mechanical strength.[39,41]

Depending on the density of the interchange current, metals may be categorized into the following three groups: Normal metals have melting values, high ($_{j0,\ dep}$ >100 A cm^{-2}) exchange current densities of metal deposition, and low catalytic activity for hydrogen evolution. Examples of these metals are Cd, Zn, Sn, and Ag. Au, Cu, and Ag are examples of intermediary metals, which have moderate melting temperatures, intermediate ($j_{0,\ dep}$ 100 A cm^{-2}) exchange current densities, and modest hydrogen evolution catalytic activity. The ability of DHBT to produce metal foams depends on the ability of hydrogen to form large enough bubbles on each of the three metal groups (this is largely an interface thermodynamic and nucleation and growth kinetics issue) and the ability of dendritic metallic complexes to outgrow a hydrogen bubble before it exits the electrode surface depends on the rate of depositing process.[42]

Dendrite production is conceivable for metals with lower mild $j_{0,\ dep}$ values if the depositing overpotential η surpasses a necessary starting overpotential.

$$\eta ini = -\frac{RT}{ZF}\frac{j_{lim.dep}}{j_{0,dep}} \tag{1.14}$$

where the actual limiting current density for metal deposition is denoted by $j_{\text{lim, dep}}$. It should be noted that the value of $j_{\text{lim, dep}}$ is highly dependent on the current hydrodynamic circumstances and the rapid mixing of the near-electrode solution brought on by HER.

The greatest size that H_2 bubbles created during the electrolysis can reach before breaking off the surface, as well as the rate at which bubble development takes place, will influence the deposit's morphology, particularly on the macroscale. According to the empirical formula, it was discovered that the break-off diameter *d* is dependent on the partial current density of hydrogen evolution j_{HER};

$$d = d_0\left(1 + aj_{\text{HER}}\right)^{\text{b}} \tag{1.15}$$

where the constants a ~ 0.2 $m^2\ A^{-1}$ and b ~0.45 were determined by Vogt and by fitting to experimental data; this should be noted that these constant values may noticeably vary depending on the system being researched. The break-off diameter in a current-free condition is represented by the parameter d_0 in eq (1.15), and its value may be calculated using a streamlined version of the Fritz equation.

$$d_0 = 1.2\vartheta\sqrt{\frac{\gamma}{g\rho}} \tag{1.16}$$

where g is the gravitational acceleration, ϑ is the bubble's contact angle with the electrode surface, 1 is the solution's density, and γ is the gas/liquid interface's interfacial stress. As a function of the applied electrode voltage (and/or current), both the contact angle # and the surface tension may change, and fluctuations in the solution's near-surface viscosity may have an impact on the break-off diameter and the trajectory of bubbles departing the electrode surface.[42]

1.4 SOL–GEL APPROACHES

Due to its ability to directly fabricate multicomponent materials in a variety of forms (monoliths, coatings, foams, and fibers) without the need for powder intermediaries or expensive processing techniques such as vacuum procedures, sol–gel methods are particularly advantageous. The sol–gel method has become a crucial synthesis pathway in many fields of study, including optics, electronics, semi- and superconductors, and biomaterials, due to the variety of materials that may be produced. Sol–gel thin film processing has several advantages, including low processing temperatures, straightforward production, and precise chemical and microstructural control. In addition to having a large SSA (which may be used as a carrier for adsorbed medicines) and a high level of biocompatibility, the sol–gel-generated film or layer also has an exterior surface with a rich chemistry that is easy to functionalize by suitable biomolecules.[43] This method can be utilized to create hybrid materials as well as materials based on phosphates, metals, and silica.[44–46] These substances work well as biosensors, multifunctional sol–gel nanocarriers for diagnostic purposes, scaffolds and matrices for tissue repair and regeneration, and nanocarriers to transport biomolecules, among other applications. The thick, homogeneous vitreous and ceramic materials may be produced at low temperatures using the sol–gel method. The synthesis process is divided into many stages. The hydrolysis (eq 1.17) and condensation (eq 1.18) reactions occur in the colloidal solution that is created in the first step when the precursor chemicals, the catalyst, the water, and sometimes a co-dissolvent are combined. The most often used precursors in the sol–gel process are metal alkoxides, which are represented in eq 1.17 as [$M(OR)_n$], where M is the metallic element and R may represent a proton or other ligands such as an alkyl or alkoxy group. Once the hydrolysis process has begun, molecules that have only partially undergone hydrolysis interact in a condensation reaction that results in the polymerization of smaller molecules. The bigger molecules randomly join one another, leading to the creation of a three-dimensional structure. The creation of the gel is now the first step in the second stage of the sol–gel procedure.[47]

$$M(OR)n + xH_2 \rightarrow M(OR)n - x + xROH \tag{1.17}$$

$$(OR)n - xM - (OH)x - M(OR)n - x \rightarrow (OR)n - xM - O - M(OR)n - x + H_2O \tag{1.18}$$

The sol–gel methods include direct assembling of nanoparticles,[48] nanosmelting to produce metal aerogels,[49] and supercritical phase synthesis of nanomaterials metal powders.[51] The latter involves heating a metal acetate suspension in methanol to supercritical temperatures, which causes the methanol to convert the metal acetate to a metal.

1.5 MICROWAVE-BASED FABRICATION OF NANOPOROUS MATERIALS MW

MWs assist in accelerating conventional reactions' time to the activation energies. The instantaneous high temperatures attained during MW irradiation are the cause of this. A combination of the following elements can increase reaction speeds up to 1000 times when compared to typical heating methods: Different transition states and reactions, an increase in heating rates, and more uniform heating.[52] Microwave-assisted synthesis is a successful method for producing NP materials such as silica, carbons, MOFs, COFs, metal oxides including ZnO, TiO_2, Al_2O_3, Fe_2O_3, and Mn_2O_3, and related nanomaterials.[53]

1.6 ION BEAM-INDUCED FABRICATION

The ion beam technique is a top–down destructive approach that bombards the target with high-energy ion beams such as Ga^+, He^+, O^+, Ar^+, or Xe^+. The potential process involved in the formation of nanopores with this technique may be explained by the combined effect of milling and sintering while being subjected to a high-energy ion beam. The ion beam technique has a number of advantages over other methods for creating NP materials, including the ability to precisely control the distribution of pore sizes and the interconnectedness of the pore network, regardless of the material used; the avoidance of hazardous chemicals; and the absence of additional steps, such as chemical dealloying. The process works in a vacuum, thus materials that are sensitive to air and water may also be employed to generate NP materials. The core of NP structures may get contaminated after being exposed to an ion beam. Ion contamination can be eliminated, nevertheless, by using thermal annealing or inert gas-based ion beams.[51]

According to Lin et al.,[54] an oblique ion beam with moderate energy levels may be used to efficiently produce high-quality nanopores with programmable geometries in graphene for a range of applications, including DNA sequencing, water desalination, and phase separation.

1.7 LASER-INDUCED FABRICATION

The fabrication of NP materials has been investigated using laser irradiation in conjunction with dealloying techniques. Laser cladding was used to create NP manganese, which was then selectively electrochemically dealloyed to show how it was made. This effort involved combining Mn and Cu elemental powder and depositing the resulting mixture on a mild steel substrate to create an Mn-Cu precursor alloy with a thickness of 1 mm. The specimen that has undergone laser processing underwent electrochemical dealloying, creating

NP MnCu. The pore size and backbone size of porous materials might be altered by adjusting the electrochemical dealloying time. It has also been shown that NP anatase TiO_2 can be created utilizing femtosecond laser ablation and chemical oxidation on a Ti-based substrate with microstructures.[1]

By using a nanosecond pulse laser to irradiate the Ti_6Al_4V surface in a nitrogen atmosphere, NP structures were successfully created. In-depth research was done on the influences of laser settings on the emergence and development of NP formations. The variation in pulse energy may be the cause of the differences in surface characteristics of the NP structures formed at different repetition frequencies (E), which can be expressed as

$$E = \frac{P}{f} \tag{1.19}$$

where P represents the typical laser power. When the average laser power remains constant, the pulse energy falls as the repetition frequency rises, resulting in variations in the surface properties of the NP structures. The advantages of this technology are minimal equipment needs, straightforward operation, good repeatability, and zero pollution. The interaction of bone cells and implants is encouraged by the proliferation and development of bone cells in porous titanium (Ti).[55]

1.8 PYROLYSIS OF METAL SALT/DEXTRAN PASTES

Macroporous metallic sponges of Ag, Au, and CuO, as well as combinations therewith, are created when pastes of the polymer dextran mixed with metal salts are heated to degrees between 500 and 900°C. Walsh et al. showed this technique. This pyrolytic process yields foams with holes ranging from 1 to 50 mm in diameter, particles/struts on the order of 1–15 mm, and surface areas on the order of 0.5–1 $m^2 g^{-1}$, depending on temperature and heat treatment time. Although the foams produced by this approach are not particularly NP or nanomaterials, they do occupy an appropriate amount of the pore size vs density parameter space between NMFs and macrocellular foams, indicating that they may be useful as NMF precursors.

1.9 COMBUSTION SYNTHESIS (CS)

In these processes, the intrinsic energy created during the burning of the precursor mixture propels high activation energy barrier forward reactions at room temperature. For a number of materials, including metal oxides, ceramics, and intermetallics, combustion synthesis (CS), also known as self-propagating high-temperature synthesis (SHS), is a process that is accessible. These processes result in the production of foams, filaments, and powdered materials. Erri et al. recently produced nickel and nickel/nickel oxide foams with holes ranging from 100 to 1 mm in diameter by burning nickel nitrates with glycine in the air. By adjusting the nickel nitrate to fuel ratio, it is possible to alter both the composition of the foams and the way the combustion wave spreads. The creation of foams over powders, which occurs when the combustion wave travels too fast, must be prevented by managing wave propagation. The procedure is far less costly and hazardous than the CVD techniques previously used to produce Ni foams with equal pore size to density ratios, and it may potentially be used for a broad variety of materials. However, the materials produced by this process have relatively modest SSAs of 50–200 m^2 mol^{-1} because they are not NP (0.8–3.5 m^2 g^{-1}). Hunt et al. have proven the use of an alternative CS method to create NiAl alloy foams. In this method, gasifying fluorinated organic ligands ($C1_3F_{27}COOH$) are used to passivate nanometer-sized Al particles. Then, the particles are combined with Al and Ni particles that are between micron and nanometer in size.[51]

As an intermetallic molecule, nitinol is a contender for the novel CS method, which offers a novel way to create porous biomaterials (CS). The exothermic chemical reaction between two or more elemental powders, which in this case results in the equiatomic TiNi combination when nickel and Ti combine, is used by the CS process to create an intermetallic complex. The TiNi compound is created from the elemental powders in a matter of seconds after the reaction is started by propagating a high-temperature reaction front across the material. Ti + Ni →TiNi reaction produces 67.8 KJ mol^{-1} of heat of formation. In an adiabatic atmosphere, this indicates that a compact of Ti and Ni particles will grow by about 940°C.[56]

1.10 BIOMEDICAL APPLICATIONS

Nanoscale-scale assembly and organization of nanomaterials make them appealing for biotechnology applications because their material topography and spatial distribution of functional groups can be exploited to regulate interactions between proteins, cells, and tissues as well as for bioseparation. The potential to create enzymatic nanomaterials that replicate biological reactions is made possible by the fact that NP materials are frequently biocompatible. Enzymes may be used in biological reactors to produce medications, eliminate trash, and do other things by being immobilized onto NP surfaces. NP substances may be used to make biosensors. Piezoelectric nanosensors with high surface area NP coatings offer enhanced detection sensitivity. Immobilized biological molecules on the surface of NP silica may be used as a biological detection technique, and piezoelectric cantilevers can be used as transducers. The cantilever's resonance frequency varies as molecules absorb on the surface. The cantilever's surface-to-volume ratio is increased by the inclusion of NP silica, which also makes the oscillator's resonant frequency more sensitive to changes in mass.[57]

1.10.1 IMPLANT

The "stress-shielding" effect, which causes bone deterioration and implant loosening, was one of the driving forces behind biomedical Ti alloy development. The considerable stiffness mismatch between metallic material and bone is what results in this phenomenon. Design solutions for numerous materials, such as low modulus β-Ti alloys, composite materials, and porous materials, have been developed to address the "stress-shielding" issue. Several low modulus porous Ti alloys with average strength have recently been produced through LMD. In this work, we used liquid metal dealloying to produce open porous TiMo alloys reinforced with dendrites. Mo was used as an alloying element for a variety of purposes, including Mo acts as the β stabilizing element in Ti alloys because Mo and Cu cannot combine, resulting in the development of TiMo-rich dendrites in the precursor alloy. Due to its dendrite-reinforced microstructure, the porous TiMo alloy exhibits a relatively high yield strength value of up to 180 MPa along with good deformability when evaluated under compression loading. The porous TiMo alloy's elastic modulus, which is less than 10 GPa, is comparable to that of human bone. This mechanical behavior and the open porosity structure make the porous TiMo alloy appealing for biomedical applications and point to potential uses for it in implant applications.[57]

Ti is significant from an applications perspective because it has the greatest strength-to-weight ratio of any elemental metal, is exceptionally corrosion resistant, and is assumed to be biologically inert. The combination of these properties makes Ti particularly beneficial for applications ranging from aerospace to medical implants. Therefore, producing Ti nanofoams would have an effect on several businesses. In the medical profession, osseointegration—the direct bonding of a structural implant and underlying live bone—is compatible with Ti. The open, porous structure of nanofoams, which are valued for their low weight, creates the prospect of even lighter stronger structural materials employing Ti nanofoams as foam cores in sandwich panels. Ti nanofoams are ideal for biomedical applications such as osseointegration, where cell penetration is a key factor, as they have a surface area of 5590 m^2 mol^{-1} (70 m^2 g^{-1}), strong monolithicity, pores in the hundreds of nanometer range, and a significant quantity of micron-diameter macroporosity. Ti nanofoams were successfully synthesized, demonstrating the adaptability of the CS method.[51]

Epoxy is injected into Ti-based NP alloys produced by liquid-metal dealloying to create interpenetrating-phase nanocomposites. Their yield strength, which can reach 260 MPa, is technologically intriguing for a deformable light material. More significantly, Young's modulus is adjustable between 4.4 and 24 GPa, allowing for bone-matching. The strength of the composite materials is also similar to bone in that it depends on the strain rate. These results imply that the innovative composite materials might serve as the foundation for potential implant materials in the future.[58]

A variety of open porous $TixZr_{100-x}$ alloys were produced by using Mg as the corrosive medium and LMD of $(TixZr_{100-x})y$ Cu_{100-y} precursors. The dealloying conditions and chemical composition of the $(TixZr_{100-x})_y$ Cu_{100-y} precursors were compared to the dealloying microstructure of the porous $TixZr_{100-x}$. In particular, increasing the dealloying time (from 5 to 20 min) and temperature (from 1073 to 1173 K) causes the microstructure of the $(TiZr)_{30}$ Cu_{70} precursor to become coarser, leading to an increase in ligament thickness. Because the Cu concentration of the $(TiZr)_y Cu_{100-y}$ precursors decreased from 70 to 40%, a higher solid fraction of the final porous TiZr may reach up to 79 vol%. The porous $TixZr_{100-x}$ alloys stand out from other porous metals due to their high yield strength of up to 480 MPa, exceptional compressive deformability, and low Young's modulus of roughly 15.1 GPa even in the case of large metal fractions of around 79 vol%. The unique combination of mechanical features of dealloying-based porous alloys and positive early biological test findings suggests opportunities for load-bearing implant applications.[59]

A possible biomedical use for magnesium and magnesium alloys in large quantities is demonstrated by the microarc oxidation (MAO) technology, which also demonstrates surface alteration with promising results for preventing corrosion. For use in bioimplant scaffolds, Ra et al.[60] created a biodegradable porous metal employing an anodic coating on AZ_{31} Mg alloy substrate. NaCl was used as a space holder during replication operations that produced the cellular Mg alloy in a controlled environment. Vacuum pressure was also used to facilitate the infiltration. Using the MAO method and a phosphate/calcium electrolyte, the Mg porous samples were coated. We were able to create a homogenous coating layer with a thickness of around 16.0 m using the MAO approach, and the surface of the foam structure had rounded pores with a diameter of less than 3.0 m. The primary components of the anodic coating are Ca, P, Mg, and O. Additionally, the Young's modulus and compressive strength of the coated and untreated porous samples are similar, measuring around 1.5 GPa and 5.0 MPa, respectively.

Zirconium titanate was uniformly NP and coated over 316L SS implants using the dip-coating procedure, according to B. Devi et al. The coating causes the production of a hydroxyapatite layer on the metal surfaces and serves as a barrier layer to the metallic implants. According to these findings, coated 316L stainless steel has better bioactivity than uncoated 316L stainless steel.

Nanostructured surfaces with a particular porous surface topography control the interactions between cells and surfaces and may be an effective tool for enhancing cell adherence and favoring the growth of some cell types over others. Bencina et al.[62] studied and evaluated the scientific literature on the anodization of stainless-steel products. Anodization is used to cause the stainless steel to oxidize for two reasons: (i) The capacity to regulate the oxide film's composition; (ii) The oxide film's numerous nanoscale morphologies, which, for example, affect how biological material reacts when it comes into touch with anodized surfaces. The creation of dense nanopores with nearly uniform diameter is facilitated by the electrolyte having a high concentration of organic components (ideally between 90 and 95 vol%).

1.10.2 DRUG DISTRIBUTION

It is enticing to use NP membranes with well-controlled pore size, porosity, and membrane thickness to create capsules with a controlled release of medicinal compounds. The effective use of gold nanoparticles with NP materials in drug delivery suggests the possibility of NPG with special features as drug carriers. The explanations are mentioned below. First, since NPG has a high effective surface area, great porosity, numerous adhesion receptors, and a strong potential for drug sorption, it may increase drug loading. Second, NPG demonstrated good biocompatibility by not being poisonous to cells or enzymes. As a result, NPG as a medicine carrier does not harm the body. Third, medications are more likely to access the target tissue or target cells because NPG's nanoscale size makes it simple to penetrate different membrane structures. Fourth, NPG's surface can be altered for various application goals, enabling medications to be delivered in a targeted manner to certain tissues or organs. Fifth, because NPG's structure, morphology, and pore size are all variable, drug loading capacity, membrane permeability, and drug targeting may all be modified using various preparation techniques.[63] The anticancer medication 5-fluorouracil (5-FU) has been loaded onto a NP MOF based on iron metal and the amino terephthalate ligand MIL-101-NH_2-Fe.[64]

Stainless steel with a NP surface could be utilized in medical equipment to regulate cellular reactions and transport medications. Stainless steel's porous surface may not only increase biocompatibility but also create an environment that makes it easier to carry biological substances and medications. The metal surface was electropolished for 10 min in an acidic atmosphere (50% H_2SO_4) at a constant voltage of 20 V and 10 A. Everolimus (EVL) was tested for its ability to load drugs onto a surface and for its kinetics of release. Surface roughness was higher in the post-polishing group than in the nonpolishing group. Inhibition of SMC adherence and migration as well as platelet adhesion was seen in the post-polish group as opposed to the pre-polish group. With half of the EVL released within 4 days as opposed to 1 day for the prepolishing group, the postpolishing group had a higher overall amount of EVL on the surface (i.e., a higher drug storage rate) and a lower drug release rate.[65]

Porous silicon is the perfect substance for medication delivery because of its high porosity and surface area. Small medicinal drugs and substances such as doxorubicin have been inserted into porous silicon holes. For drug delivery applications, a number of considerations must be made, including the pore size as the molecule must be smaller than the pore diameter to enter the pores. Porosity is important because the quantity of medication put into pores determines their capacity.[66]

Using a microwave technique, mesoporous nanosilica hollow spheres (NSHS) were created. The as-obtained NSHS had an average size of 190 nm, SSA of 330 m^2 g, and showed excellent thermal stability up to 700°C in air. The material exhibited a high ibuprofen loading capacity of up to 31%, it was also found. (assessed using UV analysis). The whole release of the ibuprofen took occurred over the course of 40 h, while only around 80% of it did so in the first 10 h. Mesoporous materials made of silica have shown to be excellent options for use in sustained drug delivery systems

(SDDSs), immediate drug delivery systems, targeted drug delivery systems, and systems that respond to stimuli (CDDSs). By including the appropriate polymers or functional groups, such as CN, SH, NH_2, and Cl, mesoporous silica's drug release rate may also be controlled. Multifunctional drug delivery systems based on MSNs (MSN = mesoporous silica nanoparticles) are now being developed to release anticancer drugs on demand and in a targeted way while minimizing the drug's premature release.[67] A class of crystalline NP materials with hundreds of unique structural variants are known as MOFs. MOFs are created by the self-assembly of metal ions that act as coordination centers and organic ligands that act as linkers between the metal centers. The distribution and storage of nitric oxide (NO), medication administration, imaging, and sensing are just a few applications for MOFs. In a review by Keskin et al.[68] they provided examples of the synthesis, structures, and properties of MOFs.

The development of hierarchical porosity in MOFs has attracted a lot of attention due to the huge potential of MOFs in a range of applications, from materials to life science. By combining perturbation-aided nanofusion (PNF) with microwave stimulation, we offer here a unique method for creating huge additional pores in the prototype MOF, Ni-MOF-74. An ideal combination of microwave irradiation, disturbance in the form of stirring, and solvent impact results in the induction of additional mesoscale porosity by fusing MOF nanoparticles. The impact of microwave is produced by altering reaction time and medium while using a range of solvents with varied dielectric constants (DMSO, DMF, DMA, acetone, EA, and THF). By applying this method, we are able to fuse nanoscale microporous MOF in a short period of time while agitating forcefully, without the usage of a template, producing wide-scale mesopores for the first time. An extra mesopore that was generated by encapsulating 4.6 mol g^{-1} of the massive biomolecule vitamin B12 (VB12) has been used.[69]

In contrast to other nanocarriers that commonly release the drug molecules with a burst effect, the drug release process from MOFs comprises delayed and controlled liberation of the medicines through matrix breakdown. Iron-containing BioMIL-1 MOFs displayed greater nicotinic acid loading of up to 75% and demonstrated regulated drug delivery as compared to native MOF structures. These methods have been combined to accomplish multimodal medication administration and imaging with the help of MOF-based delivery systems. It is interesting to note that the noncovalent strategy has a high drug-loading capacity for MOFs, as is the case for drugs with regulated drug-release profiles and no burst effects, such as cisplatin and ibuprofen. Zeolite and mesoporous silica have been shown to build strong frameworks with the advantage of being devoid of a burst-release effect in MOF complexes.[51]

1.10.3 CANCER TREATMENT

The primary focus of this review is the creation of nanoporous materials for medication delivery in lung cancer. The research looks at the many kinds of NP materials used for drug delivery today, including inorganic, organic, and hybrid porous materials for treatments including chemotherapy, radiotherapy, and phototherapy. Porous nanomaterials offer considerable advantages over their nonporous counterparts because of their large surface area, enormous pore volume, low mass density, and changeable size. One of the biggest obstacles in the delivery of cancer therapies can be overcome by using the porosity channels of the NP materials to capture and transport a significant amount of poorly soluble medicines. The increased surface area also enables a significant quantity of drug adsorption, which might lead to fewer patient administrations and medication dosing cycles. Contrarily, the size of the holes of NP materials may be altered to fit medicinal molecules of various sizes and shapes, from tiny peptides to large protein moieties. To regulate the release of the medication, several stimuli-responsive components, such as pH, temperature, redox, and magnetic factors, may be applied to the surface of the NP particles. Due to the additional property of porosity, these materials may also affect the aerosolization and impaction-related deposition of particles carrying pharmaceutical compounds. Mesoporous silicon nanoparticles, core-shell nanoparticles, porous silicon, and MOF are among the materials used.[70]

To obtain the necessary targeted impact over prolonged timeframes, applications of MOFs in cancer treatment have been carefully researched. Nano-MOFs are incredibly beneficial for treating a variety of human malignancies. Fe_3O_4-UiO_{66} MOFs have been used to deliver an anticancer agent (doxorubicin) and have improved biopharmaceutical qualities including regulated drug-release properties up to 40 days, superior anticancer activity in HeLa cells, and significantly reduced tumor volume. Taylor and colleagues reported using Mn-containing nano-MOFs, namely, $Mn(1,4\text{-}BDC)(H_2O)_2$ and $Mn_3(BTC)_2(H_2O)_6$ covered with a silica shell, for the delivery of the RGDfK peptide. By activating the Rvb3 integrin gene, the rhodamine B dye also demonstrated improved antiangiogenic capabilities in HT-29 cells. In another research on the use of nano-MOFs in ovarian cancer, the combination of cisplatin and siRNA has shown great results in reducing the development of ovarian cancer cells during cellular cytotoxicity, absorption, and apoptosis assays. Similar to this, the nano-MOFs of Gd have shown increased anticancer activity against the FITZ-HAS endothelial sarcoma cell line model by promoting cellular death of Rvb3 gene expression.[66]

1.10.4 PHOTODYNAMIC TREATMENT

Researchers have looked at using MOF in photodynamic therapy as a productive strategy for use against malignant cancer cells. The method of photodynamic treatment, which includes energy transfer from high to low energy light in the excited state, results in reactive oxygen species (ROS). With little harm to the healthy tissues, this results in the localized destruction of the sick tissues and activation of cellular apoptosis. For instance, chlorine-based nano-MOFs (DBC-UiO) have many superior photophysical characteristics than porphyrin-based nano-MOFs (DBP-UiO) owing to their crystallinity, stability, and porosity features, which promote efficient apoptosis and immunogenic cell death against colon cancer.[66]

1.10.5 BIOSENSORS

Sensory systems employ various membrane-bound protein pores to recognize substances and allow cells to respond to inputs. It has been shown that glucose oxidase immobilized in porous nanocrystalline TiO_2 film can detect blood glucose. A lot of technical fields, such as the pharmaceutical business, medical diagnostics, and the detection of dangerous biomolecules, depend on this kind of biosensing. Similar to this, cholesterol biosensors employ immobilized cholesterol oxidase enzymes present in ZnO NP thin films as sensors.[71,72]

NPG has lately been used in the creation of biosensors as a carrier for biorecognition components such as enzymes, DNA, antigens/antibodies, and whole cells due to its inherent advantages. The following are some of these advantages: The film from NPG has the following benefits: (1) its thickness (about 100 nm) makes it easy to modify on the electrode surface; (2) its high SSA can significantly increase the load of biorecognition molecules; (3) its 3D continuous NP sponge structure makes the adsorption of biorecognition molecules more robust and can speed up the diffusion of target compounds or products at the same time; and (4) its high biocompatibility can provide a safe alternative to current electrodes.

The optical and electrical properties of porous silicon play a significant role in many chemical and biological sensing applications. The majority of porous silicon-based sensors are interferometric sensors, where the optical response of the porous silicon structure is altered by the entry of the element to be detected into the pores. As the molecule to be identified is injected, the effective refractive index of the porous layers changes, moving the reflectance peaks. These sensors have been used to find organic vapors, glucose, and other compounds.[66]

Hu et al.[74] created a DNA biosensor with a 28 attomolar detection limit by first immobilizing single-stranded DNA on the NP surface, then progressively hybridizing it to target DNA, and then hybridizing it to reporter DNA coupled to a gold nanoparticle. Prostate-specific antigen concentrations as low as 0.1 ng/mL may be detected by Shulga et al.[75] using immobilized capture antibodies labeled with alkaline phosphatase on electroplated NP-Au electrodes. It is well known that DA plays a significant role as a catecholamine neurotransmitter. Devastating diseases such as Parkinson's disease, Alzheimer's disease, and schizophrenia are just a handful that may be brought on by aberrant DA levels. Yil et al.[76] developed a Pd/NPG wire DA biosensor by electrodepositing palladium (Pd) nanoparticles onto a self-supporting NPG wire. Due to the synergistic effects of the outstanding catalytic activity of Pd nanoparticles and the novel structure of NPG wire, the Pd nanoparticle decorated NPG (Pd/NPG) biosensor exhibits extraordinary superiority in the detection of DA. With a high sensitivity of 1.19 A M1, a wide detection range of 1–220 M, and a low detection limit of 1 M, the Pd/ NPG wire biosensor shows impressive performance. Additionally, the suggested dopamine biosensor had good selectivity, stability, repeatability, and reusability. The fetal bovine serum's response currents of detection were also very similar to those of the benchmark solutions. Due to its simplicity in production, tunable characteristics, optical/electrochemical properties, and exceptional durability in aqueous conditions, NP anodic alumina is also regarded as an effective material for the creation of biosensors.[77]

1.10.6 IMMUNOISOLATION

Immunoisolation is the process of preventing an immune response from reaching implanted cells or medication release mechanisms. Encapsulation utilizing an NP semipermeable membrane is typically used to achieve this. These holes are big enough to permit tiny molecules such as oxygen, glucose, and insulin to pass through yet small enough to prevent the passage of much bigger immune system chemicals such as immunoglobulin. Desai et al. studied the utilization of NP silicon surfaces created using microfabrication methods in the implanted artificial pancreas to cure diabetes.[78,79]

1.10.7 BIOMOLECULE SEPARATION AND CLASSIFICATION

The pharmaceutical business, the food industry, and biotechnology rely heavily on separation and sorting out to isolate and purify molecules from various biological feed streams. Separation science today employs various methods, such as size exclusion chromatography and biopolymer gel electrophoresis. Recently, numerous applications of biomolecular separation in more ordered pores have been investigated. The artificial NP membrane supports renal cells in the kidney application and functions as a blood filter that keeps serum proteins in while letting smaller waste materials out. Martin et al. have developed a membrane with a pore radius of less than 1 nm that is composed of a grid of cylindrical gold nanotubules. By switching the charge on the tubules from positive to negative, they demonstrated that it was feasible to reject ions with the opposite charge and enable voltage-gating of molecules with the opposing charges.[80]

1.10.8 ANTIBACTERIAL SOFTWARE

MOFs, which have lately attracted interest for usage in a variety of biological and medicinal applications, are extremely porous crystalline materials with a high loading capacity, structural variation, and biodegradability. The solvothermal synthesis of graphene oxide/cobalt metal-organic framework (GO/Co-MOF), which inhibits the development of Gram-negative *Escherichia coli* and Gram-positive *Staphylococcus aureus* bacteria, using cobalt ions and terephthalic acid. The release of cobalt ions and bacteria-damaging GO was considered as the antibacterial mechanism. At equal bacterial concentrations, colony counting results demonstrate the exceptionally high antibacterial activity of GO/Co-MOF against both bacteria, though more notably against *S. aureus*.[81]

Chlorhexidine (CHX), which is known to have antibacterial characteristics, was loaded onto Cu-BTC MOF. Significant antibacterial activity in

CHX@Cu-BTC demonstrates its potential for application as an antibacterial agent that is long-lasting, cost-efficient, and effective.[82]

Three-dimensional nanostructured Ag–Cu alloys with an atomic size of Ag to Cu ranging from zero to 1.0 were made by dealloying Mg-(Ag,Cu)-Y metallic glass predecessors in 0.04 M H_2SO_4 aqueous liquid. NP alloys with ultrafine ligament widths (down to 20 nm), a high particular surface area (up to 11.18 m^2 g), and good oxidation stability in an air environment were used to prevent the development of Gram-negative *E. coli* and Gram-positive *S. aureus*. The excellent antibacterial activity of this Ag–Cu alloy could be attributed to a very effective and long-lasting release of Cu ions.[83]

1.11 CONCLUDING REMARKS AND PROSPECTIVE VIEWS

The utilization of materials in new, high-performance applications is facilitated by NPMs with novel properties, including as large surface area, high specific strength, and unconventional functional behavior. For creating NPMFs, both electrochemical and nonelectrochemical processes have been proposed. To generate metals and metal oxides with controlled pore sizes, porous morphologies, and chemical compositions, the dealloying method has been extensively studied. Dealloying is a very straightforward process that produces mechanically strong NP materials; however, it cannot be seen as a universal technique to produce various materials, particularly soft ones. The method cannot be used to a variety of applications since the manufacturing process involves the use of dangerous chemicals, precision alloy preparation, and industrial scalability issues. Templating techniques may result in NP inorganic, polymeric, or composite materials, making them an option for dealloying techniques. However, since the withdrawal of the template may cause the nanostructures to become fragile, the mechanical performance of the NP formations is compromised and their potential practical applications are limited.

A growing range of industries, including biosensing, synthetic biology, medical implants, energy, the environment, and agriculture, are using NP materials. Due to their adaptability, advanced manufacturing methods have facilitated expansion in these fields, underscoring the fact that various applications need distinct requirements from nanostructured materials (i.e., pore size, pore structure, crystallinity, and ordered vs disordered structures). Because the frequency of the nanopores may alter how electromagnetic radiation interfaces with them, ordered NP materials perform much better in optoelectronics. For membrane and separation applications, ordered nanostructured materials are preferable over disordered ones. Contrary to ordered NP substances, disordered NP materials are mechanically robust and may be employed for applications needing great mechanical stability. Applications for microporous substances include sensing, catalysis, and medicine administration. To remove contaminants from water and gas storing systems, On the contrary, mesoporous materials may be utilized as adsorbents. The physical and chemical characteristics of NP materials might degrade over time if they are subjected to hostile conditions. A stable metal coating or metal doping into the NP structures is necessary to prevent these materials from degradation or aging.

There are still issues with conventional and environmentally acceptable fabrication techniques in industrial-scale manufacturing (capacity to make NP materials regardless of material choice without the use of harmful chemicals and materials recycling). New NP manufacturing techniques should be created and improved to reduce the dependency on hazardous and harsh solvents.

The catalytic potential and electrochemical activity of NMFs, as well as how these nanoarchitectures are similar to and different from nanoparticulate and bulk metals, still need to be described in greater detail. To fully realize the promise of NMFs for biological applications, techniques for controlling porosity at the nano, micro, and macro length scales as well as tactics for preventing monolithicity will need to be developed.

KEYWORDS

- **biomedical materials**
- **nanopores**
- **nanoscale membranes**
- **dealloying**
- **templating**
- **sol-gel**
- **combustion**
- **Ti alloys**
- **mesoporous silica**

REFERENCES

1. Hadden, M.; D. Martinez-Martin, Yong, K.-T.; Ramaswamy, Y.; Singh, G. Recent Advancements in the Fabrication of Functional Nanoporous Materials and Their Biomedical Applications. Materials 2022, 15, 2111.
2. Kim, Y. K.; Cha, S. I.; Hong, S. H. Nanoporous Cobalt Foam and a Co/Co (OH) 2 Core–Shell Structure for Electrochemical Applications. J. Mater. Chem. A 2013, 1, 9802–9808
3. Szczes´niak, B.; Choma, J.; Jaroniec, M. Major Advances in the Development of Ordered Mesoporous Materials. Chem. Commun. 2020, 56, 7836–7848.
4. Szczęs´niak, B.; Borysiuk, S.; Choma J.; Jaroniec, M. Mechanochemical Synthesis of Highly Porous Materials. Mater. Horiz. 2020, 7, 1457–1473.
5. Zhang, L.; Jaroniec, M. Strategies for Development of Nanoporous Materials with 2D Building Units. Chem. Soc. Rev. 2020, 49, 6039–6055.
6. Abdel-Karim, R. Nanoporous Metallic Foams for Energy Applications: Electrochemical Approaches for Synthesizing and Characterization. In: Handbook of Nanomaterials and Nanocomposites for Energy and Environmental Applications; Kharissova, O. V. et al., Eds.; Springer International Publishing, 2021; pp 489–511.
7. Baig, N.; Kammakakam I.; Falath, W. Nanomaterials: A Review of Synthesis Methods, Properties, Recent Progress, and Challenges. Mater. Adv. 2021, 2, 1821–1871.
8. Şeker, E.; Shih, W.-C.; Stine, K. J. Nanoporous Metals by Alloy Corrosion: Bioanalytical and Biomedical Applications MRS Bull. MRS Bull. 2018, 43 (1), 49–56.
9. Patela, P.; Bhingoleb, P. P.; Makwana, D. Manufacturing, Characterization and Applications of Lightweight Metallic Foams for Structural Applications: Review. Mater. Today: Proc. 2018, 5, 20391–20402.
10. Ortiz-Roldan, J. M.; Balestra, S. R. G.; Bueno-Perez, R.; Calero, S.; Garcia-Perez, E.; Richard, C.; Catlow, A.; Rabdel Ruiz-Salvador, A.; Hamad, S. Understanding the Stability and Structural Properties of Ordered Nanoporous Metals Towards Their Rational Synthesis. *Issue* **2022,** *2266*, 478.
11. Suvindran, N.; Servati, A.; Servati, P. Emerging Biomedical and Industrial Applications of Nanoporous Materials. In: *Advanced Functional Porous Materials: Engineering Materials*; Uthaman, A., Thomas, S., Li, T., Maria, H., Eds.; Springer, 2021.
12. Mishra, S. P.; Dutta, S.; Sahu, A. K.; Mishra K.; Kashyap, P. Chapter 3 Potential Application of Nanoporous Materials in Biomedical Field. In *Nanopores*; Ameen, S., Shaheer Akhtar, M., Shin, H.-S., Eds.; IntechOpen, 2021.
13. Zhou, Y.; Quan, G.; Wu, Q.; Zhang, X.; Niu, B.; Wu, B.; Huang, Y.; Pan X.; Wu, C. Mesoporous Silica Nanoparticles for Drug and Gene Delivery. *Acta Pharm. Sin. B* **2018,** *8*, 165–177.
14. S. Głowniak, B. Szczęśniak, Choma, J.; Jaroniec, M. Advances in Microwave Synthesis of Nanoporous Materials. *Adv. Mater.* **2021,** *33*, 2103477.
15. Pia, G.; Sogne, E.; Falqui A.; Delogu, F. Hardening of Nanoporous Au Induced by Exposure to Different Gaseous Environments. *Materials* **2022,** *15*, 2718.
16. Wang C.; Chen, Q. Reduction-Induced Decomposition: Spontaneous Formation of Monolithic Nanoporous Metals of Tunable Structural Hierarchy and Porosity. *Chem. Mater.* **2018,** *30* (11), 3894–3900.
17. Xiao, S.; Wang, S.; Wang, X.; Xu, P. Nanoporous Gold: A Review and Potentials in Biotechnological and Biomedical Applications. *Nano Select* **2021,** *2*, 1437–1458.

18. Shahbazi, P.; Kiani, A. Nanoporous Ag and Pd Foam: Redox Induced Fabrication Using Electrochemically Deposited Nanoporous Cu Foam with no Need to Any Additive. *Electrochimica Acta* **2011,** *56*, 9520–9529.
19. Yang, W.; Zheng, X.-G.; Wang, S.-G.; Jin, H.-J. Nanoporous Aluminum by Galvanic Replacement: Dealloying and Inward-Growth Plating. *J. Electrochem. Soc.* **2018,** *165* (9), C492–C496.
20. Yang, W.; Luo, Z.-P.; Bao, W.-K.; Xie, H.; You, Z.-S.; Jin, H.-J. Light, Strong, and Stable Nanoporous Aluminum with Native Oxide Shell. *Sci. Adv.* **2021,** *7*(28).
21. Gan, Y. X.; Zhang Y.; Gan, J. B. Review Nanoporous Metals Processed by Dealloying and Their Applications. *AIMS Mater. Sci.* **2018,** *5* (6), 1141–1183.
22. Erlebacher, J. An Atomistic Description of Dealloying Porosity Evolution, the Critical Potential, and Rate-Limiting Behavior. *J. Electrochem. Soc.* **2004,** *151* (10), C614–C626.
23. Erlebacher, J.; Aziz, M. J.; Karma, A.; Dimitrov, N.; Sieradzki, K. Evolution of Nanoporosity in Dealloying. *Nature* **2001,** *410* (6827), 450–453.
24. Hyun, J.-I.; Noh, H.-S.; Kong, K.; Kim, W. T.; Kim, D. H. Formation of Different Types Nanoporous Composite Structure by Dealloying of Ag and Ni Containing Al-Cu-Ti Base Amorphous Precursor Alloys. *Mater. Characterization* **2021,** *175*, 111093.
25. Abdel-Karim, R.; El-Raghy, S. Chapter 4 Electrochemical Deposition of Nanoporous Metallic Foams for Energy Applications. In: *Advanced Materials and their Applications—Micro to Nano Scale*; Ahmad, E., Ed.; One Central Press, 2017; pp 69–90.
26. Niauzorau, S.; Sharstniou, A.; Kublik, N.; Sampath, V. K.; Azeredo, B. Synthesis of Nanoporous Gold by Chemical Dealloying of Co-Sputtered Gold-Silver Thin Films and Study of Its Variability. In: *ASME 2021 16th International Manufacturing Science and Engineering Conference*, June 21–25, 2021.
27. Rahman, M. A.; Zhu, X.; Wen, C. Fabrication of Nanoporous Ni by Chemical Dealloying Al from Ni–Al Alloys for Lithium-Ion Batteries. *Int. J. Electrochem. Sci.* **2015,** *10*, 3767.
28. Barsuk, D. *Metallurgical Design of New Nanoporous Structures*; Ph. D Thesis, University of São Carlos: France, 2018.
29. Okulova, I. V.; Okulova, A. V.; Soldatov, I. V.; Luthringere, B.; Willumeit-Römere, R.; Wadab, T.; Katob, H.; Weissmüllera, J.; Markmann, J. Open Porous Dealloying-based Biomaterials as a Novel Biomaterial Platform. *Mater. Sci. Eng.: C* **2018,** *88*, 95–103.
30. Okulov, I. V.; Lamaka, S. V.; Wada, T.; Yubuta, K.; Zheludkevich, M. L.; Weissmüller, J.; Markmann, J.; Kato, H. Nanoporous Magnesium *Nano Res.* **2018,** *11* (12), 6428–6435.
31. Okulov, I. V.; Joo, S.-H.; Okulov, A. V.; Volegov, A. S.; Luthringer, B.; Willumeit-Römer, R.; Zhang, L.; Mädler, L.; Eckert, J.; Kato, H. Surface Functionalization of Biomedical Ti-6Al-7Nb Alloy by Liquid Metal Dealloying. *Nanomaterials* **2020,** *10* (8), 1479.
32. Pinna, A.; Pia, G.; Casula, M. F.; Delogu, F.; Sogne, E.; Falqui A.; Pilia, L. Fabrication of Nanoporous Al by Vapor-Phase Dealloying: Morphology Features, Mechanical Properties and Model Predictions. *Appl. Sci.* **2021,** *11*, 6639.
33. Chuang, A.; Erlebacher, J. Challenges and Opportunities for Integrating Dealloying Methods into Additive Manufacturing. *Materials* **2020,** *13*, 3706.
34. Qutaish, H. Q. *Synthesis and Characterisation of Mesoporous Transition Metal Oxides Based on Soft-Templating Method*; M.Sc. thesis, University of Wollongong: Australia, 2019.
35. Radhakrishnana, D.; Mohanana, S.; Choi, G.; Choy, J.-H.; Tiburciusa, S.; Trung, H.; Bolana, T. S.; Verrills, N.; Tanwara, P.; Karakotia A.; Vinu, A. The Emergence of

Nanoporous Materials in Lung Cancer Therapy. *Sci. Technol. Adv. Mater.* **2022,** *23* (1), 225–274.
36. Rebbecchi, T. A., Jr.; Chena, Y. Template-Based Fabrication of Nanoporous Metals. *J. Mater. Res.* **2018,** *33* (1), 2–15.
37. Dong, Y.; Ji, S.; Wang, H. V.; Linkovc; Wang, R. In-site Hydrogen Bubble Template Method to Prepare Ni Coated Metal Meshes as Effective Bi-functional Electrodes for Water Splitting. *Dalton Trans.* **2022,** *51*, 9681–9688.
38. Nørskov, J. K.; Bligaard, T.; Logadottir, A.; Kitchin, J. R.; Chen, J. G.; Pandelov, S.; Stimming, U. Trends in the Exchange Current for Hydrogen Evolution. *J. Electrochem. Soc.* **2005,** *152* (3), J23–J26.
39. Das, M.; Biswas, A.; Purkait, T.; Boruah, T.; Bhardwaj, S.; Das, S. K.; Dey, R. S. The Versatility of the Dynamic Hydrogen Bubble Template Derived Copper Foam on the Emerging Energy Applications: Progress and Future Prospects. *J. Mater. Chem. A* **2022,** *10*, 13589–13624.
40. Abdelfatah, A.; Reda, Y.; Abdel-Karim, R.; El-Raghy, S. M.; Zohdy, K. M. Electrochemical Characterization of Electrodeposited Ni–Cu Foams and Their Application as Electrodes for Supercapacitors. *Front. Mech. Eng.* **2020,** *6*, article 35.
41. Redaa, Y.; Abdel-Karim, R.; Zohdyc, K. M.; El-Raghy, S. Electrochemical Behavior of Ni–Cu Foams Fabricated by Dynamic Hydrogen Bubble Template Electrodeposition Used for Energy Applications. *Ain Shams Eng. J.* **2022,** *13* (1), 101532.
42. Vesztergom, S.; Dutta, A.; Rahaman, M.; Kiran, K.; Montiel, I. Z.; Broekmann, P. Hydrogen Bubble Templated Metal Foams as Efficient Catalysts of CO_2 Electroreduction. *ChemCatChem* **2021,** *13*, 1039–1058.
43. Owens, G. J.; Singh, R. K.; Foroutan, F.; Alqaysi, M.; Han, C.-M.; Mahapatra, C.; Kim, H.-W.; Knowles, J. C. Sol–Gel Based Materials for Biomedical Applications. *Progress Mater. Sci.* **2016,** *77*, 1–79.
44. Lei, Q.; Guo, J.; Noureddine, A.; Wang, A.; Wuttke, S.; Brinker, C. J.; Zhu, W. Sol–Gel-Based Advanced Porous Silica Materials for Biomedical Applications. *Adv. Funct. Mater.* **2020,** *30*, 1909539.
45. Ishikawa, K.; Garskaite, E.; Kareiva, A. Sol–gel Synthesis of Calcium Phosphate-based Biomaterials—A Review of Environmentally Benign, Simple, and Effective Synthesis Routes. *J. Sol–Gel Sci. Technol.* **2010,** *83* (12), 2094–2099.
46. Li, C.; Wang, M.; Luo Q.; Kim, E. J. Nanoporous Nickel Films on Glass Substrate by Sol–Gel Technique. *Mater. Res. Express* **2018,** *5* (7), 075011.
47. Hernán, J. P. F.; Torres, B.; López, A. J.; Rams, J. Review; The Role of the Sol–Gel Synthesis Process in the Biomedical Field and Its Use to Enhance the Performance of Bioabsorbable Magnesium Implants. *Gels* 2022, *8*, 426.
48. Uzun, O.; Hu, Y.; Verma, A.; Chen, S.; Centrone, A.; Stellacci, F. Water-Soluble Amphiphilic Gold Nanoparticles with Structured Ligand Shells. *Chem. Commun.* **2008,** 196.
49. Leventis, N.; N. Chandrasekaran, Sadekar, A. G.; C. Sotiriou-Leventis, and H. LuOne-Pot, Synthesis of Interpenetrating Inorganic/Organic Networks of CuO/ Resorcinol-Formaldehyde Aerogels: Nanostructured Energetic Materials, J. Am. Chem. Soc. 131(13), **2009,** 4576–4577.
50. Leventis, N.; Chandrasekaran, N.; Sadekar, A. G.; Leventis, C. S.; Lu, H. The Effect of Compactness on the Carbothermal Conversion of Interpenetrating Metal Oxide/

Resorcinol-Formaldehyde Nanoparticle Networks to Porous Metals and Carbides. *J. Mater. Chem.* **2010,** *20,* 7456–7471.
51. Tappan, B. C.; Steiner III, A. A.; Luther, E. P. Nanoporous Metal Foams. *Angew. Chem. Int. Ed.* **2010,** *49,* 4544–4565.
52. Głowniak, S.; Szczęśniak, B.; Choma, J.; Jaroniec, M. Advances in Microwave Synthesis of Nanoporous Materials. *Adv. Mater.* **2021,** *33,* 2103477.
53. Ramu G.; Jeong, H.-K.; Recent Progress on Metal-Organic Framework Membranes for Gas Separations: Conventional Synthesis vs. Microwave-Assisted Synthesis. *Membr. J.* **2017,** *27* (1), 1–42.
54. Bai, Z.; Zhang, L.; Li, H.; Liu, L. Nanopore Creation in Graphene by Ion Beam Irradiation: Geometry, Quality, and Efficiency. *ACS Appl. Mater. Interfaces* **2016,** *8* (37), 24803–24809.
55. Wanga, C.; Huang, H.; Zhang, Z.; Zhang, L.; Yan, J.; Ren, L.; Formation, Evolution and Characterization of Nanoporous Structures on the Ti_6Al_4V Surface Induced by Nanosecond Pulse Laser Iirradiation. *Mater. Design* **2022,** *223,* 111243.
56. Aihara, H.; Zider, J.; Fanton, G.; Duerig, T. Combustion Synthesis Porous Nitinol for Biomedical Applications. *Int. J. Biomater.* **2019,** *2019,* Article ID 4307461, 11 pages.
57. Berger, S. A.; Okulov, I. V. Open Porous α + β Titanium Alloy by Liquid Metal Dealloying for Biomedical Applications. *Metals* **2020,** *10,* 1450.
58. Okulov, I. V.; Weissmüller, J.; Markmann, J. Dealloying-based Interpenetrating Phase Nanocomposites Matching the Elastic Behavior of Human Bone. *Sci. Rep.* **2017,** *7,* Article 20.
59. Okulov, I. V.; Okulov, A. V.; Soldatov, I. V.; Luthringer, B.; Willumeit-Römer, R.; Wada, T.; Kato, H.; Weissmüller, J.; Markmann, J. Open Porous Dealloying-based Biomaterials as a Novel Biomaterial Platform. *Mater. Sci. Eng.: C* **2018,** *88* (1), 95–103.
60. J. M. Rúa, Zuleta, A. A.; J. Ramírez, P. Fernández-Morales, Micro-arc Oxidation Coating on Porous Magnesium Foam and Its Potential Biomedical Applications, Surface and Coatings Technology, 360, **2019,** 213- 221.
61. Devi, K. B.; Singh, K.; Rajendran, N. Sol–gel Synthesis and Characterisation of Nanoporous Zirconium Titanate Coated on 316L SS for Biomedical Applications. *J. Sol–Gel Sci. Technol.* **2011,** *59,* 513–520.
62. Ben˘cina, M.; Junkar, I.; Vesel, A.; Mozeti˘c, M.; Igli˘c, A. Review Nanoporous Stainless Steel Materials for Body Implants—Review of Synthesizing Procedures. *Nanomaterials* **2022,** *12,* 2924.
63. Xiao, S.; Wang, S.; Wang, X.; Xu, P. Nanoporous Gold: A Review and Potentials in Biotechnological and Biomedical Applications. *Nano Select* **2021,** *2,* 1437–1458.
64. Miria, B.; Motakef-Kazemib, N.; Shojaosadatia, S. A.; Morsali, A. Application of a Nanoporous Metal Organic Framework Based on Iron Carboxylate as Drug Delivery System. *Iran. J. Pharma. Res.* **2018,** *17* (4), 1164–1171.
65. Bae, I.; Lim, K.-S.; Park, J.-K.; Song, J. H.; Oh, S.-H.; Kim, J.-W.; Zhang, Z.; Park C.; Koh, J.-T. Evaluation of Cellular Response and Drug Delivery Efficacy of Nanoporous Stainless Steel Material. *Biomater. Res.* **2021,** *25,* 30.
66. Jibowu, T. A Review on Nanoporous Metals. *Front. Nanosci. Nanotech. 2* (4), 165–168.
67. Wang, Y.; Zhao, Q.; Han, N.; Bai, L.; Li, J.; Liu, J.; Che, E.; Hu, L.; Zhang, Q.; Jiang T.; Wang, S. *Nanomedicine* **2015,** *11,* 313–327.
68. Keskin, S.; Kızıle, S. Biomedical Applications of Metal Organic Frameworks. *Ind. Eng. Chem. Res.* **2011,** *50* (4), 1799–1812.

body because of their versatility and availability. The detection and treatment of diseases have been reported to aid in organ regeneration, which has led to the replacement of organs such as the heart, trachea, lungs, etc., by using specialized biomaterials.

2.1 INTRODUCTION

Sometimes genetic defects, aging, illnesses, trauma, degeneration, or accidents render human tissues and organs unable to perform their usual tasks. To address some of these diseases, people use drugs or regular medications. While some conditions can be treated with medication, others need specialized tools and materials. The inevitable result of this is the need for surgical repair, which affects anatomical components including teeth, vertebrae, knee joints, elbow joints, and other critical organs including the heart, skin, kidney, etc.

In its broadest definition, biomaterials are unique compounds or mixes of substances that are primarily anticipated to be used within an animal or a human to heal, enhance, or replace any kind of tissue. These biomaterials can be produced artificially or spontaneously by several physical and chemical methods. An interdisciplinary field is biomaterials.

In an effort to repair human bodies that have been weakened by disease or injury, metals, and other materials have been used extensively in the form of implants and other biomedical devices ever since our species first attempted to do so.[1] Biomaterials have made a significant impact on the rapidly developing pharmaceutical and medical industries during the last few decades.

Biomaterials are substances used for medicinal and diagnostic purposes that are designed to interact with biological living tissue. Any natural or synthetic material designed for implantation in living tissues, particularly as a component of a medical device, can be described as such in medical jargon.[2] Prior to now, these materials had only been employed in medical devices to treat, replace, or enhance organ functions. However, it was later discovered that they should not be given the designation "nonviable," as biomaterials have applications outside implanted devices.

Biomaterials play an important role in the routine diagnosis and treatment of many human diseases. To support, enhance, restore, or replace the biological function of damaged tissues, biomaterials are used while in continual contact with bodily fluids and they must be biologically compatible with the human body.[3]

2.2 USES OF BIOMATERIALS

Iron, cobalt, and titanium (Ti)-based systems are being used as surgical implant devices, and metallic materials have found extensive applications in this field. With relatively few devices displaying clinically significant constraints linked to material qualities, basic research, and clinical studies have unequivocally shown that alloys have their proper uses. This is, of course, in relation to the enormous number engaged.[4] Different organs and examples of biomaterials used for different purposes are summarized in Table 2.1

TABLE 2.1 Organs and Their Examples.

Organ/Tissues	Examples
Heart	Artificial valves, biventricular pacemakers, and artificial hearts
Eye	Contact lenses and synthetic intraocular lenses
Ear	Hair clips, cochlear implants, and artificial stapes
Muscle	Sutures
Kidney	Dialysis equipment
Skin	Skin substitutes, burn dressings, artificial skin, and skin wound healing
Circulation	Artificial blood vessels
Bone	Bone cement, intramedullary rods, bone screws, and plates are used to fix defects
Teeth	Replacements and fillings

2.3 DESIRED PROPERTIES OF BIOMATERIALS

Treatment, improvement, or replacement of tissue, organs, or biological functions is the ultimate goal of biomaterials in medicine (such as bone, muscle, and skin). These goals can be accomplished by integrating material properties, system properties, device architecture, and physiological requirements. The biological system's chemical and mechanical qualities must be integrated into the biomaterial application process to yield the required functional results. Many scientific and social factors are taken into account while processing biomaterials and related medical supplies.[5]

2.3.1 BIOCOMPATIBILITY

From a biological perspective, biocompatibility simply refers to the acceptance of synthetic or natural nonliving materials in a living (mammal or human) body. A material is said to be accepted when it is "able to carry out its intended tasks in relation to a therapeutic intervention, to elicit the required host response in a given setting, and to interact with living systems without injuring or poisoning the organisms involved or causing the immune system to reject it."

Since a biomaterial is intended to be used near living tissues, it must have no harmful effects on the host organs or surrounding tissues. Additionally, it is encouraged that the implanted material should stimulate a favorable cellular or tissue response rather than inhibit the functioning of normal cells or result in any unfavorable local or systemic reactions in the recipient. Depending on the many medical uses, the requirements for this biocompatibility are frequently complex and vary. For instance, a particularly crafted material (such as a screw or plate) might be acceptable for use in bone implant surgery but might not be acceptable for use on the skin.[5]

2.3.2 HOST RESPONSE

The definition of host reaction is "the local and systemic response of the host organism to the implanted substance or device." The majority of Never are things inert, and the host tissue's reaction to the alien material has a substantial impact on a biomaterial's therapeutic effectiveness. The duration, intent, and location of implantation all have a significant impact on the material establishment-host tissue interaction.[5]

2.3.3 NONTOXICITY

Elements that migrate out of biomaterials are the subject of their toxicity. A well-designed biomaterial should perform its function in the environment of the live body without having an adverse effect on other cells, organs, or the entire organism. A biomaterial shouldn't logically release or create anything from its bulk unless it is particularly intended to do so.[5]

2.3.4 MECHANICAL PROPERTIES

In addition to biocompatibility, mechanical qualities are incorporated into the design of biomaterials before use and will significantly influence the result. Materials are subject to a variety of forces, mainly under the conditions of stress, strain, shear, and combinations of these. Tensile strength, elongation at break, elongation at break, elastic modulus, resistance to corrosion and creep, and other properties of a biomaterial and hardness are some of the most crucial characteristics that need to be carefully examined and assessed before implantation. The mechanical qualities are crucial for applications involving hard tissues.

2.3.5 CORROSION, WEAR, AND FATIGUE PROPERTIES

One of the main reasons for implant failure is frequently thought to be wear. On rare occasions, it has been shown that wear accelerates the corrosion of biomedical devices and implants. The response of the material to repeated cycle stresses affects the fatigue resistance.[5]

2.3.6 DESIGN AND MANUFACTURABILITY

One of the crucial aspects to take into account for biomaterials is appropriate material design. For instance, in the early 1900s, people used bone plates to help mend lengthy bone fractures. Due to their poor mechanical design, which made them overly narrow and with a corner that concentrated force, several of these experimental plates cracked. Manufacturability is the ability to produce the product reliably, affordably, and with a level of ease that is appropriate for the purpose for which it is intended. In relation to biomaterials, the term "maneuverability" encompasses the capacity of the material to be sterilized using a validated sterilization process that is judged suitable for biomedical purposes.

In conclusion, any of the following conditions must be met for a material to be considered a biomaterial

- Be biocompatible, that is, nontoxic, noncarcinogenic, nonallergenic, etc.
- Possess necessary or appropriate physical and chemical characteristics
- Possess the necessary mechanical properties
- Hours to years, depending on the application, steady durability
- Ease of processing with extant techniques; ease of sterilization with existing facilities; cost-effectiveness and accessibility.

2.4 TYPES OF BIOMATERIALS

Based on their chemical bonding, materials can be roughly classified into three broad classes as follows:

- Polymers
- Ceramics
- Metals

These materials' varied covalent, ionic, or metallic bonding types result in diverse characteristics and, consequently, different functions in the body. There are various biomaterials and chemical linkages connected to it. Although both metals and ceramics are inorganic substances, there are differences between them in the realm of materials engineering. Every material has advantages and disadvantages of its own, and the biomedical applications of each are chosen based on their unique characteristics and intended place substitution.[5]

2.4.1 METALLIC BIOMATERIALS

As early as 1565, when Petr Onium suggested using gold plates to fix cleft palates, metals have reportedly been utilized in surgical treatments. Since then, metallic implants have been used as fixation or prosthetic devices in a number of orthopedic surgeries.

The purpose of prostheses is to restore missing body parts such as bones, joints, and plates in the skull. To regulate the bone and other tissues while they recover, fixing devices are used. The body currently uses metals the most during orthopedic procedures. A wide variety of implants are available, from simple wires and screws through fracture-fixation plates and total joint prostheses (artificial joints) for the hips, knees, shoulders, elbows, and other joints.[1]

Medical implants made of metal are quite important. Because of their mechanical qualities, biocompatibility, minimal friction, affordability, and corrosion resistance, metallic biomaterials are favored.[5] However, they are quite aggressive to the microenvironment, which can result in metal oxidation and the release of undesired metallic ions, both of which can harm and inflame the local tissues.[6] The most prevalent metallic biomaterials are Gold and gold alloys, A wide variety of metals include steels, stainless steels, Ti alloys, cobalt chromium alloys, and more. Metallic biomaterials offer a variety of inherent qualities, including strength, electrical conductivity, durability, mechanical dependability, and resistance to corrosion and wear. These characteristics of metallic biomaterials make metals more dominant than other materials in medical equipment. Nearly 70–60% of manufactured implants are discovered to be made of metal.[7]

Iron, cobalt, and Ti-based systems are being used as surgical implant devices, and metallic materials have found extensive applications in this field. With relatively few devices displaying clinically significant constraints linked to material qualities, basic research, and Clinical studies have unequivocally shown that alloys have their place in some applications. This is, of course, in relation to the enormous number employed. In part because of this background, certain metals with known biocompatibility profiles have been listed as synthetic biomaterials for tissue replacement.[4]

2.4.2 APPLICATIONS AND MECHANICAL PROPERTIES

2.4.2.1 SURGICAL STAINLESS STEEL

Since more than a century ago, metal plates have been utilized to internally treat fractures. Modern designs still have some problems, even though earlier problems such as corrosion and inadequate strength have been resolved. To create a plate that speeds up fracture healing without affecting bone physiology, more study is required.[8]

Sherman is credited for developing the iron-based alloys that are currently in use. This alloy is a relatively ductile and robust system that is easily fabricated using common machining techniques. There are plenty of plates, screws, rods, external fixators, and other equipment used in surgery that have relatively low production costs.[4]

2.4.3 COBALT-BASED ALLOYS

In comparison to systems based on iron and Ti, cast cobalt has been described as one of the least ductile alloys. The relative utility of the cobalt-based alloy systems has undoubtedly significantly enhanced as a result of recent manufacturing and alloy improvements.[4]

2.4.4 TITANIUM-BASED ALLOYS

As a means of restoring normal bodily function in a number of situations, surgical implants have been used extensively. Over 100,000 surgical implant procedures have been carried out in the field of dentistry, with Ti and Ti-based alloys accounting for the majority of these procedures in recent years. These implants are now frequently used as anchors for orofacial prostheses, pins, and plates are commonplace in orthopedic surgery, and supports for metal frameworks in edentulous patients.

It appears that a Ti implant's ability to osseointegrate with the surrounding bone is a key factor in determining whether or not it will be successful. When determining how long-lasting a prosthesis will be, "osseointegration" means that the implant is in intimate contact with the patient's living bone (at a light microscopic level). In other words, the fact that bone may grow up to the surface of Ti indicates that it has bioactive characteristics in the presence of tissue. It is possible that the osseointegration of Ti implants in the mandible will be so successful that the metal bridgework will fail due to plastic collapse and the acrylic overlay will break due to brittle failure during masticating.[9]

2.4.5 POLYMERS

The mainstays created for the delivery of therapeutic medications are polymers.[10] Due to the polymers' ability to deteriorate, polymeric materials are widely used in the biomedical industry. Different strategies are used to synthesize various polymers. Different wounded tissues are replaced using polymeric scaffolds (hard and soft tissues). Because of their subpar mechanical qualities, polymeric alternatives are less frequently used in hard tissue engineering. Thus, cross-linking via chemical processes is carried out to enhance the mechanical qualities.[11]

Bioactive substances or pharmaceuticals are entrapped inside an insoluble matrix with sub-, nano-, or micrometer-sized dimensions to offer regulated drug delivery.

The most popular option for a matrix for the regulated release of medicinal drugs is polymeric material.[12] Better drug integration, precise drug targeting, controlled drug release, improved stability, maximum distribution, and less toxicity while preserving therapeutic effectiveness should be the ideal features demanded of a biodegradable polymer.[13] Various polymers and their applications are represented in Table 2.2.

2.4.5.1 NATURAL POLYMERS

Pagarose, a marine polysaccharide extracted from red seaweed, is highly favorable due to its thermos gelling behavior, its ability to be chemically functionalized in a versatile manner, and its high bioactivity. Therefore,

TABLE 2.2 Polymers and Their Applications.

S. No.	Polymer	Application
1.	Ultrahigh-molecular-weight polyethylene	Knee, hip, shoulder, joints, dental bridges
2.	Silicone rubber	Finger joints
3.	Cells/polytetrafluoroethylene, Cells/ polyethylene terephthalate, Collagen	Vascular graft
4.	Bioglass/polyurethane, carbon fibers	Spine cages, plates, rods, screws, discs
5.	Polyethylene terephthalate/polyurethane, polyethylene terephthalate/collagen	Abdominal wall prosthesis
6.	Polyethylene terephthalate/poly(2-hydroxyethyl methacrylate), Kevlar fibers/ polymethacrylate, carbon fibers	Tendons/ligaments
7.	Polyethylene terephthalate/polyurethane, polytetrafluoroethylene/polyurethane, carbon fibers/Polytetrafluoroethylene	Cartilage replacement
8.	Polydimethyl siloxane, polyurethane, polyvinyl chloride	Facial prostheses
9.	Polymethyl methacrylate	Bone cement (2)

agarose is a key component in many different types of drug delivery systems. Most commonly known sources of the biomaterial alginate include the brown algae *Laminaria hyperborean*, *Laminaria digitate*, *Laminaria japonica*, *Ascophyllum nodosum*, and *Macrocystis pyrifera*.

The impressive mechanical qualities and enticing biological attributes of nanocellulose have made it a promising material. Hydrogel synthesis for 3D bioprinting works very well with pectin synthesized from plant cell walls because of its high molecular weight and hydrophilicity. A water-soluble polymer obtained from marine brown algae is called fucoid. PStarch is a polysaccharide derived from wheat and other tuber plants. Collagen is used as a biomaterial in wound-healing scaffolds. It is commonly utilized for skin wound healing since it is plentiful in the body and makes up most of the dermal extracellular matrix (ECM). Chitin and chitosan derivatives are polymeric polymers used as excipients, medication carriers, oral mucoadhesives, and water-resistant adhesives due to their release qualities and stickiness.[3]

2.4.5.2 SYNTHETIC POLYMERS

Research into biodegradable synthetic polymer-resistant adhesives is ongoing due to the need for new materials with properties tailored to meet the biochemical and biomechanical requirements in emerging technologies such as tissue engineering, regenerative medicine, gene therapy, novel drug delivery systems, and implantable devices.[14]

Polyesters are made by polycondensing mixtures of diols and dicarboxylic acids, or by using a catalyst that can be concentrated and segregated in the noncrystalline component to achieve a 100% polymer formation rate. In addition to the characteristics of the enzyme-catalyzed reactions mentioned above, it has been reported that di vinyl di carboxylates are efficient monomers for the enzyme-catalyzed polycondensation, making the use of enzyme in polyester synthesis noteworthy from the perspective of "green chemistry."[15]

The transformation of polymer into oriented reinforcing elements creates morphological structures out of groups of oriented polymer chains.[16]

A synthetic polymer being studied for use in biomedical applications is polyglycolide. Due to its high degree of crystallinity, this polymer has poor solubility in organic solvents and a high tensile modulus. Due to its great crystallinity, it exhibits exceptional mechanical qualities. Compared to other biodegradable polymeric systems used in medicine, polyglycolide is very rigid.[3] Several instances of synthetic polymers are discussed in the following subsections.

2.4.5.3 POLYESTERS

There are numerous families of synthetic biodegradable polymers from which to choose depending on the application. The most well-researched of them are poly (α-hydroxyl acid esters). Bioabsorbable sutures, drug delivery systems, and orthopedic fixation tools such as pins, rods, and screws are some of the main applications. These polymers continue to be appealing despite some drawbacks since it is simple to degrade them by the ester bond hydrolysis can result in breakdown products that are occasionally reabsorbed through metabolic pathways. By utilizing different copolymerization techniques, they can additionally modify the structure's mechanical and degradation rates.[14]

2.4.5.4 POLYANHYDRIDES

One of the most well-investigated groups of biodegradable polymers, polyanhydrides have proven biocompatibility and excellent controlled release properties. Recent reviews have been done on polyanhydride production, characteristics, and biodegradation. The first person to use the hydrolytic instability of aliphatic polyanhydrides for persistent drug release was Langer in 1980. Polyanhydrides are highly desirable for controlled-release applications because of their hydrophobic character, which causes surface erosion to cause surface degradation. Clinical applications of polyanhydride-based drug delivery devices have been made.[14]

2.4.5.5 POLYCARBONATES

Another family of synthetic polymers being studied for biodegradability is polycarbonate. Under physiological circumstances, aliphatic polycarbonates, such as poly(trimethylene carbonate), deteriorate. Aliphatic polycarbonates typically soften to an excessive degree, and their poor mechanical qualities make them less desirable for use in most applications. One benefit of polycarbonates is their degradation products, which are often less acidic than those created by the breakdown of polyesters such as polycarbonate (lactic acid). Targeting uses in drug delivery and tissue engineering; recent investigations have concentrated on creating aliphatic polycarbonates with functional groups that allow manipulation of the degradation rate and mechanical properties.[14]

2.4.5.6 POLYESTERAMIDES

Polyester amides are amphiphilic and biodegradable due to the presence of both amide and ester bonds. They are made to combine polyester's biodegradability with the excellent mechanical qualities of polyamides. These polymers have good thermal and mechanical properties even at low molecular weight because of the polar nature of amide groups and their capacity to form hydrogen bonds.[14]

2.4.5.7 CERAMICS

Inorganic solid materials known as ceramics are made up of metallic and nonmetallic components that are mostly connected by ionic bonding. These chemicals can be found as crystalline and noncrystalline (amorphous) compounds. Ceramics often have excellent biocompatibility, tremendous wear resistance, good corrosion resistance, high strength, extraordinarily high stiffness, and hardness. The biomedical field has focused mostly on using ceramic materials in orthopedics and dentistry. Industry has advanced. Some of the most commonly used bioceramics are bioinert ceramics such as alumina, zirconia, and pyrolytic carbon as well as bioresorbable ceramics such as calcium phosphates.[5]

2.4.5.8 *BIOACTIVE GLASS*

It has been more than 30 years since the first use of bioactive glasses (BGs) and other glass-ceramic biomaterials in the treatment of bone tissue damage. The most salient features of BGs, including those that made them special to begin with, have been extensively covered in the literature, most notably by their inventor Larry Hench.

Recent research has concentrated on ways to change their composition to impart novel traits such as antibacterial activity or further enhance their osteogenic behavior. Mounting data suggests that BGs and related glass ceramics can be engineered to introduce numerous desirable features all at once.[17]

2.4.5.9 *COMPOSITES BIOMATERIAL*

In most cases, the term "composite" refers to materials whose discrete phases have different properties, such as elastic modulus, and are separated on a scale larger than the atomic level markedly different from those of a homogeneous material. As a result, alloys such as brass are not considered composite materials, while reinforced polymers such as fiberglass and natural materials such as bone are. A composite called foam has an empty phase in it. Natural composites include skin, cartilage, dentin, wood, and bone. Wood, cancellous bone, and lung are examples of natural foams. Natural composites frequently have hierarchical structures with distinct particle, porous, and fibrous structural properties.[18]

It is crucial for every component of a composite in biomaterials to be biocompatible. Additionally, the body environment should not damage the interface between constituents. The following are a few biological uses for composites:

- Composite materials for dental fillings.
- Bone cement is made of reinforced methyl methacrylate and ultra-high molecular weight polyethylene.
- Surface-textured orthopedic implants.

Swelling is another effect of polymer components absorbing moisture. In dental composites, this swelling is advantageous since it partially compensates for shrinkage brought on by polymerization. Flexible composite bone plates work well to speed up the healing process, but their particulate debris can trigger a foreign body reaction akin to that brought on by ultrahigh molecular weight polyethylene.[18] Table 2.3 shows the application of biomaterials and their advantages and disadvantages.

TABLE 2.3 Applications of Various Types of Biomaterials, Their Benefits, and Drawbacks.

Types of biomaterials	Advantages	Disadvantages	Applications
Ceramics	Very little thermal and electrical conductivity, excellent biocompatibility, and high inertness.	Poor resistance to impacts, high manufacturing difficulty, and poor reproducibility.	Dental components, coatings, structural bone replacement, medical devices, bone fillings, and tissue regeneration are all examples of technologies related to bones.
Polymers	Low frictional qualities, simple to fabricate.	Low resistance to movement.	Implants, tissue replacement, eye lenses, sutures, and synthetic tendons.
Metals	Low friction, strong mechanical resistance, and low-cost	In a physiological environment, low biocompatibility and low resistance to corrosion are present, and mechanical qualities differ from those of biological tissues.	implants for the teeth, joint prostheses.
Biocomposites	High biocompatibility, resistance to corrosion, and inertness.	Difficult to fabricate in a similar way.	Artificial joints, knee implants, heart valves, and implants.[5]

2.4.6 APPLICATIONS OF BIOMATERIALS

Biomaterials are used in a variety of pharmaceutical and medical contexts, including as drug delivery, organ regeneration, and tissue engineering.

2.4.6.1 DENTAL APPLICATION

Resin composites, Ti alloys, zirconia, and other materials are all examples of dental biomaterials.[3] The Food and Drug Administration has authorized the use of synthetic biodegradable polymers such as polyglycolic acid (PGA), polylactic acid (PLA), and polylactic-coglycolide as drug delivery mechanisms. Due to their high reproducibility and biocompatibility, they are perfect for use in tissue engineering research. Prepared old polymers can have their shape, porosity, mechanical properties, pore size, and breakdown rate controlled. Degradation of synthetic polymers is often a simple hydrolysis process.[19]

2.4.6.2 ORGAN REGENERATION

Heart: Some examples of biomaterials used in the heart are cardiac pacemakers, artificial heart valves, total artificial heart, and blood vessels.[18]

Lung: The lungs of rats have been rebuilt ex vivo by seeding pulmonary epithelium and vascular endothelium on decellular Zed scaffolds.[3]

Knee: It was proposed that two types of ceramic-based functional biomaterials be used to reduce the risk of aseptic loosening in total knee replacements and to improve the performance of the bone prosthesis. Alumina and zircon biomaterials with functionally graded surfaces showed promising results.[3]

One of the most often used materials in orthopedics is Ti alloy. High strength, low density, strong resistance to corrosion, whole-body nontoxicity, and a mild elastic modulus make Ti alloys great materials for body implants. The fixity of the implant is dramatically improved, and micromovement is significantly reduced, by the relatively strong link that Ti and its alloys may create with the bone.[20]

2.4.6.3 REGENERATIVE MEDICINES

Regenerative medicine is an interdisciplinary field that merges the principles of materials science, conventional medicine, and the biological sciences to regenerate human organs and tissues with enhanced biological structures and functions. It is a system that incorporates tissue engineering and drug delivery. In regenerative medicine, scaffolding materials are implanted to stimulate tissue regeneration. This is because the native cells are brought into the scaffold, where they deposit ECM. To enhance tissue repair and regeneration, alginate is an exciting biomaterial with various possible applications. Due to its outstanding qualities in biocompatibility, biodegradability, nonantigenicity, and chelating ability, alginate has been widely used in a variety of biomedical applications, such as tissue engineering, drug delivery, and in some formulations to reduce stomach reflux.[21]

2.4.6.4 TISSUE ENGINEERING

The primary stage for successful tissue engineering is the construction of scaffolds. There must have been a lot of material utilized in the construction. The scaffolds can be built using a variety of natural and synthetic polymers.

When using electric fields during tissue engineering, electrically conductive polymers can be utilized in combination with other polymers to produce improved biological and physiological properties. Several tissue engineering fields use electrospun nanofibers. Although electrospinning is not a technology for making scaffolds, it can be utilized to produce electro-spun when paired with 3D printing, nanofiber can be used as a biomaterial and deliver cell-stimulating chemicals with ease.

Artificial organs can be developed using tissue engineering. It is possible to optimize remodeling and functional results for a certain development by adjusting the material design, including the pore size and degradation kinetics, and the functionalization with cell- and tissue-specific components, the intrinsic factors of the tissue constructs.[3]

2.5 CONCLUSION

Biomaterials have the potential to be the most interdisciplinary study area. The medical and pharmaceutical communities have benefited greatly from them ever since their beginnings. There are several applications for the wide variety of biomaterials that are now in use. The shape and function of tissues and organs are mimicked by a variety of biomaterials utilized in implants for organ regeneration, tissue regeneration, wound healing, disease diagnostics and treatment, and medication delivery. Recent years have also seen biomaterials used in regenerative medicine and urology. Nanocarriers, along with other drug delivery scaffolds, are showing considerable promise. The pharmaceutical and medical industries are coming to recognize the potential of biomaterials.

KEYWORDS

- **biomedical materials**
- **Nanopores**
- **Nano-scale membranes**
- **Dealloying**
- **Templating**
- **Sol-gel**
- **Combustion**
- **Titanium alloys**
- **Mesoporous silica**
- **Mechanical behavior**
- **Biocompatibility**
- **Biosensing**
- **Drug delivery**
- **Implantable materials**

REFERENCES

1. Mahapatro, A. Bio-functional nano-coatings on metallic biomaterials. Materials Science and Engineering: C. **2015,** 55:227–51.
2. Bhat, S.; Kumar, A. Biomaterials and Bioengineering Tomorrow's Healthcare. *Biomatter* **2013,** *3* (3), e24717.
3. Naidu, N. A.; Wadher, K.; Umekar, M. An Overview on Biomaterials: Pharmaceutical and Biomedical Applications. *J. Drug Deliv. Therap.* **2021,** *11* (1-s), 154–161.
4. Lemons, J.; Lucas, L. Properties of Biomaterials. *J. Arthroplasty* **1986,** *1* (2), 143–147.
5. Raghavendra, G. M.; Varaprasad, K.; Jayaramudu, T. Biomaterials: Design, Development and Biomedical Applications. In: *Nanotechnology Applications for Tissue Engineering.* Elsevier, 2015; pp 21–44.
6. Prasad, K.; Bazaka, O.; Chua, M.; Rochford, M.; Fedrick, L.; Spoor, J. et al. Metallic Biomaterials: Current Challenges and Opportunities. *Materials* **2017,** *10* (8), 884.
7. Festas, A.; Ramos, A.; Davim, J. Medical Devices Biomaterials–A Review. *Proc. Inst. Mech. Eng. Part L* **2020,** *234* (1), 218–228.
8. Sherman, W. Vanadium Steel Bone Plates and Screws. *Surg. Gynecol. Obstet.* **1912,** *14,* 629–34.
9. Sutherland, D. S.; Forshaw, P.; Allen, G.; Brown, I.; Williams, K. R. Surface Analysis of Titanium Implants. *Biomaterials* **1993,** *14* (12), 893–899.

10. Asadpour, S.; Yeganeh, H.; Ai, J.; Ghanbari, H. A Novel Polyurethane Modified with Biomacromolecules for Small-Diameter Vascular Graft Applications. *J. Mater. Sci.* **2018,** *53* (14), 9913–9927.
11. Oryan, A.; Kamali, A.; Moshiri, A.; Baharvand, H.; Daemi, H. Chemical Crosslinking of Biopolymeric Scaffolds: Current Knowledge and Future Directions of Crosslinked Engineered Bone Scaffolds. *Int. J. Biol. Macromol.* **2018,** *107*, 678–688.
12. Wadher, K. J.; Kakde, R. B.; Umekar, M. J. Study on Sustained-Release Metformin Hydrochloride from Matrix Tablet: Influence of Hydrophilic Polymers and In Vitro Evaluation. *Int. J. Pharm. Investig.* **2011,** *1* (3), 157.
13. Roy, S. M.; Sahoo, S. K. Controlled Drug Delivery: Polymeric Biomaterials for Encyclopedia of Biomedical Polymers and Polymeric Biomaterials. **2015,** *11*, 2135–2146.
14. Gunatillake, P.; Mayadunne, R.; Adhikari, R. Recent Developments in Biodegradable Synthetic Polymers. *Biotechnol. Annu. Rev.* **2006,** *12*, 301–347.
15. Okada, M. Chemical Syntheses of Biodegradable Polymers. *Progress Polym. Sci.* **2002,** *27* (1), 87–133.
16. Törmälä, P. Biodegradable self-Reinforced Composite Materials; Manufacturing Structure and Mechanical Properties. *Clin. Mater.* **1992,** *10* (1–2), 29–34.
17. Fernandes, J. S.; Gentile, P.; Pires, R. A.; Reis, R. L.; Hatton, P. V. Multifunctional Bioactive Glass and Glass-Ceramic Biomaterials with Antibacterial Properties for Repair and Regeneration of Bone Tissue. *Acta Biomater.* **2017,** *59*, 2–11.
18. Parida, P.; Behera, A.; Mishra, S. C. Classification of Biomaterials Used in Medicine, 2012.
19. Alshehadat, S. A.; Thu, H. A.; Hamid, S. S. A.; Nurul, A. A.; Rani, S. A.; Ahmad, A. Scaffolds for Dental Pulp Tissue Regeneration: A Review. *Int. Dental Med. J. Adva. Res.* **2016,** *2* (1), 1–12.
20. Ayatollahi, M. R.; Davari, M. H.; Shirazi, H. A.; Asnafi, A. To Improve Total Knee Prostheses Performance Using Three-Phase Ceramic-Based Functionally Graded Biomaterials. *Front. Mater.* **2019,** *6*, 107.
21. Sun, J., Tan, H. Alginate-Based Biomaterials for Regenerative Medicine Applications. *Materials* **2013,** *6* (4), 1285–1309.

CHAPTER 3

Metallic Nanocarrier for Bone Tissue Engineering

AJAYKUMAR CHITTIPOLU

Vision College of Pharmaceutical Sciences and Research, JNTUH, Hyderabad, Telangana, India

ABSTRACT

Tissue engineering (TE) strives to create integrated solutions that use technical, biological, and medical notions to provide effective replacements for damaged tissues. Bone regeneration is one of the areas where it remains difficult to create a model that accurately matches all tissue characteristics. Due to its hierarchical nature and extensive vascularization of bone, particularly in big bone defects, in conjunction to the tremendous mechanical stress to which it is confronted the regeneration of bone remains challenged. With the advancement in technology permitting the creation of nanostructures that are similar in size to the structures found in natural bone, nanotechnology has the potential to usher in a new age for TE. Nanomaterials have garnered a lot of interest in biomedical applications due to their exceptional qualities, including their favorable biosafety, huge specific surface area, tenability, porosity, and diverse applications. Among them, metal-based nanomaterials show significant bone tissue regeneration potential, advanced drug delivery utilities, and antibacterial properties, making them essential development platforms for bone tissue engineering and medication therapy for orthopedic diseases. The nanoscale metallic carrier's structure and topological characteristics also improve the physiochemical characteristics of scaffolds; increase drug-loading and ion-releasing proficiency; and regulate the stem cell adhesion, proliferation, and differentiation. In this book chapter we

Metals in Medicine, Volume 1: Metals for Tissue Engineering and Pharmaceutical Applications.
Sonali Sundram, Rishabha Malviya, and GSN Koteswara Rao

harness features of conductive nanometallic carrier polymers are emphasized; highlighted the new perspectives, challenges and future research direction for this emerging technology.

3.1 INTRODUCTION

Tissue engineering and regenerative medicine (TERM) is a field that uses both biological and engineering methods to make replacements for sick or damaged tissues that can work. One of TERM's biggest difficulties is the regeneration of bone tissue. Bone is unique and it is very hard to copy due to its complicated anatomical structure and exposure to extreme mechanical stress. However, several tactics have been employed, with fruitful outcomes.[1,2] In a perfect world, these structures, such as stem cells, scaffolds, and growth factors, would be able to improve, maintain, or even restore tissue function.[3] The scaffolds provide support so tissues can develop and form. Stem cells are given in efficient forms; these cells later develop into many types of tissues. The growth factors are further incorporated since they allow processes of proliferation and differentiation.

Because articular cartilage does not have blood vessels or nerves, it can't heal itself very well, so a good way to fix it is needed. Additionally, mild osteoarthritis can develop from minor articular cartilage defects if they are not addressed and result in impairment. It is vital to create new approaches for its restoration. To heal damaged tissue, including bone, cartilage, skin, muscle, liver, and heart, tissue engineering (TE) has become a powerful discipline. The development of innovative ways for the healing of injured cartilage is a major focus of this research project due to the alarmingly high frequency of illnesses linked with damaged cartilage in both the general population and the younger population.

A new era for TERM has begun with the development of structures that are the same size as those seen in naturally occurring bones. Nanomaterials are different from other materials because of how they behave physically, chemically, and biologically. For example, nanomaterials are small, have magnetic effects, have high surface energy, have a large specific surface area, and are resistant to corrosion. Nanomaterials may be categorized into three dimensions based on their structure and morphology: nanoparticles (NPs), nanowires, and nanolayers. NPs can directly transport biologically active compounds and mimic natural nanoscale extracellular matrix components based on their distinct characteristics and dimensions.[4] NPs can penetrate cell membranes and aid in protein absorption by cells. The aforementioned factors allow for the construction and application of nanomaterials with natural qualities or functionalized with other relevant features in TE, gene therapy, bioimaging, drug delivery, and other domains.[5]

Additionally, NPs deliver medications in a dependent manner, either locally or systemically. In a different method, stem cells, specifically, can be labeled using NPs. This adaptability is largely due to the variety of functionalization methods for NPs. Some of the molecules that can be attached to NPs include labeling probes, oligonucleotides, antibodies, hydrophobic or hydrophilic molecules, DNA, and/or molecules that enable a customized application for the intended use. Although bone TERM applications utilizing NPs are not yet commercially available, the volume of in vitro and in vivo studies conducted over the past few years indicates the technology's enormous potential.[5,6]

3.2 TYPES OF NANOPARTICLES

The current research looks at how targeted drug delivery using NPs has changed and talks about the pros and cons of different ways to give drugs. NPs are capable of delivering conventional medicines, recombinant proteins, nucleotides, and vaccinations effectively. Lipids, proteins, synthetic and natural polymers, metals, and other organic and inorganic materials can all be used to create NPs Figure 3.1. Based on the ingredients used for synthesis or the structural characteristics of the NP, NPs can be divided into several categories, including polymeric NPs, liposomes, dendrimers, micelles, and inorganic NPs. Its use and utility would also be determined by the production processes and the characteristics of the NPs. There are a variety of synthesis techniques, such as physical, chemical, and biological ones, each of which has its own unique strengths. Several procedures are used to functionalize the nanomaterials. Additionally, new techniques are continually updated, giving consumers a more precise grasp of nanomaterials, which include the product's antigenicity, drug release behavior, biodegradability, biocompatibility, toxicity, the physical and chemical characteristics of the size of the drug, NPs, and surface charge distribution.[5,7]

3.2.1 METALLIC-BASED NANOPARTICLES

Magnetic organic framework NPs, metal NPs, and metal oxide NPs are the three main categories of metallic-based NPs. The unique antibacterial properties, catalytic activity, mechanical properties, and electrical

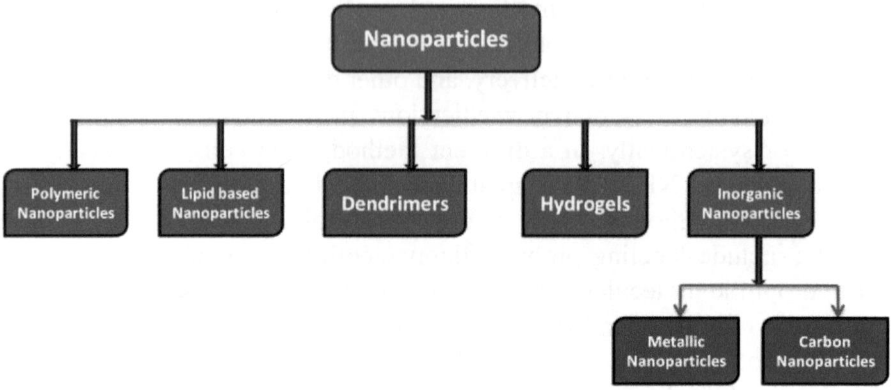

FIGURE 3.1 Types of nanomaterials

conductivity of metal NPs make them ideal for use in TE.[8,9] Because of the aforementioned natural characteristics, metal NPs made of precious metals are often employed extensively in the sectors of cosmetics and medicine Figure 3.2. Gold nanoparticles (AuNPs) have been extensively utilized in cancer detection and therapy, biological probes, and drug administration, among other applications, because of their excellent biocompatibility and simple production.[10] created AuNPs with a diameter of around 20 nm, which were shown to be effective antiangiogenic, blocking various heparin-binding growth factors, and decreasing the development of ovarian and pancreatic tumors; Similar to this, silver nanoparticles (AgNPs) are widely used in the biosensing, food, and dental TE fields. AgNPs are used to create a unique hybrid coating.[10] Xie et al. also looked at how the NPs affected antibacterial activity. Testing both in vivo and in vitro revealed that the hybrid coating's combination of AgNPs' photodynamic and physical properties may effectively and safely destroy bacteria.[11] In addition, several additional metal-based NPs have been extensively created for drug delivery, vaccine administration, immunological modulation, etc., all of which profited from their natural characteristics outlined. Magnetism is prominently displayed in magnetic nanomaterials and is strongly correlated with the applied magnetic field. It has been used for a variety of purposes, including directing and regulating medication delivery, promoting tissue development, preventing implant infection, etc.[12] Maghemite (Fe_2O_3), spinel ferrites (AFe_2O_4), and magnetite (Fe_3O_4) deliver medications such as docetaxel and doxorubicin (DOX) to particular sites.

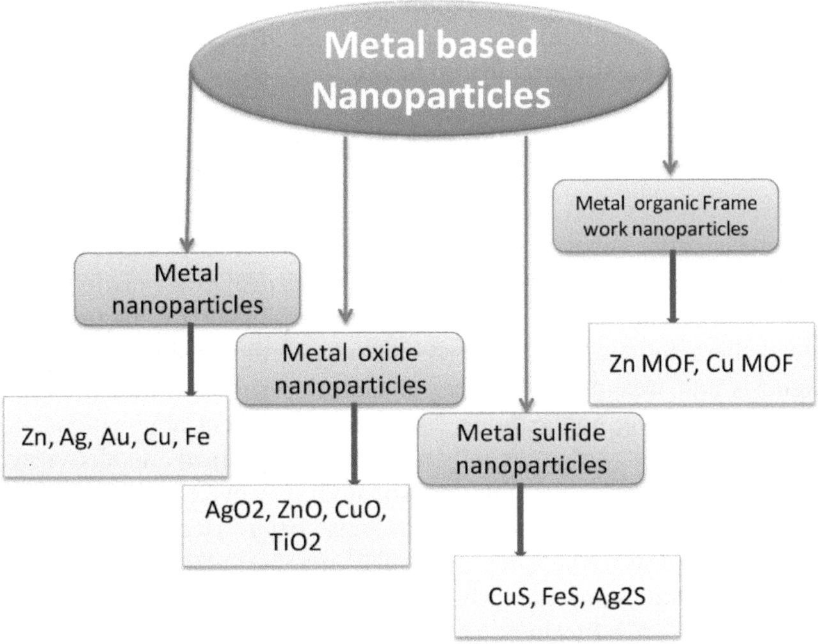

FIGURE 3.2 List of metals used in the preparation of metal-based NPs

3.2.2 METALLIC OXIDE-BASED NANOPARTICLES

Different types of metal oxide NPs are important in many parts of physics, chemistry, and materials science right now. The various metals may produce a wide variety of metal oxides. Metal oxide NPs are employed in technical applications such as optoelectronics, the construction of micro-electronic circuits, sensors, fuel cells, and piezoelectric devices. Metal oxide NPs come in a variety of forms, including MgO, ZnO, NiO, TiO_2, ZrO_2, and CuO NPs.[8] Making nanoarrays or nanostructures with unique features in comparison to those of bulk or single particle classes is an aim in the emerging subject of nanotechnology.[9,11] Due to their high density and small size at the corner or edge of the surface, metal oxide NPs display distinctive chemical and physical characteristics. NPs need to have a low surface free energy to show mechanical stability. This need has the effect of making phases that are poorly stable in bulk materials that are highly stable in nanostructures.

Examples of NPs having size-induced structural changes linked to changes in cell characteristics include those made of CuO, ZrO2, AgO, SnO_2,

ZnO, TiO_2, MgO, CeO_2, Al_2O_3. As the size of the NPs decreases, the growing number of atoms at the surface and interface produces strain or stress, which causes concurrent structural disturbances.

3.2.3 METAL SULFIDE–BASED NANOPARTICLES

Numerous studies have been conducted into the special characteristics of NPs and are the subject of ongoing research in the biomedical sciences, a vibrant field of study in molecular and translational medicine.[12] Their advantageous and readily adjustable physical, chemical, magnetic, and/or optical characteristics can be partly credited for their rising relevance in the diagnosis and treatment of cancer and other disorders, drug delivery, and in vitro biosensing applications.[14] For many different applications, copper sulfide (CuS), a *p*-type semiconductor with good optical and electrical characteristics, has been thoroughly investigated. However, until the last several years, information on its biological uses has been essentially absent.[13] As a potential platform for sensing, molecular imaging, photothermal treatment, drug administration, and multifunctional agents that may combine imaging and therapy, CuS NPs have just begun to gain popularity. Various uses of metal-based nanocarriers are shown in Figure 3.3.

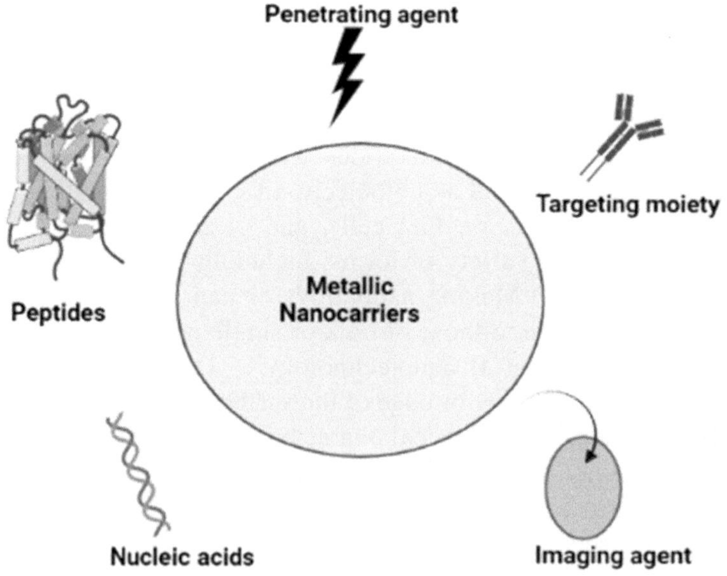

FIGURE 3.3 Uses of matal-based nanocarriers.

3.2.4 METAL-ORGANIC FRAMEWORKS

"Metal–organic frameworks (MOFs)" refers to a type of crystalline nanoporous material that is not very old. This is one of the most interesting new developments in the field of porous coordination, which is also called hybrid organic–inorganic coordination networks.[15] MOFs are more useful than other porous materials[16] because they have a high surface area and a high porosity, which is usually between 1000 and 10,000 m^2/g. Metal–organic frameworks have been studied a lot as potential drug delivery systems because they break down quickly, can be made to do different things, can hold a lot of drugs, and don't react badly with the body. MOFs are recognized as the best material for drug delivery applications due to pore size modulation and the potential to control functional groups.[17]

3.3 CLASSIFICATION OF METALLIC-BASED NANOPARTICLES (MNPs)

NPs are important for many medical research applications, and they often come in a few basic forms. The metal-based NPs, also known as metal NPs, are present in the nanomaterials pure form. The other categories of nanomaterials include metal oxide NPs, such as zinc oxide (ZnO), titanium dioxide, and others. Moreover, due to their promising qualities and potential uses in several biological sectors, metal–organic frameworks (MOFs) and metal sulfide nanomaterials have also attracted a great attention. Although the metallic nanoparticle carriers are biocompatible and stable, these inorganic metal components are found in humans and vital for survival, such as Ti, Cu, Fe, Zn, Zr, Mg, and Co. In addition to this, they are useful in many chemical catalysis, and enzymatic mediators and provide magnetic properties, ionic interactions, pH responsiveness, photothermal responses, and antibacterial properties.[18,19] The following sections describe the metallic-based NPs specific to treating bone disease.

3.3.1 Zn-BASED NANODELIVERY PLATFORM

Nano-Zn MOFs have pores of different diameters in the range of 3.8–28.8 and connect Zn (II) ions using organic ligands such as imidazolate or its derivatives.[20] MOFs made from Zn metal are made to be pH-dependent drug carriers that can be used in the medical field. The anticancer medication DOX, which is more easily loaded into the polyacrylic acid@zeolitic imidazolate framework-8, enhances the loading capacity. This is attributable to the coordination relationship between Zn^{2+}-DOX and electrostatic interactions. The drug loaded with MOF releases more quickly at a buffer solution's pH of 5.5 than it does at a neutral pH of about 7.4. Researchers have recently focused on modifying MOFs to increase their stability, and in this context, the creation of nano-MOFs or modifications to MOFs using metal NPs is a significant step forward. Such MOFs' activity is influenced by the characteristics of the nanoparticles and the specific kind of linkers.[21] The ZIF-8, which uses particles of a regulated size, is an illustration of a nanoparticle-based MOF. By employing PEG as a capping agent to regulate the particle size of ZIF-8. These MOFs demonstrated effective drug release against cancer cells that were pH dependent.[22,23]

The ZIF-8 nanoplatform has been used to distribute biologically active substances or medicines in bone disorders or bone TE regeneration. ZIF-8 is a space-filling packing with a pore size of 11.6 and a structure made up of truncated octahedrons.[24] Alendronate (Ald), indocyanine green (ICG), dexamethasone,[25] risedronate,[26] 5-fluorouracil, and simvastatin are among the small-molecule medications that have been seen.[27] Zn-based MOFs have the potential to transport both medicines and genes concurrently. In addition to Zn-based MOFs, they carry viral vectors for delivering tiny non-coding RNAs such as micro-RNAs (miRNAs)[28]; BMP-2; and cisplatin for bone regeneration.

There are several types of ZnO, including nanosheets, nanospheres, nanowires, and nanorods.[29] Zn ions successfully promote migration, tube formation of vascular endothelial cells, osseointegration of implants, mineralization of bone marrow mesenchymal stem cells' extracellular matrix, and antibacterial effects.[30] ZnO is a well-known potential material for angiogenesis and bone regeneration, as well as impacts on infection and bacterial resistance. ZnO also offers a wide range of potential as nanocarriers. Simple and efficient approaches may be used to load ZnO with different medicines. The drugs such as DOX, docosahexaenoic acid, and curcumin are effectively loaded by ZnO-based nanodelivery.

3.3.2 Fe-BASED NANODELIVERY PLATFORM

In general, organic solvents and water are stable for Fe-MOFs. In contrast to conventional porous materials, Fe-MOF allows for the modification of the interior pore environment and pore size, which increases the potential for and capacity for loading guest molecules. Due to their high drug loading and superior biocompatibility, Fe-MOFs are therefore thought to have several potential applications in the field of drug administration. Materials of Institute Lavoisier (MIL)-n family are Fe-based MOFs (Zhong et al., 2021). MIL-100(Fe), MIL-88B(Fe), MIL-88A(Fe), MIL-53(Fe), and MIL-101(Fe) are typical examples of Fe-based MOFs. Due to its superior characteristics, including low biodegradability, toxicity, pore volume, biocompatibility, and a large surface area, Fe-based MIL has received much research attention in antibacterial, bioimaging, biosensing, and drug delivery[31] due to their active metabotropic properties, such as Ald.[32] Fe MOFs can thus be employed in diagnostics and treatment to overcome difficulties in bone repair and regeneration.

FeO NPs are multifunctional nanomaterials that are important for bone disease detection, distribution, and bone replacement material modification. They can effectively reach target regions using an external magnetic force, which has tremendous applications as nanocarriers. This increases the bioavailability of medicinal chemicals. A number of medications, including docetaxel, DOX, lauric acid, mitoxantrone, 10-hydroxycamptothecin, artemisinin, dopamine, paclitaxel, cisplatin, docetaxel, rifampicin, and tetracycline hydrochloride, can be successfully delivered by FeONPs.[33]

3.3.3 Zr-BASED NANODELIVERY PLATFORM

Due to their mechanical, and low toxicity in aqueous and acidic media, Zr MOFs are regarded as potential MOFs for bone disease-related applications and bone TE.[34] The first Zr MOF was created by Cavka in 2008, known as Uio-66[35] made up of Zr and 1,4-benzene dicarboxylic acid. Other popular Zr-based MOFs are made, including MOF-525, MOF-545, and NU-902.[36] Zr MOFs porosity, size, and delivery characteristics are controlled by synthesizing various functional groups such as NH2 and NO2.[37] Different medications or active components can be delivered via Zr MOFs to treat various bone disorders. Additionally, PCN-222 may be used to transport a few single metal atoms (Cu, Au, Pt, Au, and Ru).[36,37] Additionally, it has been observed that UiO-66 can successfully transport such molecules as cytosine-phosphate-guanosine (immunostimulatory oligonucleotides).[38]

3.3.4 Cu-BASED NANODELIVERY PLATFORM

Cu is one of the important trace metals that all living things need. Compared to Au and Ag, it is cheap and easy to get. Cu's superior chemical, electrical, physical, and optical capabilities[39,40] are capable of killing germs and accelerating wound healing. Since the doped Cu^{2+} could trap electrons, electron-hole recombination was reduced. This increased the ROS output and sped up carrier transport. The findings showed that when the level of metalation grew, the photooxidation ability of MOFs initially rose and then fell; MOFs' capacity to produce heat was improved by the Cu^{2+} dd transition. The MOF's antibacterial effectiveness was 99.71% against *Staphylococcus aureus* and 97.14% against *Escherichia coli.* Such research offers a suitable model for the efficient use of copper-doped MOFs in the fight against bacterial infection. Additionally, the size-switchable nanosystem has excellent potential for killing tumor cells with high selectivity and little invasiveness since it can precisely inject medicine into the deeper area of the tumor.[41] The Cu^{2+}/Cu^{+} ion combination has a stronger catalytic activity and a lower redox potential than the conventional Fe^{2+}-based Fenton's reagent. It was discovered that, after being ingested by cancer cells, the Cu^{2+}/Cu^{+} ion pair demonstrates better catalytic capacity to quicken wound healing compared to conventional iron-based kinetic reagents.

Recently, there has been a lot of study done on nanoscale Cu MOFs in the domains due to their various advantages. They can promote angiogenesis by simulating hypoxia and stimulating endothelial cell proliferation and differentiation, Cu-based MOFs have been used to successfully load small-molecule medications into nanodrug delivery systems, including DOX,[42] chlorhexidine.[43] As a result, nano-Cu MOFs have lately attracted the greatest interest as a platform for nanodrug delivery.

3.3.5 Ti-BASED NANODELIVERY PLATFORM

Ti MOFs have tremendous applications due to their higher biocompatibility and photocatalytic activity when compared to other metals. The first report of a Ti-based formulation by MIL-125(Ti), which consists of terephthalate dianions and Ti octahedra with reachable pore diameters of 6.13 and 12.55,[44] but has the capability to load small molecules, includes aspirin,[45] and DOX[46] makes a good option for platform materials for nanodelivery.

The Ti metal has outstanding osteointegration and biocompatibility properties, which are widely recognized and extensively used as implant materials in meshes, fracture repair screws, implants, and bone substitutes. TiO_2) NPs have caught the interest of researchers due to the remarkable characteristics of Ti. Numerous TiO_2 nanostructures, including TiO_2 nanotubes, NPs, matrices, rods, and whiskers, are finding new uses as delivery systems for various medications or active ingredients. TiO_2 nanomaterials, for instance, are capable of effectively delivering a variety of small-molecule medications, including curcumin, dexamethasone, valproic acid, gambogic acid, temozolomide, DOX, cisplatin, and daunorubicin; and biologically active proteins such as human recombinant BMP-2.[47]

3.3.6 Ag-BASED NANODELIVERY PLATFORM

The synthesis of NPs and NPs uses silver, the precious metal with the highest profit orientation and anti-fungal, antibacterial, antiviral, and antioxidant activities. These are well-known for having exceptionally increased physicochemical characteristics relative to the bulk material, such as electrical, thermal, optical, and catalytic capabilities. AgNPs are employed in many industries and in daily life. Environmentally friendly synthesis techniques must be developed to meet the growing demand for AgNPs. Furthermore, AgNPs interact with bacteria and release a silver ion that delays membrane penetration while deactivating cellular-based enzymes. A variety of cell types have been shown to be susceptible to cytotoxicity caused by AgNPs via apoptosis and necrosis.[48] Additionally, they show results against side effects of conventional therapies such as DNA damage, the production of reactive oxygen species (ROS), an increase in lactate dehydrogenase leakage, and inhibition of stem cell development.[49] With about 10 million new cases each year, cancer is one of the main causes of death in the contemporary era. The anticancer properties of AgNPs are also the subject of research. ROS are able to be produced when AgNPs are stimulated, which kills cancer cells' mitochondrial respiratory chain. According to certain studies, AgNPs cause a cytotoxic impact on leukemic cells.[50] The colon cancer Caco-2 cells were treated using the produced nanocarrier. They reported that a 60% reduction in Caco-2 cell growth was achieved with the produced AgNPs at concentrations up to 39 g/mL, which allowed for safe usage.[51] MCF-7 breast cancer cells were shown to be cytotoxic to AgNPs at a concentration of 20 g/mL for 48 hours, as well as H1299 lung cancer cells, where 50% of the cells were destroyed at a concentration of 5 g/mL. AgNPs have demonstrated efficient kills of 5 to 28 g/mL in colon cancer cells in cell lines including $Caco^{-2}$, HCT116, and HT-29, and it has also been demonstrated that AgNPs have a significant potential to operate as a nanocarrier to carry anticancer medications to cancer cells.[52,53] The possibility of using AGNPs for cancer treatment is highly supported by this research.

S. aureus has been demonstrated to be diminished by the extracellular silver ions in Ag NPs, indicating that these particles have antibacterial potential against Gram-positive and Gram-negative bacteria.[54] The findings demonstrated that the aggregation of NPs caused damage to the tested bacteria's cell walls. Following disc diffusion experiments, the antibacterial action of Ag NPs against *E. coli* was also noted.[55]

3.3.7 Au-BASED NANODELIVERY PLATFORM

One of the well-known systems that have been widely researched for the administration of different medications is AuNPs. The complex chemistry of the creation of AuNPsThese NPs are now in the spotlight for assessment for the delivery of various medications, including DOX—thanks to their subsequent application in material development, synthetic chemistry, drug delivery, and other domains.[56] Dox has been joined to a polymer molecule deposited over the AuNPs by several types of covalent bonding.[57]

Amine-functionalized polyethylene glycol was used to coat the AuNPs (PEG-NH2). To integrate terminal thiol groups into the polymer (forming PEG-SH), the surface amine groups were functionalized.[58] PEG-SH was then employed to couple with the thiol-modified Dox through disulfide bonds. Dox was found on the terminal ends of the PEG coating and all over the surface of the AuNPs. Due to their exceptional biocompatibility, antibacterial capability, physicochemical properties, and osseointegration capacity, AuNPs have a wide range of applications, including, biocoatings, and targeted drug carriers. A variety of pharmaceutical substances, including proteins, peptides, pDNA, and siRNA.[59] Ginsenoside Rg3,[60] and gemcitabine have all attracted significant interest because of their extraordinary properties.[61]

3.3.8 ADDITIONAL METAL MOF NANODELIVERY SYSTEMS

Other platforms, including Mg-, Ca-, and Co-based MOFs, have potential uses in bone regeneration in addition to the other MOFs that were already discussed. These MOFs have been gaining more research interest recently, even though further study is needed to increase their capabilities for nanodrug delivery. Mg MOFs are capable of loading small molecules such as icariin, ibuprofen, curcumin, and alpha-cyano-4-hydroxycinnamate. Co MOFs were employed to load enzymes, pharmaceuticals, and biologically active compounds, including benzamide, olsalazine, and glucose oxidase.[62,63]

Among the metal components primarily found in bones, Ca is also seen to form MOFs that act as nanocarriers for medications. Overall, due to their great potential to address bone-related issues, more research and study of Co, Ca, and Mg MOFs are needed.

3.4 MNPs ARE USED TO TREAT BONE DISEASES

3.4.1 BONE REGROWTH

The specifically designed materials are needed to accompany basic diseases such as diabetes, osteoporosis, infection, hyperlipidemia, and vascular necrosis. MNPs, especially Zn-based NPs, have potential in these difficult bone-repair scenarios and are frequently used as bone TE materials. Additionally, ZIF-8 can deliver bisphosphonates (BP) to prevent osteoclast behavior in the treatment of osteoporosis and other disorders of bone immune behavior.[26] Metals such as Ti that are compatible with bone implants are frequently used in the design of MNPs. Saha et al.[64] created a new bone implant with drug release and supporting virtues by modifying the surfaces of Ti6Al4V implants with curcumin-loaded TiO_2 nanotubes. Notably, MNPs are recommended because of their high loading capacity and steady distribution ability. The capacity of MNPs to release drugs or deliver regulated releases of substances makes it possible for bones to regenerate and mend at several levels and stages and for a variety of purposes.[65] Additionally, the metal components in MNPs have an impact on the physiological functions of bones. First, a small number of metal elements, including zinc, directly promote osteogenic differentiation.

A new multifunctional bone adhesive gel uses ZIF-8 NPs to upregulate alkaline phosphate, osteocalcin, and extended bone remodeling. For instance,[66] prepared a multifunctional bone adhesive hydrogel using nano-ZIF-8, which upregulated the production and secretion of collagen 1, promoted osteogenic differentiation, alkaline phosphatase, and osteocalcin, and expedited bone remodeling. Similar to this, the nano-ZnO particles directly support bone healing. Studies have shown that increasing the Wnt/-catenin pathway can cause these Zn-based nanomaterials to have an osteogenic impact.[67] NPs produced from Fe, Cu, and Mg have been used to speed vascularized bone repair in addition to direct osteogenesis,[68] offering benefits for designed MNPs for bone repair. Researchers are also interested in how the osteoclast process could be hampered. In their investigation of the impact of AuNPs on osteoclasts without the addition of any drugs, Bai et al.[69] concluded that the use of MNPs in the field of bone regeneration is considerably facilitated by the active control of osteogenesis-related processes employing metal elements. Bone regeneration by metal-based NPs is shown in Figure 3.4.

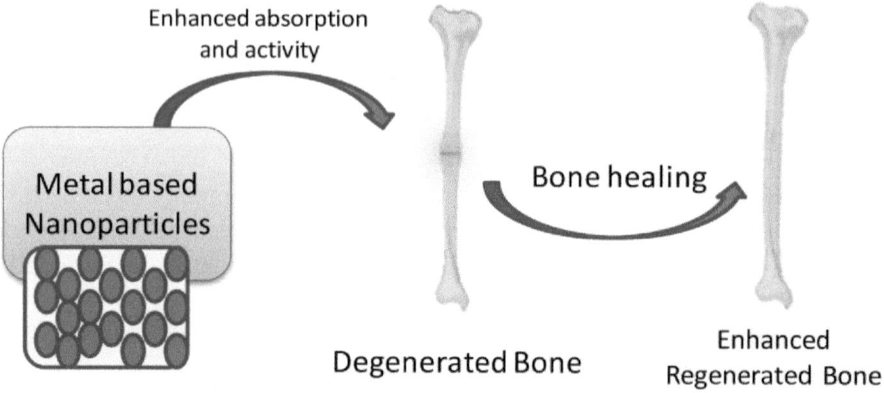

FIGURE 3.4 Enhanced bone regeneration by metal-based nanoparticles.

3.4.2 BONE TUMOR

Bone tumors can take many different forms, including bone metastases and osteosarcoma from different cancers. Bone tumors frequently present with pathological fractures, hypocalcemia, severe pain, and bone marrow aplasia, all of which cause the patients to experience a great deal of agony.[70] The most commonly used non-surgical techniques for treating bone cancers are computed tomography (CT), radiation, and ablation.[71] Commonly used CT medicines for bone cancers include mesna, tetracycline, ifosfamide, cabozantinib, cisplatin, BP, DOX, methotrexate, and denosumab.[72] Drugs must pass across the blood-bone marrow barrier to reach bone tissues when administered systemically.[73] MNPs are, therefore, preferred by experts in bone tumors due to their tiny diameters and great loading capabilities. A few researchers[74] successfully administered the drug riluzole using two distinct iron oxide NPs and dramatically increased tumor tissue death in mice using the osteosarcoma model. Methotrexate into the tunnels of Cu-MOF by[75] to create Cu-MOF/MTX nanodelivery, these two-dimensional tunnels' suitability for targeted anticancer drug delivery was further shown by inserting Cu-MOF/MTX into a series of synthesis experiments to create Cu- to create multifunctional MNPs (Au@MMSN), metal manganese (Mn) was in situ doped into Au core mesoporous silica NPs, according to a publication.[76]

Ultrafine W-doped TiO_2 (W-$Ti_2$2) combined for tumor treatment.[77] They found that W doping increases the acoustodynamic properties of TiO_2 by reducing the band gap; W-TiO_2 improves improve elimination of tumors and alters the microenvironment. A composite nanoplatform was recently created by Zou et al.[78] employing ZIF-8-capped Cu^2-XSe and employed for CDT and PTT of bone cancers. With the breakdown of ZIF-8 in the tumor's acidic microenvironment, Cu^2-XSe was produced, and it subsequently degraded into Cu^+ and Cu^{2+} to start a Fenton-like reaction that caused CDT. Cu^2-XSe can also inhibit osteoclasts and tumor cells while inducing the PTT effect. Effectively demonstrating the potential benefit of MNPs for cutting-edge treatment of bone cancers is this ZIF8-capped nanomedicine.

3.4.3 OSTEOMYELITIS

Osteomyelitis has a significant impact on patients' everyday lives. It frequently affects elderly adults, diabetics, and people in poor overall health. Fungal infections frequently lead to osteomyelitis because of pyrogenic bacteria. It could also be a side effect of facial cosmetic surgery, tooth extraction, or orthopedic surgery. Systemic antibiotic administration, which is the main mode of therapy currently used, is less efficient for treating localized infection sites. Ag-based nanodelivery systems have been thoroughly verified for their potent antibacterial, antifungal, and osteoinductive characteristics, making them by far the most widely used commercial NPs.[79] Additionally, there is strong proof that a variety of nanomaterials, including those based on copper, titanium, zinc, palladium, iron, cobalt, and others, have effective antibacterial characteristics.[45] MNPs with focused functions or antibiotic-encapsulated MNPs can be applied topically to improve osteomyelitis treatment, delay medication action, lessen systemic adverse effects, and prevent osteonecrosis. Ag–Cu–Boron (ACB) alloy NPs coupled with cadherin antibodies can target the osteoblast and inhibit the *S. aureus*-based infection.[80] Ti oxide based MTF loaded with gentamicin conjugated with BMP-2 on their surface reduce the *S. aureus* infection and successfully stop the proliferation and differentiation of preosteoblastic cells.[81]

Also, compared to traditional antibiotics, MNPs can get around the problems caused by drug resistance. To sterilize alginate/hydroxyapatite composite scaffolds against both Gram-positive and Gram-negative bacterial strains, researchers[82] created scaffolds incorporating AgNPs. They then showed that this did not alter the scaffold's capacity to encourage osteoblastic growth. MIL-125(Ti)NH_2 Ag NPs composites[83] demonstrate a good impact against *S. aureus* biofilm along with a threefold increase in antibacterial activity. This research offers strong support for the use of MNPs to prevent the growth of biofilms around bone implants and cure osteomyelitis brought on by bacterial infections. TiO_2 can be employed as an efficient antibacterial coating material[84] because of its special photocatalytic capabilities, which can efficiently decrease *E. coli*. Additionally, raising the Co^{2+} level increased the antibacterial activity.[85] New approaches to treating deep osteomyelitis are occasionally developed through the collaboration of several metal NPs. An engineered macrophage with a nuclear-membrane structure was created, and the nuclear component was made out of Fe_3O_4 and Au NPs. Under microwave irradiation, the nuclear component may generate large amounts of ROS and heat, which suppress inflammatory reactions, kill bacteria in place, and simultaneously promote osteoblast development for osteomyelitis.[86]

3.4.4 OSTEOARTHRITIS

Osteoarthritis is a chronic condition marked by synovial inflammation, abnormally reduced joint lubrication and the gradual deterioration of articular cartilage. The main clinical signs of osteoarthritis are joint discomfort, joint deterioration, and joint dysfunction.[87] Osteoarthritis is treated using a variety of typical medications, such as NSAIDs, antirheumatics, glucocorticoids, and other agents such as intra-articular medication injections for arthritis, but these medications have low bioavailability. This has led to a lot of research on MNPs as a medicine delivery system for osteoarthritis.

Li et al.[88] that concurrently supplied anti-inflammatory anti TNF-siRNA and antioxidant -TOS. In arthritic mice models, the complex may greatly increase macrophages' antioxidant capacity and suppress inflammatory cytokines, leading to a combination of antioxidant and anti-inflammatory treatment for joint inflammation. Additionally, MNPs have a special contribution to make to osteoarthritis stem cell treatment. The metformin-loaded CuS@MnO_2 NPs may be employed as a target for MSCs, which are then used in osteoarthritis stem cell treatment. The potential of MSCs transformed with these MNPs to demonstrate improved anti-inflammation and chondrogenesis, as well as successfully alleviate osteoarthritis symptoms, has been verified. Similar to this, MNPs provide new therapy options for osteoarthritis because of their outstanding light responsiveness, robust flexibility, and self-anti-inflammatory characteristics.

3.5 CHALLENGES OF MNPs

A few MNPs are entered into the market despite the fact that they are efficient in bone TE. The transition of MNPs from fundamental studies to clinical applications in orthopaedics, which may come from several aspects and domains, still faces a number of difficulties. A deeper comprehension of the molecular processes underlying NPs' biological features, particularly their antibacterial ones, is necessary for future study. The focus on nanotoxicological research must be conducted to prevent the negative effects of NPs. Designing nanoparticle-based pharmaceuticals with extremely favorable pharmacological/toxicological profiles will be made possible by detailed knowledge of the interactions in terms of cytotoxicity between live cells and NPs. Unquestionably, NPs are an effective tool, but more work needs to be done before we can say that using them is risk-free.

3.6 TOXICOLOGY

MNP toxicity has long been a popular area of study. MNP toxicity can be attributed to a number of factors, including the agglomeration phenomena already discussed. MNPs have a high surface reactivity due to their large specific surface area, which is a double-edged sword that might result in unforeseen toxicological pathways.[89] Because of their tiny sizes, MNPs encourage cellular absorption, which raises their bioavailability and intensifies their toxicity.[90] The MNPs released a large quantity of metal ions that caused a bactericidal effect, and along with that effect, they damaged the balance of the electrolyte, which led to cytotoxicity.[91] Build-up of MNP-based metal ions and dysfunction of enzymes by replacing the missing portions of enzymes, which increase the risk for osteoarthritis and osteoporosis.[91] Toxicities caused by organic linkers, metal ions, solvents, and chemical residues created during MNP synthesis are additional issues that should be addressed. Although some researchers have functionally changed MNP surfaces by targeting ligands in an effort to lessen systemic toxicity by targeting MNPs, MNP toxicity still poses a significant challenge and restricts its clinical applicability.

3.7 COMPLICATIONS IN CREATING MNPs

The collaboration of substances such as scaffolds, gels, and biofilms is frequently necessary in preparing MNPs Comprehensive consideration should be given to the resistance to treatment, type of illness, treatment

7. Mughal, S. S.; Hassan, S. M. Comparative Study of AgO Nanoparticles Synthesize Via Biological, Chemical and Physical Methods: A Review. *Am. J. Mater. Synth. Process.* **2022,** *7* (2), 15–28.
8. Salem, W.; Leitner, D. R.; Zingl, F. G.; Schratter, G.; Prassl, R.; Goessler, W.; Reidl, J.; Schild, S. Antibacterial Activity of Silver and Zinc Nanoparticles Against Vibrio Cholerae and Enterotoxic *Escherichia coli*. *Int. J. Med. Microbiol.* **2015,** *305* (1), 85–95.
9. Pratiwi, F. W.; Kuo, C. W.; Chen, B. C.; Chen, P. Recent Advances in the Use of Fluorescent Nanoparticles for Bioimaging. *Nanomedicine* **2019,** *14* (13), 1759–1769.
10. Zheng, X.; Zhang, P.; Fu, Z.; Meng, S.; Dai, L.; Yang, H. Applications of Nanomaterials in Tissue Engineering. *RSC Adv.* **2021,** *11* (31), 19041–19058.
11. (a) Gao, X.; Zhai, M.; Guan, W.; Liu, J.; Liu, Z.; Damirin, A. Controllable Synthesis of a Smart Multifunctional Nanoscale Metal–Organic Framework for Magnetic Resonance/ Optical Imaging and Targeted Drug Delivery. *ACS Appl. Mater. Interfaces* **2017,** *9* (4), 3455–3462. Li, Z.; Zhang, Y.; La, H.; Zhu, R.; El-Banna, G.; Wei, Y.; Han, G. Upconverting NIR Photons for Bioimaging. *Nanomaterials* **2015,** *5* (4), 2148–2168.
12. Ayodhya, D.; Veerabhadram, G. Green Synthesis, Characterization, Photocatalytic, Fluorescence and Antimicrobial Activities of *Cochlospermum gossypium* Capped Ag2S Nanoparticles. *J. Photochem. Photobiol. B: Biol.* **2016,** *157*, 57–69.
13. Asri, R. I.; Harun, W. S.; Samykano, M.; Lah, N. A.; Ghani, S. A.; Tarlochan, F.; Raza, M. R. Corrosion and Surface Modification on Biocompatible Metals: A Review. *Mater. Sci. Eng.: C.* **2017,** *77*, 1261–1274.
14. Argueta-Figueroa, L.; Martinez-Alvarez, O.; Santos-Cruz, J.; Garcia-Contreras, R.; Acosta-Torres, L. S.; De la Fuente-Hernandez, J.; Arenas-Arrocena, M. C. Nanomaterials Made of Non-Toxic Metallic Sulfides: A Systematic Review of Their Potential Biomedical Applications. *Mater. Sci. Eng.: C.* **2017,** *76*, 1305–1315.
15. Khan, I.; Saeed, K.; Khan, I. Nanoparticles: Properties, Applications and Toxicities. *Arab. J. Chem.* **2019,** *12* (7), 908–931.
16. Bushra, R.; Shahadat, M.; Ahmad, A.; Nabi, S. A.; Umar, K.; Oves, M.; Raeissi, A. S.; Muneer, M. Synthesis, Characterization, Antimicrobial Activity and Applications of Polyaniline Ti (IV) Arsenophosphate Adsorbent for the Analysis of Organic and Inorganic Pollutants. *J. Hazard. Mater.* **2014,** *264*, 481–489.
17. Di, S.; Ning, T.; Yu, J.; Chen, P.; Yu, H.; Wang, J.; Yang, H.; Zhu, S. Recent Advances and Applications of Magnetic Nanomaterials in Environmental Sample Analysis. *TrAC Trends Analyt. Chem.* **2020,** *126*, 115864.
18. Fernandes, C. S.; Nordin, N. A.; Bilad, M. R.; Matsuura, T.; Putra, Z. A.; Wirzal, M. D.; Jaafar, J. Explication of Hydrophobic Silica as Effective Pore Former for Membrane Fabrication. *Appl. Surf. Sci. Adv.* **2021,** *3*, 100051.
19. Fardjahromi, M. A.; Nazari, H.; Tafti, S. A.; Razmjou, A.; Mukhopadhyay, S.; Warkiani, M. E. Metal-Organic Framework-Based Nanomaterials for Bone Tissue Engineering and Wound Healing. *Mater. Today Chem.* **2022,** *23*, 100670.
20. Liu, Y.; Xu, Z.; Qiao, M.; Cai, H.; Zhu, Z. Metal-Based Nano-Delivery Platform for Treating Bone Disease and Regeneration. *Front. Chem.* **2022,** *10*.
21. Deng, X.; Liang, S.; Cai, X.; Huang, S.; Cheng, Z.; Shi, Y.; Pang, M.; Ma, P. A.; Lin, J. Yolk–Shell Structured Au Nanostar@ Metal–Organic Framework for Synergistic Chemo-Photothermal Therapy in the Second Near-Infrared Window. *Nano Lett.* **2019,** *19* (10), 6772–6780.

22. Safdar Ali, R.; Meng, H.; Li, Z. Zinc-Based Metal-Organic Frameworks in Drug Delivery, Cell Imaging, and Sensing. *Molecules* **2021,** *27* (1), 100.
23. He, S.; Wu, L.; Li, X.; Sun, H.; Xiong, T.; Liu, J.; Huang, C.; Xu, H.; Sun, H.; Chen, W.; Gref, R. Metal-Organic Frameworks for Advanced Drug Delivery. *Acta Pharm. Sinica, B* **2021,** *11* (8), 2362–2395.
24. Ran, J.; Zeng, H.; Cai, J.; Jiang, P.; Yan, P.; Zheng, L.; Bai, Y.; Shen, X.; Shi, B.; Tong, H. Rational Design of a Stable, Effective, and Sustained Dexamethasone Delivery Platform on a Titanium Implant: An Innovative Application of Metal Organic Frameworks in Bone Implants. *Chem. Eng. J.* **2018,** *333*, 20–33.
25. Cheng, X.; Zhu, Z.; Liu, Y.; Xue, Y.; Gao, X.; Wang, J.; Pei, X.; Wan, Q. Zeolitic Imidazolate Framework-8 Encapsulating Risedronate Synergistically Enhances Osteogenic and Antiresorptive Properties for Bone Regeneration. *ACS Biomater. Sci. Eng.* **2020,** *6* (4), 2186–2197.
26. Qiao, M.; Xu, Z.; Pei, X.; Liu, Y.; Wang, J.; Chen, J.; Zhu, Z.; Wan, Q. Nano SIM@ ZIF-8 Modified Injectable High-Intensity Biohydrogel with Bidirectional Regulation of Osteogenesisand Anti-Adipogenesis for Bone Repair. *Chem. Eng. J.* **2022,** *434*, 134583.
27. Feng, H.; Li, Z.; Xie, W.; Wan, Q.; Guo, Y.; Chen, J.; Wang, J.; Pei, X. Delivery of Therapeutic miRNAs Using Nanoscale Zeolitic Imidazolate Framework for Accelerating Vascularized Bone Regeneration. *Chem. Eng. J.* **2022,** *430*, 132867.
28. Carofiglio, M.; Barui, S.; Cauda, V.; Laurenti, M. Doped Zinc Oxide Nanoparticles: Synthesis, Characterization and Potential Use in Nanomedicine. *Appl. Sci.* **2020,** *10* (15), 5194.
29. Nakamura, T.; Yoshida, E.; Hara, T.; Fujie, T.; Yamamoto, C.; Fujiwara, Y.; Ogata, F.; Kawasaki, N.; Takita, R.; Uchiyama, M.; Kaji, T. Zn (ii) 2, 9-Dimethyl-1, 10-Phenanthroline Stimulates Cultured Bovine Aortic Endothelial Cell Proliferation. *RSC Adv.* **2020,** *10* (69), 42327–42337.
30. Zhong, Y.; Liu, W.; Rao, C.; Li, B.; Wang, X.; Liu, D.; Pan, Y.; Liu, J. Recent Advances in Fe-MOF Compositions for Biomedical Applications. *Curr. Med. Chem.* **2021,** *28* (30), 6179–6198.
31. Golmohamadpour, A.; Bahramian, B.; Shafiee, A.; Ma'mani, L. Slow Released Delivery of Alendronate Using β-Cyclodextrine Modified Fe–MOF Encapsulated Porous Hydroxyapatite. *J. Inorg. Organomet. Polym. Mater.* **2018,** *28*, 1991–2000.
32. Vangijzegem, T.; Stanicki, D.; Laurent, S. Magnetic Iron Oxide Nanoparticles for Drug Delivery: Applications and Characteristics. *Exp. Opin. Drug Deliv.* **2019,** *16* (1), 69–78.
33. Lazaro, I. A.; Haddad, S.; Sacca, S.; Orellana-Tavra, C.; Fairen-Jimenez, D.; Forgan, R. S. Selective Surface PEGylation of UiO-66 Nanoparticles for Enhanced Stability, Cell Uptake, and pH-Responsive Drug Delivery. *Chemical* **2017,** *2* (4), 561–578.
34. Cavka, J. H.; Jakobsen, S.; Olsbye, U.; Guillou, N.; Lamberti, C.; Bordiga, S.; Lillerud, K. P. A New Zirconium Inorganic Building Brick Forming Metal Organic Frameworks with Exceptional Stability. *J. Am. Chem. Soc.* **2008,** *130* (42), 13850–13851.
35. Yu, K.; Won, D. I.; Lee, W. I.; Ahn, W. S. Porphyrinic Zirconium Metal-Organic Frameworks: Synthesis and Applications for Adsorption/Catalysis. *Korean J. Chem. Eng.* **2021,** *38*, 653–673.
36. Li, Z.; Guo, R.; Gu, Z.; Wang, X.; Wang, Y.; Xu, H.; Wang, C.; Liu, X. Identification of a Promoter Element Mediating Kisspeptin-Induced Increases in GnRH Gene Expression in Sheep. *Gene* **2019,** *699*, 1–7.

37. Pang, Y.; Fu, Y.; Li, C.; Wu, Z.; Cao, W.; Hu, X.; Sun, X.; He, W.; Cao, X.; Ling, D.; Li, Q. Metal–Organic Framework Nanoparticles for Ameliorating Breast Cancer-Associated Osteolysis. *Nano Lett.* **2020,** *20* (2), 829–840.
38. Ramalingam, G.; Nagapandiselvi, P.; Priya, A. K.; Rajendran, S. A Review of Graphene-Based Semiconductors for Photocatalytic Degradation of Pollutants in Wastewater. *Chemosphere* **2022,** 134391.
39. Cordeiro, J. M.; Nagay, B. E.; Dini, C.; Souza, J. G.; Rangel, E. C.; da Cruz, N. C.; Yang, F.; van den Beucken, J. J.; Barão, V. A. Copper Source Determines Chemistry and Topography of Implant Coatings to Optimally Couple Cellular Responses and Antibacterial Activity. *Biomater. Adv.* **2022,** *134*, 112550.
40. Sun, Y.; Jiang, X.; Liu, Y.; Liu, D.; Chen, C.; Lu, C.; Zhuang, S.; Kumar, A.; Liu, J. Recent advances in Cu (II)/Cu (I)-MOFs based nano-platforms for developing new nano-medicines. Journal of Inorganic Biochemistry. 2021 Dec 1;225:111599.
41. Golmohamadpour, A.; Bahramian, B.; Shafiee, A.; Ma'mani, L. Slow Released Delivery of Alendronate Using β-Cyclodextrine Modified Fe–MOF Encapsulated Porous Hydroxyapatite. *J. Inorg. Organomet. Polym. Mater.* **2018,** *28*, 1991–2000.
42. Soltani, S.; Akhbari, K. Cu-BTC Metal–Organic Framework as a Biocompatible Nanoporous Carrier for Chlorhexidine Antibacterial Agent. *J. Biol. Inorg. Chem.* **2021,** 1–7.
43. Dan-Hardi, M.; Serre, C.; Frot, T.; Rozes, L.; Maurin, G.; Sanchez, C.; Férey, G. A New Photoactive Crystalline Highly Porous Titanium (IV) Dicarboxylate. *J. Am. Chem. Soc.* **2009,** *131* (31), 10857–10859.
44. Rojas-Andrade, M. D.; Chata, G.; Rouholiman, D.; Liu, J.; Saltikov, C.; Chen, S. Antibacterial Mechanisms of Graphene-Based Composite Nanomaterials. *Nanoscale* **2017,** *9* (3), 994–1006.
45. Rengaraj, A.; Puthiaraj, P.; Heo, N. S.; Lee, H.; Hwang, S. K.; Kwon, S.; Ahn, W. S.; Huh, Y. S. Porous NH2-MIL-125 as an Efficient Nano-Platform for Drug Delivery, Imaging, and ROS Therapy Utilized Low-Intensity Visible Light Exposure System. *Colloids Surfaces B: Biointerfaces.* **2017,** *160*, 1–0.
46. Han, T.; Xue, P.; Ju, S.; Zhang, Z.; Zeng, J.; Zhang, Y.; Jiang, Q. RNA-seq Reveals Correlations Between Cytoskeleton-Related Genes and the Osteogenic Activity of Mesenchymal Stem Cells on Strontium Loaded Titania Nanotube Arrays. *Mater. Sci. Eng.: C.* **2021,** *122*, 111939.
47. Zhang, X. F.; Gurunathan, S. Combination of Salinomycin and Silver Nanoparticles Enhances Apoptosis and Autophagy in Human Ovarian Cancer Cells: An Effective Anticancer Therapy. *Int. J. Nanomed.* **2016,** *11*, 3655.
48. Emami Nejad, A.; Najafgholian, S.; Rostami, A.; Sistani, A.; Shojaeifar, S.; Esparvarinha, M.; Nedaeinia, R.; Haghjooy Javanmard, S.; Taherian, M.; Ahmadlou, M.; Salehi, R. The Role of Hypoxia in the Tumor Microenvironment and Development of Cancer Stem Cell: A Novel Approach to Developing Treatment. *Cancer Cell Int.* **2021,** *21* (1), 1–26.
49. Jabeen, S.; Qureshi, R.; Munazir, M.; Maqsood, M.; Munir, M.; Shah, S. S.; Rahim, B. Z. Application of Green Synthesized Silver Nanoparticles in Cancer Treatment—A Critical Review. *Mater. Res. Express* **2021,** *8* (9), 092001.
50. Chandrakala, V.; Aruna, V.; Angajala, G. Review on Metal Nanoparticles as Nanocarriers: Current Challenges and Perspectives in Drug Delivery Systems. *Emergent Mater.* **2022,** 1–23.

51. Bharadwaj, K. K.; Rabha, B.; Pati, S.; Sarkar, T.; Choudhury, B. K.; Barman, A.; Bhattacharjya, D.; Srivastava, A.; Baishya, D.; Edinur, H. A.; Abdul Kari, Z. Green Synthesis of Gold Nanoparticles Using Plant Extracts as Beneficial Prospect for Cancer Theranostics. *Molecules* **2021,** *26* (21), 6389.
52. Thakur, R.; Arora, V. Comprehensive Review on Polymeric and Metal Nanoparticles: Possible Therapeutic Avenues. *Int. J. Polym. Mater. Polym. Biomater.* **2022,** 1–21.
53. Nanda, A.; Saravanan, M. Biosynthesis of Silver Nanoparticles from *Staphylococcus aureus* and Its Antimicrobial Activity Against MRSA and MRSE. *Nanomed.: Nanotechnol. Biol. Med.* **2009,** *5* (4), 452–6.
54. Ghiuță, I.; Cristea, D. Silver Nanoparticles for Delivery Purposes. In: *Nanoengineered Biomaterials for Advanced Drug Delivery*; Elsevier, 2020; pp 347–371.
55. Saratale, R. G.; Karuppusamy, I.; Saratale, G. D.; Pugazhendhi, A.; Kumar, G.; Park, Y.; Ghodake, G. S.; Bharagava, R. N.; Banu, J. R.; Shin, H. S. A Comprehensive Review on Green Nanomaterials Using Biological Systems: Recent Perception and Their Future Applications. *Colloids Surfaces B: Biointerfaces* **2018,** *170*, 20–35.
56. Shi, L.; Ding, P.; Wang, Y.; Zhang, Y.; Ossipov, D.; Hilborn, J. Self-Healing Polymeric Hydrogel Formed by Metal–Ligand Coordination Assembly: Design, Fabrication, and Biomedical Applications. *Macromol. Rapid Commun.* **2019,** *40* (7), 1800837.
57. Jia, C.; Guo, Y.; Wu, F. G. Chemodynamic Therapy via Fenton and Fenton-Like Nanomaterials: Strategies and Recent Advances. *Small* **2022,** *18* (6), 2103868.
58. Mallakpour, S.; Azadi, E.; Hussain, C. M. Recent Advancements in Synthesis and Drug Delivery Utilization of Polysaccharides-Based Nanocomposites: The Important Role of Nanoparticles and Layered Double Hydroxides. *Int. J. Biol. Macromol.* **2021,** *193*, 183–204.
59. Zhang, W.; Zhao, X.; Yuan, Y.; Miao, F.; Li, W.; Ji, S.; Huang, X.; Chen, X.; Jiang, T.; Weitz, D. A.; Song, Y. Microfluidic Synthesis of Multimode Au@ CoFeB-Rg3 Nanomedicines and Their Cytotoxicity and Anti-Tumor Effects. *Chem. Mater.* **2020,** *32* (12), 5044–5056.
60. Wang, Z.; Chen, L.; Chu, Z.; Huang, C.; Huang, Y.; Jia, N. Gemcitabine-Loaded Gold Nanospheres Mediated by Albumin for Enhanced Anti-Tumor Activity Combining with CT Imaging. *Mater. Sci. Eng.: C* **2018,** *89*, 106–118.
61. Sun, Y.; Bao, B.; Zhu, Y.; Shen, J.; Liu, X.; Gao, T.; Lin, J.; Huang, T.; Xu, J.; Chai, Y.; Zheng, X. An FPS-ZM1-Encapsulated Zeolitic Imidazolate Framework as a Dual Proangiogenic Drug Delivery System for Diabetic Wound Healing. *Nano Res.* **2022,** *15* (6), 5216–5229.
62. Li, D.; Li, L. F.; Zhang, Z. F.; Xue, D.; Pan, L.; Liu, Y. Ultrasound-Assisted Synthesis of a New Nanostructured Ca (II)-MOF as 5-FU Delivery System to Inhibit Human Lung Cancer Cell Proliferation, Migration, Invasion and Induce Cell Apoptosis. *J. Coord. Chem.* **2020,** *73* (2), 266–281.
63. Saha, S.; Pramanik, K.; Biswas, A. Antibacterial Activity and Biocompatibility of Curcumin/TiO_2 Nanotube Array System on Ti_6Al_4V Bone Implants. *Mater. Technol.* **2021,** *36* (4), 221–232.
64. Karimi, M.; Ghasemi, A.; Zangabad, P. S.; Rahighi, R.; Basri, S. M.; Mirshekari, H.; Amiri, M.; Pishabad, Z. S.; Aslani, A.; Bozorgomid, M.; Ghosh, D. Smart Micro/Nanoparticles in Stimulus-Responsive Drug/Gene Delivery Systems. *Chem. Soc. Rev.* **2016,** *45* (5), 1457–1501.

65. Liu, G.; Lovell, J. F.; Zhang, L.; Zhang, Y. Stimulus-Responsive Nanomedicines for Disease Diagnosis and Treatment. *Int. J. Mol. Sci.* **2020,** *21* (17), 6380.
66. Gao, X.; Xue, Y.; Zhu, Z.; Chen, J.; Liu, Y.; Cheng, X.; Zhang, X.; Wang, J.; Pei, X.; Wan, Q. Nanoscale Zeolitic Imidazolate Framework-8 Activator of Canonical MAPK Signaling for Bone Repair. *ACS Appl. Mater. Interfaces*. **2020,** *13* (1), 97–111.
67. Zhu, Z.; Jiang, S.; Liu, Y.; Gao, X.; Hu, S.; Zhang, X.; Huang, C.; Wan, Q.; Wang, J.; Pei, X. Micro or Nano: Evaluation of Biosafety and Biopotency of Magnesium Metal Organic Framework-74 with Different Particle Sizes. *Nano Res*. **2020,** *13*, 511–526.
68. Bai, X.; Gao, Y.; Zhang, M.; Chang, Y. N.; Chen, K.; Li, J.; Zhang, J.; Liang, Y.; Kong, J.; Wang, Y.; Liang, W. Carboxylated Gold Nanoparticles Inhibit Bone Erosion by Disturbing the acidification of an Osteoclast Absorption Microenvironment. *Nanoscale* **2020,** *12* (6), 3871–3878.
69. Ferguson, J. L.; Turner, S. P. Bone Cancer: Diagnosis and Treatment Principles. *Am. Fam. Phys*. **2018,** *98* (4), 205–213.
70. Cazzato, R. L.; Auloge, P.; De Marini, P.; Boatta, E.; Koch, G.; Dalili, D.; Rao, P. P.; Garnon, J.; Gangi, A. Spinal Tumor Ablation: Indications, Techniques, and Clinical Management. *Techn. Vasc. Intervent. Radiol*. **2020,** *23* (2), 100677.
71. Chindamo, G.; Sapino, S.; Peira, E.; Chirio, D.; Gonzalez, M. C.; Gallarate, M. Bone diseases: Current Approach and Future Perspectives in Drug Delivery Systems for Bone Targeted Therapeutics. *Nanomaterials* **2020,** *10* (5), 875.
72. Sarin, H. Physiologic Upper Limits of Pore Size of Different Blood Capillary Types and Another Perspective on the Dual Pore Theory of Microvascular Permeability. *J. Angiogen. Res*. **2010,** *2*, 1–9.
73. Raghubir, M.; Rahman, C. N.; Fang, J.; Matsui, H.; Mahajan, S. S. Osteosarcoma Growth Suppression by Riluzole Delivery Via Iron Oxide Nanocage in Nude Mice. *Oncol. Rep*. **2020,** *43* (1), 169–176.
74. Nezhad-Mokhtari, P.; Arsalani, N.; Javanbakht, S.; Shaabani, A. Development of Gelatin Microsphere Encapsulated Cu-Based Metal-Organic Framework Nanohybrid for the Methotrexate Delivery. *J. Drug Deliv. Sci. Technol*. **2019,** *50*, 174–180.
75. Sha, Z.; Yang, S.; Fu, L.; Geng, M.; Gu, J.; Liu, X.; Li, S.; Zhou, X.; He, C. Manganese-Doped Gold Core Mesoporous Silica Particles as a Nanoplatform for Dual-Modality Imaging and Chemo-Chemodynamic Combination Osteosarcoma Therapy. *Nanoscale* **2021,** *13* (9), 5077–5093.
76. Geng, B.; Yang, X.; Li, P.; Shi, W.; Pan, D.; Shen, L. W-doped TiO2 nanorods for multimode tumor eradication in osteosarcoma models under single ultrasound irradiation. ACS Applied Materials & Interfaces. 2021 Sep 17;13 (38), 45325–34.
77. Zou, B.; Xiong, Z.; He, L.; Chen, T. Reversing Breast Cancer Bone Metastasis by Metal Organic Framework-Capped Nanotherapeutics Via Suppressing Osteoclastogenesis. *Biomaterials* **2022,** *285*, 121549.
78. Hauser, M.; Nowack, B. Probabilistic Modelling of Nanobiomaterial Release from Medical Applications into the Environment. *Environ. Int*. **2021,** *146*, 106184.
79. Abdulrehman, T.; Qadri, S.; Skariah, S.; Sultan, A.; Mansour, S.; Azzi, J.; Haik, Y. Boron Doped Silver-Copper Alloy Nanoparticle Targeting Intracellular, *S. aureus* in Bone Cells. *PLoS One* **2020,** *15* (4), e0231276.
80. Escobar, A.; Muzzio, N.; Coy, E.; Liu, H.; Bindini, E.; Andreozzi, P.; Wang, G.; Angelomé, P.; Delcea, M.; Grzelczak, M.; Moya, S. E. Antibacterial Mesoporous Titania Films with Embedded Gentamicin and Surface Modified with Bone Morphogenetic

Protein 2 to Promote Osseointegration in Bone Implants. *Adv. Mater. Interfaces* **2019,** *6* (9), 1801648.

81. Marsich, E.; Bellomo, F.; Turco, G.; Travan, A.; Donati, I.; Paoletti, S. Nano-Composite Scaffolds for Bone Tissue Engineering Containing Silver Nanoparticles: Preparation, Characterization and Biological Properties. *J. Mater. Sci.: Mater. Med.* **2013,** *24,* 1799–1807.
82. Arenas-Vivo, A.; Amariei, G.; Aguado, S.; Rosal, R.; Horcajada, P. An Ag-Loaded Photoactive Nano-Metal Organic Framework as a Promising Biofilm Treatment. *Acta Biomaterialia* **2019,** *97,* 490–500.
83. Krumdieck, S. P.; Boichot, R.; Gorthy, R.; Land, J. G.; Lay, S.; Gardecka, A. J.; Polson, M. I.; Wasa, A.; Aitken, J. E.; Heinemann, J. A.; Renou, G. Nanostructured TiO_2 Anatase-Rutile-Carbon Solid Coating with Visible Light Antimicrobial Activity. *Sci. Rep.* **2019,** *9* (1), 1883.
84. Žalnėravičius, R.; Paškevičius, A.; Mažeika, K.; Jagminas, A. Fe (II)-Substituted Cobalt Ferrite Nanoparticles Against Multidrug Resistant Microorganisms. *Appl. Surface Sci.***2018,** *435,* 141–148.
85. Fu, J.; Li, Y.; Zhang, Y.; Liang, Y.; Zheng, Y.; Li, Z.; Zhu, S.; Li, C.; Cui, Z.; Wu, S. An Engineered Pseudo-Macrophage for Rapid Treatment of Bacteria-Infected Osteomyelitis via Microwave-Excited Anti-Infection and Immunoregulation. *Adv. Mater.* **2021,** *33* (41), 2102926.
86. Litwic, A.; Edwards, M. H.; Dennison, E. M.; Cooper, C. Epidemiology and Burden of Osteoarthritis. *Br. Med. Bull.* **2013,** *105* (1), 185–199.
87. Li, J.; Chen, L.; Xu, X.; Fan, Y.; Xue, X.; Shen, M.; Shi, X. Targeted Combination of Antioxidative and Anti-Inflammatory Therapy of Rheumatoid Arthritis Using Multifunctional Dendrimer-Entrapped Gold Nanoparticles as a Platform. *Small* **2020,** *16* (49), 2005661.
88. Mahana, A.; Guliy, O. I.; Mehta, S. K. Accumulation and Cellular Toxicity of Engineered Metallic Nanoparticle in Freshwater Microalgae: Current Status and Future Challenges. *Ecotoxicol. Environ. Saf.* **2021,** *208,* 111662.
89. Wang, D.; Lin, Z.; Wang, T.; Yao, Z.; Qin, M.; Zheng, S.; Lu, W. Where Does the Toxicity of Metal Oxide Nanoparticles Come from: The Nanoparticles, the Ions, or a Combination of Both? *J. Hazard. Mater.* **2016,** *308,* 328–334.
90. Krizkova, S.; Kepinska, M.; Emri, G.; Rodrigo, M. A.; Tmejova, K.; Nerudova, D.; Kizek, R.; Adam, V. Microarray Analysis of Metallothioneins in Human Diseases—A Review. *J. Pharm. Biomed. Anal.* **2016,** *117,* 464–473.
91. Chandrakala, V.; Aruna, V.; Angajala, G. Review on Metal Nanoparticles as Nanocarriers: Current Challenges and Perspectives in Drug Delivery Systems. *Emerg. Mater.* **2022,** , 1–23.
92. Sengul, A. B.; Asmatulu, E. Toxicity of Metal and Metal Oxide Nanoparticles: A Review. *Environ. Chem. Lett.* **2020,** *18,* 1659–1683.
93. Nolte, T. M.; Hartmann, N. B.; Kleijn, J. M.; Garnæs, J.; Van De Meent, D.; Hendriks, A. J.; Baun, A. The Toxicity of Plastic Nanoparticles to Green Algae as Influenced by Surface Modification, Medium Hardness and Cellular Adsorption. *Aqua. Toxicol.* **2017,** *183,* 11–20.

CHAPTER 4

Metallic Foams for Biomedical Application

DEVDHAR YADAV[1], GSN KOTESWARA RAO[2], ROJA RANI BUDHA[3], and NARESH BABU REKHA[4]

[1]*Department of Pharmacy, School of Medical and Allied Sciences, Galgotias University, Greater Noida, India*

[2]*Shobhaben Pratapbhai Patel School of Pharmacy & Technology Management, SVKM's NMIMS, Vile Parle, Mumbai, India*

[3]*H.K. College of Pharmacy, Oshiwara, Jogeshwari (W, Mumbai, India*

[4]*Nirmala College of Pharmacy, Atmakur, Mangalagiri, Guntur, India*

ABSTRACT

Metal foams are now the preferred material in many fields, including transportation, construction, and biomaterials, due to their strength, lightweight, and ability to retain shape. By studying bubble formation, foam nucleation, growth, stability, and the regions where the foam structure is growing, scientists are working to improve the quality of all foams. Metal foams can have open pores, closed pores, or a combination of the two. The pores of an open pore structure are in constant contact with one another and the surrounding medium. The pores in a closed pore structure are not only separated from one another but also from their external surroundings. Having two different kinds of pores in the same mixed pore structure is a unique and interesting arrangement. A variety of biological uses are included in this chapter that involve the intentional insertion of metal foams into living creatures. The first requirement is that it be biologically compatible with its live tissue (it should be nontoxic, nonallergenic, and not have any cancer-causing components).

Metals in Medicine, Volume 1: Metals for Tissue Engineering and Pharmaceutical Applications.
Sonali Sundram, Rishabha Malviya, and GSN Koteswara Rao

Lastly, the material should have good mechanical and physical characteristics, such as enough strength, toughness, fatigue strength, resistance to abrasion, and a low density.

The biomaterial's open porosity structure, which allows blood and bodily fluids to flow through but does not impede the growth of live tissue, is essential for increasing biocompatibility and ensuring the material lasts for a long time. In this chapter, we also see how the application of metal foams, which are now in advanced development, may be applied to the bone-implant interface to possibly address postoperative issues including bone fracture and stress shielding. With all of these good qualities, metal foams could make a big difference in the biomaterials industry.

4.1 INTRODUCTION

Cellular materials are rapidly expanding in use because of their many desirable properties, including low densities, high strength-to-weight ratios, structural properties, thermal and mechanical characteristics. Cellular materials can be acquired naturally or manufactured, and they must be constituted of two stages, one solid and one gaseous.[1] A few instances of spontaneously occurring cellular materials can be seen in Figure 4.1 In response to the unusual mix of features displayed by these types of materials, scientists were intrigued to artificially replicate similar structures, resulting in the production of artificial cellular structures for instance metallic foams. They have a cellular construction that is created by injecting air into melted metal, generating gaps that cool to form a porous structure.

Metal foams provide a high stiffness-to-weight ratio and unique blends of physiological, mechanical, thermodynamic, electrical, and acoustic material characteristics like high heat conductivity, and gas permeability.[2] Amazing performance may be achieved with these materials in applications that seek lightweight and rigid constructions, effective energy absorption, and thermal management.[3]

When the cell structure is taken into consideration, metal foams may be roughly divided into two categories: open and closed-cell foams. Comparatively speaking to a loofah sponge, Metal foams with open cells are constructed from a mesh of pores which are linked to one another. On the other hand, the pores in closed-cell metal foams[4,5] are not interconnected; rather, they are sealed off in a manner analogous to a cellulose kitchen sponge, where each cell is separated by a very thin metal cell wall. The choice of the material structure should be made dependent on the application being used for it. Closed-cell metallic foams have outstanding mechanical qualities, nevertheless because the pores are separated, it is not possible to access the interior surface of the material. As a result, they are used for applications that need load-bearing and structural support.[6] Due to their permeability, open porous foams find usage in filters, catalyst carriers, and biological applications. Various metallic foams manufactured from a variety of metals have found use in recent years. The structural similarity between metallic open porous foam structures and bone tissue suggests that they may have important medicinal uses.[7]

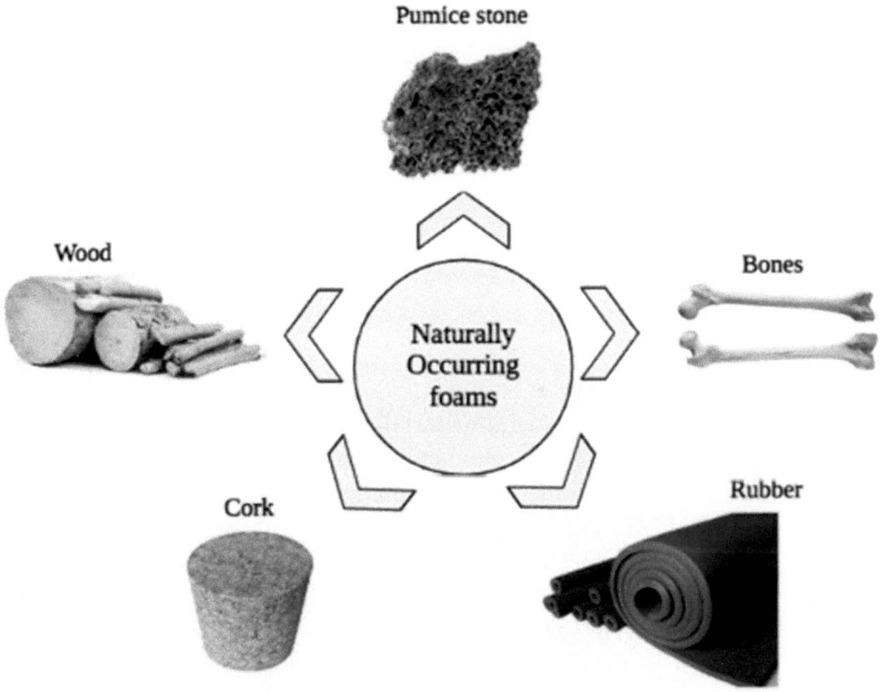

FIGURE 4.1 Naturally occurring cellular material.

4.2 SUITABILITY OF METAL FOAMS

Metallic foams remain utilized in the bone implants or dental implants since they are biocompatible and provide the required durability, stiffness, and strength. Dental implants, for example, require the same strength as the jaw. Titanium or cobalt–chromium foams are suitable for this. Metal foams with open permeability enhance bone formation in biomedical implants in general because of the strong relationship between density and modulus of metal foams, as well as better stiffness and biological compatibility. Figure 4.2 illustrates the functional bone replacement device that is biologically compatible.[8] Magnesium foams can also be used to create biodegradable implants. Metal foams are also increasingly being used as protective gear in the sports sector due to their great energy absorption capability.[9,-11]

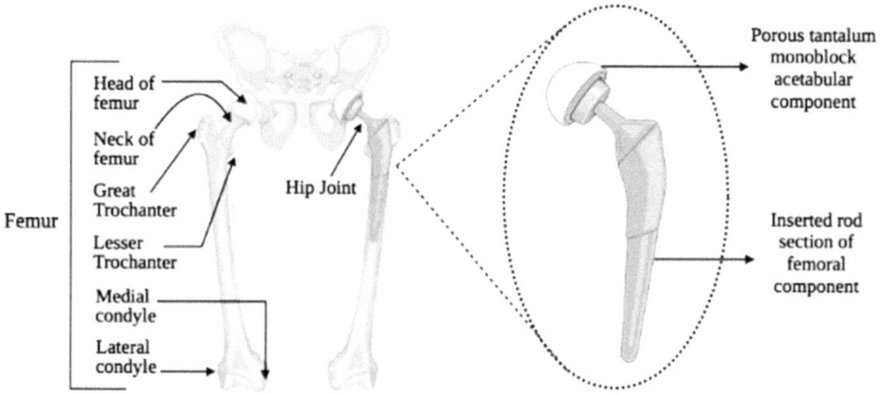

FIGURE 4.2 Inserted rod section of femoral metal implant with acetabular component in complete hip replacement.

In order to function as a biomaterial, a substance must possess some fundamental qualities. These characteristics, as well as the compliance of metallic foams with some of these characteristics, are discussed in this section.

4.2.1 BIOCOMPATIBILITY

A poisonous, bioinert, bioactive, or biodegradable response from living tissue is possible depending on the biomaterial utilized. When implant material is introduced to the body, the tissues there either entirely reject it or tolerate it. The objective of an ideal implementation is to implant the component into the body with no problems or adverse consequences. Toxic metals include nickel, aluminum, and vanishingly rare vanadium. Materials like titanium and stainless steel (316 L, 17-4 PH) are bioinert, whereas magnesium and zinc are biodegradable.

Used metal should not cause any adverse reactions in muscle, bone, or fluids. Toxic by-products, allergens, carcinogens, and metallic ions should not be formed or released. Biocompatible behavior is shown by foams made from titanium, stainless steel, cobalt chrome, and magnesium.[12] Metallic foam's porous structure, which is comparable to bone's, allows it to transport bodily fluids and promote adherence to the tissue to which it is implanted.[13]

4.2.2 MECHANICAL PROPERTIES

It is preferable for the material that is going to be utilized as a biomaterial to have mechanical qualities (strength, hardness, elastic modulus, toughness, and wear resistance etc.) that are compatible with the properties of bone. To begin, it is vital to have an understanding of the characteristics of the bone in order to be able to select the suitable material. Cortical bone has an elasticity modulus within the range of 15–20 GPa and a compression yield strength which falls within the range of 30–150 Mpa. Cancellous bone has an elasticity modulus in the range of 0.09–2 GPa, and its compression yield strength falls between 10 and 70 MPa.[14] The establishment of a stress shielding effect is brought on by the fact that the mechanical characteristics of the implant and the bone are incompatible with one another. Some of the metals used in implants are illustrated with their mechanical properties in Table 4.1.[15] In the event that the mechanical characteristics of the implant and the bones are incompatible, the implant will bear the load. In this scenario, stress shielding will take place, and the load will not be communicated to the bone, causing the bone to deteriorate over time.[16]

4.2.3 REPRODUCIBILITY

Sterilization and reproducibility of the material utilized are two requirements that must be met in order to comply with international standards. Coating or the manufacturing process itself might be used to create the pores in the material. Additionally, production expenses need to be within a fair range. The implantation process needs to be straightforward, accurate, and repeatable.[17]

4.2.4 ELECTRICAL PROPERTIES

The inverse of electrical resistivity is electrical conductance. Because of gas-filled nonconducting pores, Metallic foams have a lower conductivity than solid metals. Foams made of metal can have different properties depending

TABLE 4.1 Mechanical Characteristics of Some of the Alloys Used for Implants.

S. no.	Metals	Composition	Mechanical characteristics			
			Yield strength (Mpa)	Ultimate tensile strength (Mpa)	Young's modulus (GPa)	Max elongation (%)
1	316 L type of Stainless steel	Iron, 16–18.5 Chromium, 10–14 Nickel, 2–3 Molybdenum, <2 mn;<Isi; <0.003°C	190	490	193	40
2	CoCrWNi	Cobalt, 19–21 chromium; 14–16 tungsten, 9–11 nickel	310	860	210	20
	and	and				
	CoNiCrMo	Cobalt, 33–37 nickel, 19–21 chromium, 9–10.5 molybdenum	241	793	232	50
3	Pure titanium grade 4 (F67)	Titanium, 0.05 nitrogen, 0.1 carbon, 0.5 iron, 0.015 hydrogen, 0.4 oxygen	485	550	110	15
	and	and				
	Ti_6Al_4V (F136)	Titanium, 5.5–6.75 Aluminum, 3.5–4.5 Vanadium, 0.08 carbon, 0.2 oxygen	795	860	116	10
4	Pure iron WE43 magnesium alloy	99.8 Iron	150	210	200	40
		and				
		Magnesium, 3.7–4.3 Yttrium, 2.4–4.4 neodymium; 0.40–1.0 zirconium	150	250	44	4

on whether or not their shells are open or closed. As shown in Figure 4.3, electrical resistivity (ρ) is measured in metallic foams with a four-point probe technique. The sample of foam used in the trials was created sufficiently thick so that it would act as a semi-infinite medium. Two of the probes (P1 and P4) introduce direct current (I) to the foam sample, while the voltage differential (V) between the other pair of probes (P2 and P3) is measured.[18]

If the test sample is sufficiently thick, the electrical resistivity of metal foam (unit μΩcm) may be expressed as[19]

$$\text{ñ} = 2\pi\left(V / I\right)$$

$$1 + 1 - 1 - 1$$

$$S1 \quad S3 \quad S1{+}S2 \quad S2{+}S3$$

In which S1, S2, and S3 denote the distance between probes.

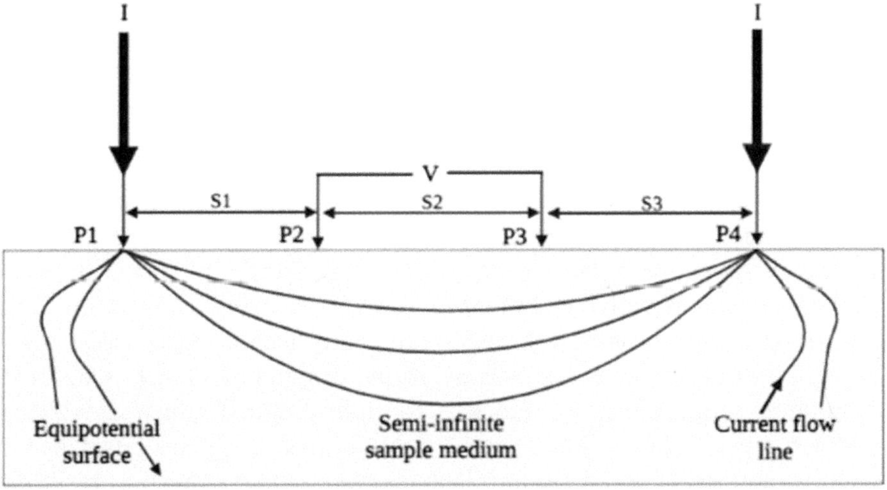

FIGURE 4.3 Evaluation of metal's conductivity by four-point probe method.

4.2.5 *PHYSICAL AND CHEMICAL PROPERTIES*

Biomaterials' physical qualities include things like density, porosity, and pore size. Intruding implant materials, especially those that are bulky, can be annoying to the host. As a result, titanium implants have replaced the more cumbersome platinum implants. The lightweight design and energy-absorbing characteristics of porous materials would be useful in this regard. Also, the porous design allows for nutrition transfer and tissue ingrowth, which promotes osseointegration and long service life.[20] A porous material's linked structure, pore size and shape, and porosity characteristics are all crucial for bone tissue regeneration. According to a research, biomaterial with porous architectures designed to be inserted into body tissues needs to have a pore size of at least 200 m. Because the cells cannot pass through the holes if they are too tiny.[21] Further, large pore diameters have a detrimental effect on mechanical characteristics, while porosity is the more crucial factor in determining such qualities. Porosity affects both permeability and elastic modulus; as porosity rises, permeability rises but elastic modulus falls.[22]

Metallic foams have an advantage in biomedical applications due to their porous structure, which allows for customization of pore size, porosity, and open/closed pore shape throughout the manufacturing process. Porous metals also have other useful qualities, like high resistance to corrosion and heat conduction. Higher electrochemical activity and lower density. Due to the fact that the specific surface areas of foams exceed those of even the densest metals.[23]

4.3 SOME COMMON METALS USED IN BIOMEDICAL FIELD

Cobalt–chromium alloys, Ti-alloys, and stainless steel are the top 3 metals currently utilized for the purpose of implants. Since the initial implant-grade stainless steel had around 18 wt% Cr and around 8 wt% Ni, it was much more durable and resistant to corrosion than standard steel. Type 316 stainless steel, so named because of its increased resistance to corrosion thanks to the inclusion of molybdenum (Mo), is one such material. Later on, it had its carbon composition of 0.03 wt%, eventually increasing its resistance to corrosion in cl^- solution, and was given the designation 316 L. One of the titanium's defining characteristics is its lightweight. Compared with 316 stainless steel (7.9 g/cm^3) and cast CoCrMo alloys (8.3 g/cm^3), its density is significantly lower at 4.5 g/cm^3.[24] The tensile strength as well as resistance to corrosion of Ti as well as its alloys like Ti_6Al_4V are familiar. Nitinol, a titanium–nickel alloy, has the shape-memory characteristic that makes it useful in many contexts, including the wiring of dental restorations.

In dentistry, expensive metals and alloys, such as gold, silver, and platinum, as well as their respective alloys, are commonly utilized. They do have excellent castability and ductileness, as well as resistance to corrosion, among other desirable characteristics. The AuAgCu system, in which the AuAgCu with the inclusion of Zinc and Sn, which is referred to as orthodonture solder, and AuPtPd system are all types of dental alloys. The AuAgCu system is utilized for porcelain merged with metal for dental repairs. The use of cobalt–chromium alloys in the manufacturing of artificial joints dates back to few decades. which have a stellar reputation for withstanding wear.

4.4 BIOMEDICAL APPLICATIONS

The usage of various metals in medical implants is context-dependent. From the field of cardiovascular surgery to that of otorhinolaryngology, 316 L stainless steel (ss) implants continue to reign supreme. In cases where extreme wear resistance is needed, implants of CoCrMo alloys are well suited for uses including such artificial joints. Materials like titanium and stainless steel, which are widely utilized in the applications, are discussed in this section, along with their application domains and the benefits and drawbacks associated with their use.

4.4.1 *STAINLESS STEEL*

One of its kind, bioinert metals to be employed in orthopedic implant applications was stainless steel. The essential components of stainless steel are iron, carbon, nickel, and chromium. However, the addition of additions like molybdenum can increase the quality of stainless steel. 316 L. This has a lesser strength but a stronger corrosion resistance and a higher level of hardness when compared with other utilized metals. However, 316 L offers resistance to corrosion because it is protected by a thin oxide layer that acts as a passivation barrier. 316 L has a higher resistance to corrosion when it has a porosity that is increased. The geometry of the surface as well as the pore distribution are both essential characteristics. Because the open pore structure makes it easier for oxygen to move through the material, it makes the production of a passive layer possible. Titanium and the alloys made from it are more favorable in applications thanks to their high hardness.[25]

4.4.2 *IRON FOAM*

Despite the fact that the vast majority of metallic foams are constructed out of Al-alloys, Fe-based metallic foams provide a number of benefits that aluminum alloy-based metal foams do not. These benefits include high strength, high ability to absorb energy, cheap price, and improved weld-ability. Because iron has a high melting point and other traditional foaming ingredients are not as effective, it is difficult to create iron-based foams.[26] By using carbon monoxide and carbon dioxide as foaming gases rather than the more traditional foaming agents, iron-based foams were effectively developed. This recently invented method of manufacturing consisted of creating a parent form by cold-pressed powdered Fe, graphite as well as hematite. The procedure was created in the United States. Following the heating of the precursor, a reduction process caused foam to form in the molten iron. At a temperature of 1350°C, spherical pores with a maximum porosity of 57% were produced.[27,28]

4.4.3 MAGNESIUM

In the realm of bone-related biological applications, magnesium is an essential component. It is necessary for human nutrition as well as the health of the bones. Advantages for applications involving biomaterials include the substance's capacity to biodegrade and the compatibility of its mechanical qualities with the structure of bone. After it has been implanted, the tissue will recover thanks to its capacity to biodegrade, and then it will either be absorbed by the body or removed from the body. Therefore, there is no need for a further procedure. In addition, the preparation of porous magnesium only needs to be done at a low temperature, and it also requires a reduced number of spacing agents to be used. These are both benefits. Porous magnesium, on the other hand, does not get a lot of favor due to the fact that its corrosion resistance is inadequate in vitro, that it has several phases in its structure, and that it does not have enough porosity.[29]

4.4.4 TITANIUM AND ITS ALLOYS

Porous titanium is a material that is commonly utilized in biomaterial applications, and it has been shown to generate effective outcomes in these applications. Because of its great chemical stability and superior mechanical qualities, it is the material of choice. The great chemical resistance and high mechanical strength of CoCrMo alloys, titanium (Ti) metal, and its many alloys have made them particularly useful in a variety of applications. Ti metal and its alloys are especially noteworthy for their greater biological compatibility with live tissue, in addition to their possessing elastic modulus that is comparable to that of bone tissue.[30,31] In particular, their mechanical compatibility is enhanced by the incorporation of pores, which reduces their elastic modulus to levels similar to bone tissue. The osteoconductivity of titanium metal and alloys was also confirmed, which refers to on-surface bone growth in contact with bone, and osteoinductivity, which refers to ectopic bone formation, when subjected to certain chemicals as well as heat treatments. As a result, it is anticipated that titanium foam will be essential in the procedure of creating bone tissue as well. Furthermore, Fiber sintering,[32] plasma spraying of Ti particles, and other techniques can all be used to create a porous coating on Ti or its alloys. This porous coating grows on medical devices like hip joints which can be used to help secure the device to the patient's bone via a mechanical interlocking system. To strengthen the hip joint's attachment to the bone around it, the porous layer is treated with chemicals and heat to induce bioactivity. In Japan, such bioactive hip replacements have already been used in patients since 2007.

4.4.5 COBALT-CHROMIUM ALLOYS

On account of its inertness and resistance to wear, CoCr alloys are a popular choice for implants. The acetabular cup, femoral stem, and other components of total knee arthroplasty are made from it because of its high abrasion resistance. However, a little fibrous ingrowth is seen upon closer inspection of the tissue ingrowth. This might prevent any permanent results from being achieved and there is a lot of nickel in alloys made from the CoCr base metal. As a result, it might trigger allergic reactions. Mo-containing alloys are recommended above Ni-based ones.[33]

4.4.6 TANTALUM

When compared with other metals, tantalum emerges as a very exceptional biomaterial. It has potential value in the biomedical field, since it is biocompatible and has adequate biomechanical characteristics. It is favored because it is very porous, has a low elastic modulus, and has a strong resistance to friction. Studies have demonstrated that despite its significant porosity nature, it is robust to physiological stresses and may sustain bone ingrowth under even these conditions. In addition, its corrosion resistance exceeds that of titanium, the metal often used for such purposes. However, the production cost is greater. Tantalum was shown to promote superior extracellular matrix production, cell adhesion, and proliferation in vitro. Numerous orthopedic procedures now make use of it, including complete hip replacement (acetabular component) (Fig. 4.2),[34] knee replacement (patellar component),[35] foot and ankle surgery, spine fusion, etc.

Despite its great benefits, its manufacture and processes are constrained by its high melting point (2996°C) and strong affinity to oxygen. The positive result of a total hip arthroplasty (THA) is based on a number of elements, including the implant's design, manufacturing method, surface structure, and bone integration characteristics. There are three types of tantalum acetabular components available: a Monoblock component with direct compression molded polyethylene, a Monoblock cup with peripheral screw fixation, and a modular component covered with a porous tantalum framework.[36]

4.5 MANUFACTURERS OF METALLIC FOAMS

Some of the manufacturers that are known for the production of metallic foams are listed below in Table 4.2.

TABLE 4.2 List of Manufacturers of Metallic Foam with Their Native Countries.[6]

S. no.	Company	Country	Website
1	Aritech Chemazone Pvt. Ltd.	India	http://www.nanochemazone.org/
2	M-Pore	Germany	https://www.mayser.com/en
3	VIM Technology, Ltd.	China	http://www.vim-metalfoam.com/
4	Alantum Corporation	Korea	http://www.alantum.com/
5	Porometal	China	http://www.porometal.com/
6	Recemat Bv	Netherlands	www.recemat.nl/
7	Havel metal foam GmbH	Germany	https://havel-mf.com/
8	Integran Technologies Inc.	Canada	www.integran.com/
9	Alusion	Canada	www.alusion.com
10	AlCarbon	Germany	http://www.alcarbon.de/startseite
11	Aluinvent Inc.	Hungary	http://aluinvent.com/
12	Composite Materials, Ltd.	Russia	https://alupor.com/
13	Exxentis	Switzerland/ Austria	http://www.exxentis.com/
14	Alcarbon GmbH	Switzerland	https://www.alcarbon.de/
15	Corex Honeycomb	UK	https://corex-honeycomb.co.uk/
16	Alveotec	France	http://www.alveotec.fr/fr/
17	Ultramet	USA	https://ultramet.com/
18	American Elements	USA	https://www.americanelements.com/
19	Chand Eisenmann Metallurgical	USA	http://www.porvairfiltration.com/
20	Cymat	Canada	http://www.cymat.com/

4.6 FUTURE PROSPECTS

The outlook for metal foams in the future is quite positive. It is not at all difficult to see that the application of cutting-edge metal foams is rapidly expanding. Their usefulness in a diversity of industries, which includes aerospace, automotive industries, construction, as well as biomedical sectors is driving the desire for them to be manufactured in mass. Recent years have seen significant technological developments, which have contributed to an increase in manufacturing capacity. When compared with the costs of producing traditional materials, the cost of producing metal foams might be significantly lower. The creation of models will be of additional assistance in boosting manufacturing rates, as well as improving characteristics, quality, and durability. The decline in the price of foam structures is the final but no less important factor; it is this factor that will assure the rapid expansion of the market in terms of both quantity and quality in the years to come.

4.7 CONCLUSION

Since metallic foams may have their qualities enhanced, they find applications in many fields and have great promise for many others. Since the pore structure is so analogous to that of cancellous bone, it finds significant application in the biological field. Over the years, a wide variety of metals have been evaluated for potential application here. This review discussed the compatibility of metallic foam qualities in bioimplant applications, as well as the varieties of metallic foam employed in these contexts and the locations where they are implanted. Foams, especially particularly those made of tantalum and titanium, have found widespread use. Problems arise, though, its porous form reduces corrosion resistance and triggers ion release. Hence, it is better to use a coating in certain areas than all over, rather than as a totally porous structure. As manufacturing techniques advance and component strengths rise, metallic foams are predicted to play a more important role in biomaterials.

KEYWORDS

- **metallic foams**
- **stainless steel**
- **iron foam**
- **mg foam**
- **titanium foam**
- **tantalum**
- **iron foam**

REFERENCES

1. Gibson, L. J. Cellular Solids. *Mrs Bull.* **2003,** *28* (4), 270–274.
2. Banhart, J. Manufacture Characterization and Application of Cellular Metals and Metal Foams. *Progress Mater. Sci.* **2001,** *46*, 599–632.
3. Ashby, M. F.; Evans, T.; Fleck, N. A.; Hutchinson, J. W.; Wadley, H. N.; Gibson, L. J. *Metal Foams: A Design Guide*; Elsevier, 2000.
4. Guden, M.; Celik, E.; Cetiner, S.; Aydin, A. Metals Foams for Biomedical Applications: Processing and Mechanical Properties. In: *Biomaterials*; Springer: Boston, 2004; pp 257–266.
5. Rajak, D. K.; Gupta, M. *An Insight Into Metal Based Foams*; Singapore: Springer, 2020.
6. Lefebvre, L. P.; Banhart, J.; Dunand, D. C. Porous Metals and Metallic Foams: Current Status and Recent Developments. *Adv. Eng. Mater.* **2008,** *10* (9), 775–787.
7. Beköz, N. Microstructural and Mechanical Properties of Iron Based Foamed Metals Obtained by Powder Metallurgy Method; Doctoral Thesis, Istanbul University, 2011.
8. Murr, L. E.; Gaytan, S. M.; Medina, F.; Lopez, H.; Martinez, E.; Machado, B. I.; Hernandez, D. H.; Martinez, L.; Lopez, M. I.; Wicker, R. B.; Bracke, J. Next-Generation Biomedical Implants Using Additive Manufacturing of Complex, Cellular and Functional Mesh Arrays. *Phil. Trans. R. Soc. A: Math. Phys. Eng. Sci.* **2010,** *368* (1917), 1999–2032.
9. Dukhan, N. (Eds.). *Metal Foams: Fundamentals and Applications*; DEStech Publications, Inc, 2013.
10. Banhart, J. Light-Metal Foams—History of Innovation and Technological Challenges. *Adv. Eng. Mate.* **2013,** *15* (3), 82–111.
11. Banhart, J. Aluminium foams for lighter vehicles. *Int. J. Veh. Design* **2005,** *37* (2–3), 114–125.
12. Mutlu, İ. Microstructural and Mechanical Properties of Porous Martensitic Stainless Steel Obtained by Powder Metallurgy Method; Doctoral Thesis, Istanbul University, 2011.

13. Nouri, A. Titanium Foam Scaffolds for Dental Applications. In: *Metallic Foam Bone* **2017,** ; Woodhead Publishing, 2017; pp 131–160.
14. Matsushita, T.; Fujibayashi, S.; Kokubo, T. Titanium Foam for Bone Tissue Engineering. In: *Metallic Foam Bone*; Woodhead Publishing, 2017; pp 111–130.
15. Hermawan, H.; Ramdan, D.; Djuansjah, J. R. Metals for Biomedical Applications. Biomedical Engineering-From Theory to Applications. **2011,** *1*, 411–430.
16. Joshi, M. G.; Advani, S. G.; Miller, F.; Santare, M. H. Analysis of a Femoral Hip Prosthesis Designed to Reduce Stress Shielding. *J. Biomech.* **2000,** *33* (12), 1655–1662.
17. Matassi, F.; Botti, A.; Sirleo, L.; Carulli, C.; Innocenti, M. Porous Metal for Orthopedics Implants. *Clin. Cases Miner. Bone Metabol.* **2013,** *10* (2), 111.
18. Dharmasena, K. P.; Wadley, H. N. Electrical Conductivity of Open-Cell Metal foams. *J. Mater. Res.* **2002,** *17* (3), 625–631.
19. Ashby, M. F.; Evans, T.; Fleck, N. A.; Hutchinson, J. W.; Wadley, H. N.; Gibson, L. J. *Metal Foams: A Design Guide*; Elsevier, 2000.
20. Karageorgiou, V.; Kaplan, D. Porosity of 3D Biomaterial Scaffolds and Osteogenesis. *Biomaterials* **2005,** *26* (27), 5474–5491.
21. Xue, W.; Krishna, B. V.; Bandyopadhyay, A.; Bose, S. Processing and Biocompatibility Evaluation of Laser Processed Porous Titanium. *Acta Biomater* **2007,** *3* (6), 1007–1018.
22. Wu, S.; Liu, X.; Yeung, K. W.; Liu, C.; Yang, X. Biomimetic Porous Scaffolds for Bone Tissue Engineering. *Mater. Sci. Eng.: R: Rep.* **2014,** *80*, 1–36.
23. Qin, J.; Chen, Q.; Yang, C.; Huang, Y. Research Process on Property and Application of Metal Porous Materials. *J. Alloys Compd.* **2016,** *654*, 39–44.
24. Smithells, C. J.; Brandes, E. A. *Smithells Metals Reference Book*, 1992.
25. Beköz Üllen, N.; Karabulut, G. The place of Metal Foams in Biomaterial Applications. In: *2nd International Eurasian Conference on Science, Engineering and Technology* (EurasianSciEnTech 2020); Gaziantep: Turkey, 2020; pp 473–479.
26. Murakami, T.; Akagi, T.; Kasai, E. Development of Porous Iron Based Material by Slag Foaming and Its Reduction. *Procedia Mater. Sci.* **2014,** *4*, 27–32.
27. Murakami, T.; Ohara, K.; Narushima, T.; Ouchi, C. Development of a New Method for Manufacturing Iron Foam Using Gases Generated by Reduction of Iron Oxide. *Mater. Trans.* **2007,** *48* (11), 2937–2944.
28. Murakami, T.; Omameuda, G.; Kasai, E. Effect of Cr_2O_3 and WO_3 addition on Pore Formation and Microstructure in Iron Foam. *ISIJ Int.* **2010,** *50* (2), 307–313.
29. Zhuang, H.; Han, Y.; Feng, A. Preparation, Mechanical Properties and In Vitro Biodegradation of Porous Magnesium Scaffolds. *Mater. Sci. Eng.: C.* **2008,** *28* (8), 1462–1466.
30. Niinomi, M.; Hattori, T.; Morikawa, K.; Kasuga, T.; Suzuki, A.; Fukui, H.; Niwa, S. Development of Low Rigidity β-Type Titanium Alloy for Biomedical Applications. *Mater. Trans.* **2002,** *43* (12), 2970–2977.
31. Ozaki, T.; Matsumoto, H.; Watanabe, S.; Hanada, S. Beta Ti Alloys with Low Young's Modulus. *Mater. Trans.* **2004,** *45* (8), 2776–2779.
32. Weiss, M. B. Titanium Fiber-Mesh Metal Implant. *J. Oral Implantol.* **1986,** *12* (3), 498–507.
33. Cömert, I. Using Powder Metallurgy Process on Applications of the Biomaterials; Master's Thesis, Yıldız Technical University, 2005.
34. George, N.; Nair, A. B. Porous Tantalum: A New Biomaterial in Orthopedic Surgery. In: *Fundamental Biomaterials: Metals*; ; Woodhead Publishing, 2018; pp 243–268.

35. Solarino, G.; Carlet, A.; Moretti, L.; Miolla, M. P.; Ottaviani, G.; Moretti, B. Clinical Results in Posterior-Stabilized Total Knee Arthroplasty with Cementless Tibial Component in Porous Tantalum: Comparison Between Monoblock and Two Pegs vs. Modular and Three Pegs. *Prosthesis* **2022,** *4* (2), 160–168.
36. Foran, J. R. H.; Miller, M. D. Osteonecrosis of the Hip, **2018**. https://orthoinfo.aaos.org/en/diseases--conditions/osteonecrosis-of-the-hip (accessed on 18 Aug 2020).

CHAPTER 5

Role of Metal–Organic Framework in Therapeutic Delivery

ROHIT RAJ[1], UMA SANKAR GORLA[2], APARNA BADWANE[1], MADHURA TIWARI[1], KOMAL SHARMA[1], PARTH JOSHI[1], DARSHAN PATEL[1], ARYAN PATEL[1], and GSN KOTESWARA RAO[1]

[1]*Shobhaben Pratapbhai Patel School of Pharmacy & Technology Management, SVKM's NMIMS, Vile Parle, Mumbai, India*

[2]*Viswanadha Institute of Pharmaceutical Sciences, Mindivanipalem, Visakhapatnam, India*

ABSTRACT

Metal–organic frameworks are porous frameworks made up of endless metal nodes connected by organic linkers. The study of MOFs is now a quickly expanding field of research. There have been reports of around 90,000 different MOF structures so far, and the number increases daily. The MOFs structure and characteristics depend upon the selection of metallic nodes and organic nodes linker. Their application is expanding to several fields like physical, chemical, pharmaceutical, and medical fields. In this chapter, their role in therapeutic delivery will be discussed with additional emphasis on their biocompatibility, process parameters, preparation, etc.

5.1 INTRODUCTION

Metal–organic frameworks (MOFs) are a versatile group of advanced crystalline porous compounds that integrate a network of metal ions with polydentate organic molecules to form three-dimensional structures. MOFs are hybrid materials with distinctive structure design and tunability that

Metals in Medicine, Volume 1: Metals for Tissue Engineering and Pharmaceutical Applications.
Sonali Sundram, Rishabha Malviya, and GSN Koteswara Rao

are made of two major components: an inorganic metal cluster (secondary-building unit or SBU) and an organic molecule (linker) (Fig. 5.1).[1,2]

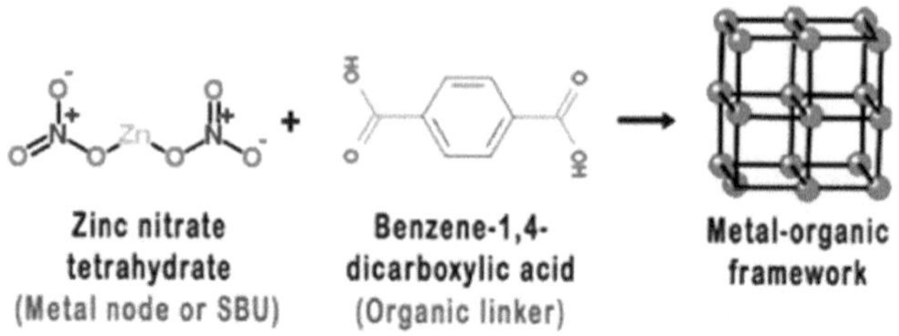

FIGURE 5.1 Diagrammatic representation showing the formation of MOF.

The study of MOFs is now a quickly expanding field of research. There have been reported around 90,000 different MOF structures so far, and the number increases daily. The MOF structure and characteristics depend on the selection of metallic nodes and organic node linkers. With their unmatched high surface area (more than 6000 m^2/g), high porosity (a maximum of 90% free volume), tunable pore sizes, robustness, and structural diversity, MOFs are well-suited for an extensive range of applications, covering heterogenous catalysis, the breakdown of harmful organic dyes from aqueous mediums, proton conductivity, magnetic separation, drug delivery, biomedical imaging, gas storage, and separation (Table 5.1).[2–5]

5.2 BIOCOMPATIBILITY AND TOXICITY

Delivery of any drug is always supported by vehicles or called excipients and MOFs. Considering MOFs to be acceptable and useful clinical drug delivery vehicles, the MOFs must be biocompatible and have very little or no toxic effect on the body systems.[6–9] Biocompatibility is impacted by the type of coordination which is among the metal element vs. organic linker; overall, this coordination is dependent upon the physical properties, such as structure, the charge on the surface, and the side of the molecules. Biocompatibility of the MOFs is an important aspect and factor that influences the bioavailability range of any drug.[10]

Toxicity and cytotoxicity and the MOFs are dependent upon the built structure of the MOFs that is the metal (basically these metals are essential body metals such as iron, zinc, and magnesium) and the ligands used for their formation. To get the toxicity data of the MOFs, the comparative assessment of the individual metals and the ligands and the assembled MOF

TABLE 5.1 List of Various MOFs with Applications.

Metal node	Organic linker	MOF	Applications
Zn^{2+}	2-methylimidazole	ZIF-8	Drug delivery Tumor therapy
$Cr_3O(OH)_3$	Terephthalic acid	MIL-101 (Cr)	Adsorption Photocatalysis Sensor design Drug delivery
MgOH	2,5-dihydroxy-terephthalic acid	MOF-74 (Mg)	Sensing, storage, and separation of gases
$Zr_6O_4(OH)_8(H_2O)_4$	Tetrakis (4-carboxyphenyl) porphyrin (Fe)	PCN-222 (Fe)	Adsorptive removal of dyes from water
$Zr_6O_4(OH)_4$	4,4'-biphenyldicarboxylic acid	Zr-UiO-67	Gas adsorption and separation, catalyst support
$Zr_6O_4(OH)_4$	Terephthalic acid	Zr-UiO-66	Gas adsorption and separation, catalysis, sensors
$Fe_3O(OH)_3$	Tetrakis (4-carboxyphenyl) porphyrin	PCN-600(Fe)	Catalysis, storage of gas and adsorption, adsorption of liquid phase
$Zr_6O_4(OH)_8(H_2O)_4$	4,4',4",4'"-(pyrene-1,3,6,8-tetryl)tetrabenzoic acid	NU-1000 (Zr)	Gas adsorption and separation, catalyst support
Zn^{2+}	Terephthalic acid	MIL-96 (AI)	Gas adsorption and separation, drug delivery

can be helpful as opinion can be formed by getting the direct correlation with the study.[11,12] This can lead to the fact that cytotoxicity of the individual component and the assembled MOFs can be complicated and dependent on each other, that is, while formulating a MOF let us suppose cubic-zeotype mesoporous MIL-100 and MIL-101 solids are being used for the preparation of MOF and there can be possibilities like[13]:

i. Both materials can show toxicity individually.
ii. The toxicity can be seen while in combination.

So, the conclusion can be derived that individually the elements and MOF in assembled form should be biocompatible with the body, tissues, and its environment and should not leach to bodily fluid and tissue with due course of time.[14–16] And toxicity depends on many factors like degradation kinetics of the materials, the biodistribution, deposition in tissues and organs, elimination, and excretion of the MOFs from the body and these factors are cell type-dependent.[17–19] Method of preparation of MOF is shown in Figure 5.2.

5.3 METHODS OF PREPARATION

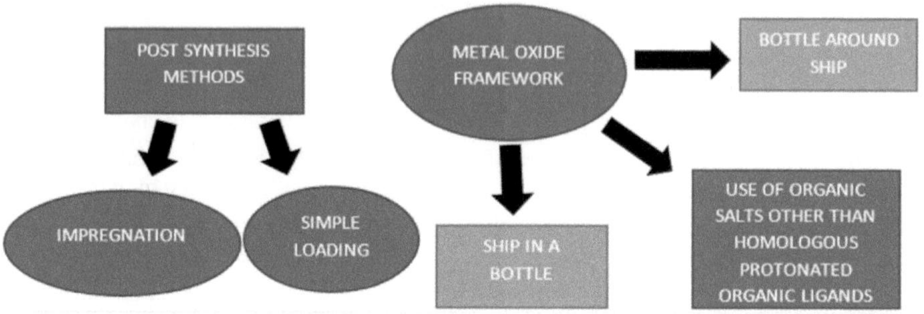

FIGURE 5.2 Methods of preparation of MOFs.

5.3.1 BOTTLE AROUND SHIP (BAS)

In one of the techniques, composing elements that have already been made are combined with MOF precursors before the synthesizing process is carried out.

Graphite oxide/MOF (GO/MOF) is one of these types of materials that has been widely reported for various applications.[20–23] Bandosz et al. published reports on GO/MOF composites prepared using this procedure and successfully applied them in gas phase adsorptive removal of toxic gases, such as NH_3, H_2S, NO_2, and so on.[20–23]

The planar cage structure of MOF's acts as the base structure where the GO layers are stacked to produce the composites of MOF. The composing material particles are also entangled within the MOF pores resulting in the stabilization or immobilization. The overall model is termed "Bottle Around Ship" (BAS).

5.3.2 SHIP IN A BOTTLE (SIB)

The MOF composite is also produced from the predecessors of the composing components and the previously formed MOF. According to Gascon et al.,[24] this method is occasionally referred to as the "ship in a bottle" (SIB) method.

It involves the development of composing materials within the MOF cages and a solvent system often facilitates the precursors' diffusion within the cages. The particles inside the cages, as a result of their larger size, remain stable. Typically, the composing components' precursors are introduced as solutions and dispersed into the pores. The composing moiety is then stabilized within the MOF pores, either chemically or thermally, to create the composite. One of the top instances of this is the direct encapsulation of different porphyrines into ZMOFs, and this composite was successfully applied in catalytic oxidation.[25] Although SIB techniques are widely known for zeolite composites,[26] their study within the MOF field has recently started and there are vast opportunities for utilizing this encapsulation method for MOFs.

The composing material grows within the MOF cages, and a solvent solution frequently speeds up the diffusion of precursors there. Because of their improved size, the particles get entrapped and stay stable within the cages. Precursors to those composing elements are typically injected as solutions which are disseminated within the apertures. The composing moiety is then chemically or thermally stabilized inside the MOFs' pores to produce the composite. Direct encapsulation of various porphyrines into ZMOFs is one of the best examples of this, as illustrated in Figure 5.3, and this composite was successfully used in catalytic oxidation.[25] Despite the fact that SIB approaches are well known for zeolite composites,[26] their study within the MOF sector has just begun, and there are numerous prospects for this encapsulating technique for MOFs has a wide range of applications.

For liquid phase adsorptions, Jhung's group loaded polyoxometalates (POM) and soluble salts onto these materials.[27,28] The insolubilized elements or loaded metal oxides inside the pores, which are produced chemically, are one of the greatest examples of these materials happening via a change of the oxidation state. Metal oxide MOFs, such as Cu_2O, have been prepared using this technique.[29] Moreover, research on the insolubilization of composing materials has shown that precipitates were created by altering the oxidation state of the soluble salts.[30] A controlled encapsulation technique involving the trap of surfactant-capped nanostructured objects produced a zeolitic imidazolate framework (ZIF-8). The objects can be of different shapes, sizes, and compositions. This approach was successful in incorporating several functions into the MOF pores with nanoparticles. The ZIF-8 crystals contain the integrated nanoparticles completely and with good dispersion.[31]

Post-synthesis techniques can be used to carry out the composing process if the solubility of the composing components does not pose a problem for applications. Straightforward loading, also known as impregnation, is a commonly used technique of this kind.

Due to the large variety of ions and ligands that can be used to create MOFs, an extensive range of chemical and physical characteristics are feasible. By using reticular chemistry (structure-guided synthesis), MOF frameworks can be developed to address the need of a certain application without requiring extensive empirical research. The ligand can be changed later on while still preserving the MOF framework's general shape (aka isoreticular chemistry). These alterations can be utilized to gradually alter pore size, surface area, and void volume. Changing the framework's chemistry and structure also affects how the medicinal compounds are stored and released. Many times, this control was obtained through stable MOFs and improved properties have been found in biological fluids, using several isoreticular MOF series. With the use of reagents, solvent ratios, reaction kinetics, temperature, equilibrium, and modulating agents, the macroscopic order can be tailored by controlled synthesis.[13,15] Modulating agents can function as competing ligands favoring the process of controlled synthesis or can act as deprotonating reagents that change the nucleation process followed by the development of the MOF.[6] These agents are chemically identical to the MOF ligand. Additionally, to achieve larger pore sizes or greater empty space, modifying agents might introduce flaws into the MOF structure. Flexible MOF manufacturing is made possible by a variety of synthesis techniques. The MOF determines the type of synthesis, with certain MOFs requiring numerous techniques. MOFs are frequently synthesized using solvothermal and non-solvothermal processes. To dissolve the material, solvothermal synthesis is typically done at high pressures or above the boiling point.

Flexible MOF manufacturing is made possible by a range of synthesis techniques. The MOF determines the type of synthesis, with some MOFs requiring numerous techniques.[32] MOFs are frequently synthesized using solvothermal and non-solvothermal processes. To decompose the material, solvothermal synthesis is typically done at high temperatures or above the boiling point to facilitate synthesis and disperse the reactants. Non-solvothermal synthesis takes place below the solvent's boiling point and is typically conducted under circumstances that encourage nucleation. For medication distribution uses, unconventional synthesis techniques, such as microwaving, sonicating, or mechanical grinding are used.[33,34] Numerous of these techniques involve the use of organic liquids, which can persist in MOFs after their production and can then be eliminated through the "activation" process.

Synthesis techniques have been created in aqueous circumstances and using light alcohol solvents to prevent solvent problems for biological uses.[35–39] Additionally, techniques for mechanical synthesis without fluid have been researched.[40,41] MOFs are defined using a range of methods after synthesis. For instance, the crystalline structure of medi-MOF-1, a curcumin and zinc-based MOF, was confirmed using powder X-ray diffraction (PXRD) analysis before and after contact with various liquids.[42] TGA analysis revealed that medi-MOF-1 retained structural integrity at temperatures as high as 300°C. Bonding and ibuprofen accumulation were subsequently confirmed using Fourier transform infrared (FTIR) analysis.[42] The properties of medi-MOF-1's porous structure, including Brunauer–Emmett–Teller (BET) surface area (3002 m^2/g) and pore volume (0.902 cm^3/g), were determined using nitrogen adsorption.[42] Molecular simulation was employed while medi-MOF-1's size (80–100 m) was determined using light-based imaging, its coordination scheme, SBU, pore sizes (9.2–11), free volume (1.51 cm^3/g), and simulated X-ray diffraction pattern were all revealed by molecular modeling.[42] Depending on their size, transmission electron microscopy (TEM) and scanning electron microscopy (SEM) are also frequently used to view the visible shape of MOF particles.[43]

5.4 AMORPHOUS AND POROUS NATURE OF MOFS

Crystalline MOFs are porous frameworks with endless number of metal nodes linked by organic linkers. The complexity of constituent parts and molecular networks has massively increased; however, there are still more than 6000 novel MOF structures documented year. Because of their propensity for sorption and separation, their frequently occurring structures result in chemically variable porous designs that have attracted extensive research. Recently, catalytic uses based on their chemical tunability have been suggested, and accounts of negative linear compressibility and negative thermal expansion have increased interest in the area.[44,45]

Amorphous MOFs have the nature of lacking long-range periodic order but maintain fundamental building elements and connectivity of their crystalline cousins. Atoms arranged periodically have wide "humps" from diffuse scattering ruling their X-ray diffraction patterns, making it difficult to differentiate between them. Although the field is largely unexplored, amorphous MOFs offer many intriguing possibilities for practical application, either as new functional materials themselves or enabling other processes (total amorphous MOF reported structures amounting to under 30).[46] While there is potential that heat amorphization creates super strong glasses and hybrid liquids, the ion-carrying capability of crystalline MOFs may be enhanced during partial structural failure. As amorphous MOFs are frequently more mechanically resilient than crystalline materials, which is important for industrial uses, it may be feasible to tune the release times of MOF drug delivery carriers by partial structural failure.[47]

Amorphous MOF frameworks are commonly difficult to characterize. Single crystal diffraction methods, which are frequently used in the characterization of crystalline compounds, are not possible to use because there is no structural periodicity. Since the atomic-scale structure of materials determines usefulness frequently regardless of the level of long-range order, the relatively limited knowledge of amorphous MOFs stops their rational design and subsequently impedes their advancement toward potential applications.[48,49] The structural modeling of amorphous MOFs is still in its youth in contrast to models of amorphous inorganics, which have been around for more than 50 years and include amorphous silicon and germanium.[50,51] The amorphous ZIF-4 ($Zn(C_3H_3N_2)_2$) is one of the important members of the zeolitic imidazolate framework (ZIF) family, which has received the bulk of attention in research. In reality, among the 205 models, amorphous ZIF-4 was the only one that had MOF inclusion with a catalog of rigid, porous, amorphous materials. This article was taken from a study of amorphous ZIF-4 to show a reconstructive transition upon heating from the ZIF-4 crystal and the topological resemblance of aZIF-4 to the continuous random network structure of silica.[52] The research used neutron and X-ray total scattering studies alongside modeling of reverse Monte Carlo (RMC). The melt quenching process was simulated along with conventional molecular dynamics in later attempts to create amorphous ZIF-4 atomistic models, or mechanistic understanding was obtained using ab initio molecular dynamics. Both of these latter two methods are presently restricted to small configuration sizes and neither is easily generalizable to other MOF designs; the former requires reactive force fields while the latter is still very computationally demanding.[51,53]

5.5 CHARACTERIZATION OF MOFS

MOFs are characterized for several properties, such as crystallinity (powder XRD), size and morphology (SEM, TEM), surface characterization (X-ray photon electron spectroscopy/absorption spectroscopy), hydrodynamic diameter (dynamic light scattering, nanoparticle tracking analysis), MOF degradation, drug-loading, surface modification (FTIR), elemental composition (ICP-MS), thermal decomposition (TGA), homogeneity (Raman microscopy) etc.[54]

5.6 PROCESS PARAMETERS

Process parameters that influence the characteristics of MOF include temperature, pressure, source of heat, and duration of reaction. Microwave-assisted synthesis as well as sonochemical method are reported to produce small crystals with homogeneity in comparison with conventional synthesis.[55]

Nano-MIL-88A was synthesized by these methods to produce crystals of varying sizes. Traditional hydrothermal synthesis produced crystals of about 250 nm; sonochemical synthesis produced crystals of 100 nm; microwave-aided synthesis produced homogenous crystals of size less than 100 nm. Within these methods, it was reported that the temperature and duration of reaction played key in the production of crystals with varying crystal shapes and size.[55]

Similar to this, by lowering the reaction period from 90 to 10 min, the crystal size of $Zn_3(BTC)_2 \cdot 12H_2O$ MOFs reduced to 100 nm which is otherwise 900 nm.[55] Solvents, pH, temperature, and reaction time are four critical parameters that are frequently described in terms of crystal size and shape among many other contributing factors.[55]

Alterations in macroscopic order can also be tailored through control of temperature in addition to solvent–reagent ratio, reaction kinetics, equilibrium, and modulating agents which was described in the earlier section.[54]

Since particle size plays a key role in interaction with tissues at the cellular level, the tailoring of size is of prime value to offer profound biomedical applications. It also influences the drug loading, need for surface tailoring, and selection of route of administration. As a result, it is crucial to prepare stable, monodispersed, and homogenous nanoparticles. It is difficult to manage the crystallization process that could produce particles with controlled morphology and narrow size distribution, regardless of the synthesis technique used. Controlling composition and process conditions, adding additives, using nanoscale templates, and shrinking the particles via mechanical or mechanochemical processes are the main tactics for achieving this goal.[55]

During selective adsorption and separation of gases, with a raise in temperature from 25 to 75 degrees Celsius, the CO_2 uptake capability drastically dropped. The reduction in CO_2 sorption was caused by the increase in temperature (energy). In other words, during the adsorption process, CO_2 escaped the amine due to the greater sorption temperature. Furthermore, high temperatures may have reduced the ability of porous NEU-2's PEI absorption by evaporating and/or degrading it. The pseudo-kinetic regime's

CO_2 absorbing capability increased logically as the temperature rose from 25 to 75 degrees Celsius. Yet, when the temperature increased, the CO_2 capture capacity in the pseudo-diffusive regime dropped proportionally with overall CO_2 intake. The effectiveness of using a relatively low-temperature sorption supported-amine system to capture CO_2 was shown to be realistic by the discovery that a high uptake temperature reduced the amine efficiency.[56]

5.7 APPLICATIONS OF MOFs

Several applications of MOFs are represented in Figure 5.3 and discussed in detail in the following sections.

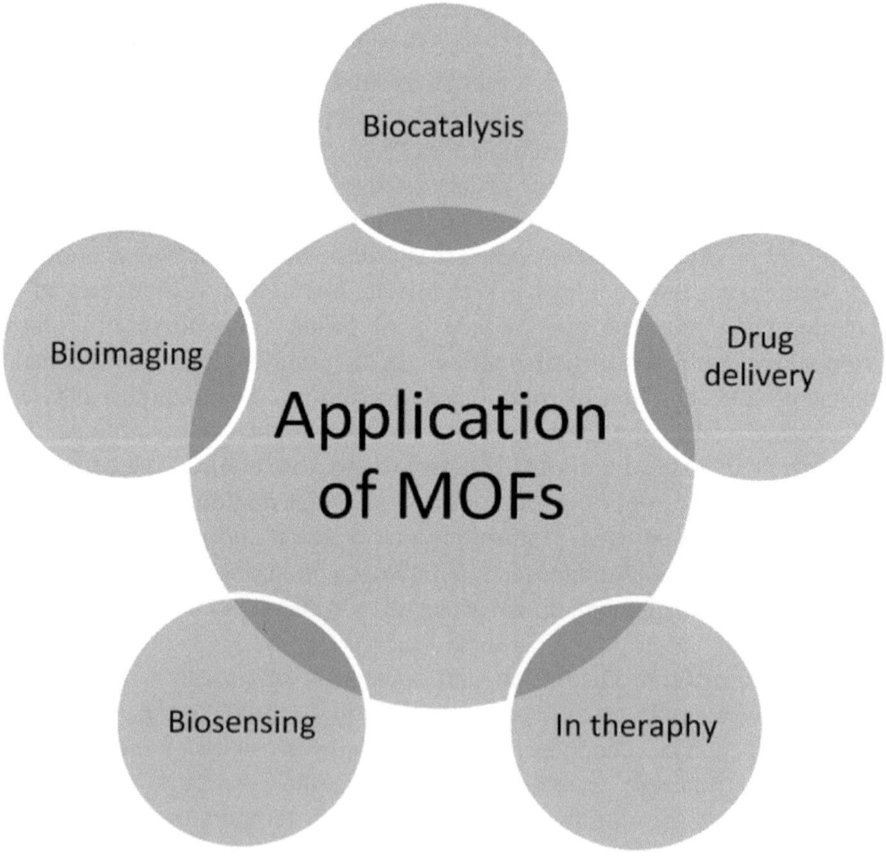

FIGURE 5.3 Applications of MOFs.

5.7.1 BIOSENSING

Recognizing the possibility of employing fluorescent MOF composites, EAUC was developed for the preliminary diagnosis of asthma. Application of MOFs include biocatalysis, drug delivery, therapy, biosensing,[57–59] bioimaging,[60] biomarker in biological systems. According to studies, for in situ detection of H_2S, the EAUC (Eu^{3+}/Ag^{+}@UiO-66- $(COOH)_2$) sensor has a fast response, with high sensitivity and excellent selectivity, which is relatively better than the reported best materials. Based on the EAUC, an INHIBIT logic gate was created using inputs of Ag^{+} and H_2S and output as the intensity of the fluorescent signal. The EAUC logic platform, with its nanoscale size, great biocompatibility, and minimal cytotoxicity, has been successfully employed for H_2S detection in both PC12 cells and diluted blood samples, confirming its sensing potential in vivo.[57] Nucleic acid sensing because DNA and RNA are essential for physiological regulation, nucleic acid levels aid in illness detection and the observation of biological systems. One example of this method is the incorporation of the triplex-forming oligonucleotide with H_2dtoaCu MOFs to detect HIV DNA sequences.[58] Research that intracellular pH sensing the expression of physiological environment changes. F-UiO MOFs were created by conjugating fluorescein isothiocyanate with Zr-based MOFs for real-time intracellular pH monitoring.[59]

5.7.2 BIOIMAGING

Potential possibilities for the application of Mn, Fe, and Gd-based MOFs in magnetic resonance imaging (MRI) as a diagnostic tool were reported.[5] Positron emission tomography (PET) provides 3D pictures of human metabolic processes with high resolution. This was happened by monitoring positron emission from radioactive materials accumulating at the target organs or tissues. PET imaging was performed using Zr-based MOFs.[61]

5.7.3 BIOCATALYSIS

Certain MOFs have both high catalytic efficiency and low toxicity that favor catalysis based on biomimetic principles. Hence, they are paving the path as suitable candidates for illness diagnosis and testing. The inherent peroxidase-like catalytic activity of the nanometric MIL-100 was used for ascorbic acid colorimetric sensing.[62]

5.7.4 *MOFS IS THERAPEUTIC DELIVERY*

MOFs because of their superior physicochemical qualities, MOFs and their derivative materials are rapidly being explored as nanocarrier systems for drug delivery, bioimaging or diagnostic agents, and therapeutic agents. Liposomes, nanoparticles, and micelles, suffer from low drug loading which may count to around 5%, and rapid release of drug in several instances. On the other end, MOFs were found to offer high drug-loading capacity due to their huge surface area. The prerequisites for selection as competent drug carriers include a high drug load, control over matrix degradation and drug release, and minimal toxicity. The pharmaceuticals can be loaded into MOFs by noncovalent encapsulation into the MOF via physisorption, post-synthetic alteration of the organic ligands after the MOF's production, or by using the medications as catalysts.[60] MOFs were investigated as promising carriers for drug delivery addressing a variety of disorders, including infections, lung disease, diabetic mellitus, ophthalmic disease, and malignancies, because of their superior drug delivery characteristics. Table 5.2 depicts the examples of MOFs as carriers for drug delivery.

TABLE 5.2 List of Few MOFs Used for Drug Delivery Systems.

MOF	Organic linker	Metal node	Therapeutic agent
MIL-53 (Fe)	Benzene-1,4-dicarboxylic acid	$FeCl_3.6H_2O$	Ibuprofen
			Caffeine
MIL-100 (Fe)	Benzene-1,3,5-tricarboxylic acid	Fe_3O (trimer)	Doxorubicin
			Caffeine
Mi-UiO-68	Maleimide-attached H_2L ligand	$ZrCl_4$	Doxorubicin
			Folic acid
ZIF-8	Imidazolate-4	$Zn(NO_3)_2.6H_2O$	5-Flurouracil
UiO-66-NH_2	Amino terephthalic acid	Zr_6O_8 cluster	5-Flurouracil
MIL-88A (Fe)	Fumaric acid	$FeCl_3.6H_2O$	Cidofovir

When a free drug is administered directly inside the body, delivery of drugs is uncontrolled and non-specific, which would be associated with a significant number of adverse effects. Researchers have put forth considerable effort to create techniques for controlled, systemic, and targeted drug administration. A quick and efficient solution to this challenge has been delivered by nanocarriers. It has been suggested that both organic and inorganic nanocarriers could be used as efficient drug delivery systems. When administered, organic nanocarriers are less steady and quickly engulfed by the vascular endothelial system whereas inorganic nanocarriers have been reported to be cytotoxic. Porous MOFs are an example of an inorganic–organic hybrid nanocarrier that has several benefits in comparison to its pure organic and inorganic equivalents and has become the ideal drug delivery system. Formerly, MOFs have been used to deliver small molecules, however, recent studies have focused on supra-molecular cargos such as proteins and nucleic acids.[3–5]

Biocompatible MOFs with their special characteristic properties have shown potential applications in the field of medicine. Moreover, MOFs have distinctive qualities that are essential for regulating drug loading and release, including breathing, linker rotation, swelling, and sub-network displacements. Many researchers have created numerous low-toxicity MOFs and investigated how they can be used to load and release multiple therapeutic medications for possible clinical applications. In addition to general applications, MOFs have several other biomedical uses, such as targeted drug delivery, molecular imaging, and biological sensing, and have also been identified. The very well-porous crystalline MOFs excelled in more conventional nanometric carrier systems such as quantum dots, liposomes, and inorganic nanoparticles in terms of instability, drug loading, systemic complications, and toxicity.[3–5]

5.8 MODIFICATION OF MOFS FOR THERAPEUTIC DRUG DELIVERY

A vast range of therapeutic small molecules and macromolecules can be encapsulated by MOFs. They are especially helpful for encapsulation of the poorly water-soluble cancer therapies and gasotransmitter molecules. Even bigger cargos, such as cells and vaccines, have been investigated. In biological environments, alteration of MOFs with an objective of improving drug delivery and release kinetics is possible. It is also made possible to modify MOFs to boost loading by the addition of moieties that produce beneficial interfaces. As part of the modification of MOF structures, mechanical and thermal alterations have also been used. Mechanical grinding and ball milling have been employed to reduce MOF size to enhance permeability, retention, or biocompatibility.[3–5]

5.9 MOF VACCINES

The biocompatible polymer framework of MOF vaccines helps to work by "refrigerating" the proteins within the vaccines. The proteins dissolve after being administered to human skin. This innovation could benefit healthcare professionals who administer vaccines in remote areas with sporadic electricity. MOFs perform better at ambient conditions than synthetic silica encasings in view of their structural configuration. Since MOFs are porous, they can act as a semi-permeable barrier for the movement of proteins or vaccine antigens.

Even though employing MOFs for medication delivery has made great progress, there are still a lot of challenges to overcome. Initially, only a minimal amount of research on drug loading and release kinetics was available. Recent studies have shown that the accessibility of cages in MOFs controls the drug-loading process, whereas the hydrophobic or hydrophilic nature of the drug molecules/MOFs influences the loading capacity and drug release. It is challenging to compare the outcomes because there have been several in vitro cell line toxicity studies conducted so far. Recent toxicity studies have also been assessed using zebrafish embryos. According to the findings, MOFs were found to show little acute toxicity and were quickly taken up by the reticuloendothelial system.[3–5]

The exploration of MOFs as suitable nanocarrier systems for the delivery of drugs has garnered considerable attention over the past several years. Nowadays, numerous compounds, including anticancer medications, nucleic acids, and proteins, are being researched as therapeutic agents for treating diseases. In conclusion, MOFs act as therapeutic agents for drug delivery based on functional molecules that serve as the building blocks of pore encapsulation, surface adsorption, covalent binding, and other processes. MOFs are distinctive and offer promising scope for the intracellular delivery of drugs for the therapy of several diseases.[3–5]

5.10 MOFS IN CANCER

The alpha-fetoprotein (AFP) quantification test was used in research[63] to apply magnetic MOF-based platform (Cu-MOF-NPs) as biosensor for the early detection of hepatocellular carcinoma with 1.18 ng/mL as a detection limit of 3.58 ng/mL as a quantification limit using serum samples. There was no evidence of competitive cancer biomarkers. According to the Fenton reaction, the anticancer therapeutic strategy includes the formation of OH radicals from H_2O_2, catalyzed by Fe^{3+} ions as well as Mn^{2+}, Cu^{2+}, and Cr^{4+}. The uncontrolled development of the tumor and metabolic dysfunction create O_2, H_2O_2, OH, ClO, and others as reactive oxygen species (ROS). More than any other ROS, hydroxyl radicals are capable of causing harm to tumor cells. The foregoing investigations have led to the development of the latest anticancer therapies such as chemodynamic therapy (CDT), photodynamic therapy (PDT), and sonodynamic therapy (SDT). Over the previous decade, MOFs have been used in PDT, SDT, and CDT.[64] MOFs have been extensively studied as theragnostic systems for cancer diagnosis and treatment,[64] for example, the simultaneous MRI and administration of drug through investigated Fe_3O_4@UiO-66 core shell composites. Because of the amphiphilic nature, metal sites, open cavities, and Zr–O clusters, of the UiO-66 shell, significant coordination contacts were established among the Zr (IV) centers of UiO-66 with hydroxyl groups in doxorubicin. On the other hand, the Fe_3O_4 core, was employed as an MRI contrast agent. In vitro and in vivo investigations revealed increased cancer cell death (around 60%), good inhibition of tumor growth, and a significant reduction in tumor size. Nanospheres of [Zn(bix)] (bix = 1,4-bis(imidazole-1-ylmethyl)benzene) can encapsulate and release known anticancer drugs, such as doxorubicin, camptothecin, SN-38, and daunomycin, and show very strong cytotoxic effects against human promyelocytic leukemia cells (HL60) due to the release of doxorubicin from the MOF spheres, causing the death of cancer cells.[63–65]

5.11 MOFs FOR ANTIBACTERIAL THERAPY

Antibacterial–antifungal-MOFs have been studied for their antibacterial and antifungal properties. BioMIL-5, for example, is made from Zn(II) and azelaic acid and has remarkable dermatological and antibacterial activities against Gram-positive bacteria *S. aureus* and *S. epidermidis*.[66] Antibacterial activity of Ag(I)-MOFs against *S.aureus* and *E. coli* was demonstrated,[67] and the first antibacterial Co-MOF, Co-TDM (TDM = tetrakis[(3,5-dicarboxyphenyl)- oxam- ethyl]methane), inactivates the Gram-negative bacterium *E. coli*.[57,68] $[Cu_3(BTC)_2(H_2O)_3]$ (BTC = 1,3,5-benzenetricarboxylate) was tested against *Aspergillus oryzae, Candida albicans, Fusarium oxysporum*, and *Aspergillus niger* and shown strong antifungal action due to its capacity to diminish oxygen gas and the creation of ROS, which harm cells and inhibit microorganisms.[69]

High-resolution STEM-EDS elemental mapping was used to investigate the effective loading of ceftazidime in ZIF-8. During the first day, ~70% of the ceftazidime was released at pH 5.0, whereas 50% was released at pH 7.0.

Pristine ZIF-8 and ceftazidime@ZIF-8 particles were investigated for their antibacterial effect against *E. coli* was tested. Interestingly, no difference was observed after 24 h, but ceftazidime@ZIF-8 inhibited nearly all *E. coli* growth at 50 g/mL, whereas pristine ZIF-8 showed no antibacterial

18. Grall, R.; Hidalgo, T.; Delic, J.; Garcia-Marquez, A.; Chevillard, S.; Horcajada, P. In Vitro Biocompatibility of Mesoporous Metal (III; Fe, Al, Cr) Trimesate MOF nanocarriers. *J. Mater. Chem. B* **2015,** *3* (42), 8279–8292. DOI: 10.1039/c5tb01223f
19. Alsaiari, S. K.; Qutub, S. S.; Sun, S.; Baslyman, W.; Aldehaiman, M.; Alyami, M.; Khashab, N. M. Sustained and Targeted Delivery of Checkpoint Inhibitors by Metal-Organic Frameworks for Cancer Immunotherapy. *Sci. Adv.* **2021,** *7* (4), eabe7174. DOI: 10.1126/sciadv.abe7174.
20. Petit, C.; Huang, L.; Jagiellom J.; Kenvin, J.; Gubbins, K. E.; Bandosz, T. J. Toward Understanding Reactive Adsorption of Ammonia on Cu-MOF/Graphite Oxide Nanocomposites. *Langmuir* **2011,** *27* (21), 13043–13051. DOI: 10.1021/la202924y.
21. Petit, C.; Mendoza, B.; Bandosz, T. J. Hydrogen Sulfide Adsorption on MOFs and MOF/Graphite Oxide Composites. *Chemphyschem* **2010,** *11* (17), 3678–3684. DOI: 10.1002/cphc.201000689.
22. Petit, C.; Bandosz, T. J. Synthesis, Characterization, and Ammonia Adsorption Properties of Mesoporous Metal–Organic Framework (MIL (Fe))–Graphite Oxide Composites: Exploring the Limits of Materials Fabrication. *Adv. Funct. Mater.* **2011,** *21*, 2108–2117.
23. Petit, C.; Bandosz, T. J. Exploring the Coordination Chemistry of MOF-Graphite Oxide Composites and Their Applications as Adsorbents. *Dalton Trans.* **2012,** *41*, 4027–4035.
24. Juan-Alcaniz, J.; Gascon, J.; Kapteijn, F. Metal–Organic Frameworks as Scaffolds for the Encapsulation of Active Species: State of the Art and Future Perspectives. *J. Mater. Chem.* **2012,** *22*, 10102–10118.
25. Alkordi, M. H.; Liu, Y.; Larsen, R. W.; Eubank, J. F.; Eddaoudi, M. Zeolite-Like Metal-Organic Frameworks as Platforms for Applications: On Metalloporphyrin-Based Catalysts. *J. Am. Chem. Soc.* **2008,** *130*, 12639–12641.
26. Corma, A.; Garcia, H. Supramolecular Host–Guest Systems in Zeolites Prepared by Ship-in-a-Bottle Synthesis. *Eur. J. Inorg. Chem.* **2004,** *2004*, 1143–1164.
27. Khan, N. A.; Jhung, S. H. Adsorptive Removal of Benzothiophene Using Porous Copper-Benzenetricarboxylate Loaded with Phosphotungstic Acid. *Fuel Process. Techn. 100*, 49–54.
28. Ahmed, I.; Khan, N. A.; Hasan, Z.; Jhung, S. H. Adsorptive Denitrogenation of Model Fuels with Porous Metal-Organic Framework (MOF) MIL-101 Impregnated with Phosphotungstic Acid: Effect of Acid Site Inclusion. *J. Hazard. Mater.* **2013,** 250–251, 37–44.
29. Khan, N. A.; Jhung, S. H. Low-Temperature Loading of Cu+ Species Over Porous Metal-Organic Frameworks (MOFs) and Adsorptive Desulfurization with Cu+-Loaded MOFs. *J. Hazard. Mater.* **2012,** *237–238*, 180–185.
30. Sánchez-Sánchez M, Getachew N, Díaz K, Díaz-García M, Chebude Y, Díaz I. Synthesis of Metal–Organic Frameworks in Water at Room Temperature: Salts as Linker Sources. *Green Chem.* **2015,** *17* (3), 1500–1509.
31. Ahmed, I.; Jhung, S. H. Composites of Metal–Organic Frameworks: Preparation and Application in Adsorption. *Mater. Today* **2014,** *17* (3), 136–146.
32. Butova, V. V.; Soldatov, M. A.; Guda, A. A.; Lomachenko, K. A.; Lamberti, C. Metal-Organic Frameworks: Structure, Properties, Methods of Synthesis and Characterization. *Russ. Chem. Rev.* **2016,** *85* (3), 280–307. https://doi.org/10.1070/rcr4554.
33. Nadizadeh, Z.; Naimi-Jamal, M. R.; Panahi, L. Mechanochemical Solvent-Free in Situ Synthesis of Drug Loaded {Cu2 (1,4-Bdc)2 (Dabco)}n MOFs for Controlled

Drug Delivery. *J. Solid State Chem.* **2018,** *259,* 35–42. https://doi.org/10.1016/j.jssc.2017.12.027.
34. Bennett, T. D.; Cao, S.; Tan, J. C.; Keen, D. A.; Bithell, E. G.; Beldon, P. J.; Friscic, T.; Cheetham, A. K. Facile Mechanosynthesis of Amorphous Zeolitic Imidazolate Frameworks. *J. Am. Chem. Soc.* **2011,** *133* (37), 14546–14549. https://doi.org/10.1021/ja206082s.
35. Horcajada, P.; Chalati, T.; Serre, C.; Gillet, B.; Sebrie, C.; Baati, T.; Eubank, J. F.; Heurtaux, D. et al. Porous Metal-Organic-Framework Nanoscale Carriers as a Potential Platform for Drug Delivery and Imaging. *Nat. Mater.* **2010,** *9* (2), 172–178. https://doi.org/10.1038/nmat2608.
36. El-Massaoudi, M.; Radi, S.; Mabkhot, Y. N.; Al–Showiman, S. S.; Ghabbour, H. A.; Ferbinteanu, M.; Adarsh, N. N.; Garcia, Y. Cu (II) and Mn (II) Coordination Complexes Constructed by C Linked Bispyrazoles: Effect of Anions and Hydrogen Bonding on the Self Assembly Process. *Inorganica Chimica Acta.* **2018,** *482,* 411–419. https://doi.org/10.1016/j.ica.2018.06.041
37. Yang, X.; Tang, Q.; Jiang, Y.; Zhang, M.; Wang, M.; Mao, L. Nanoscale ATP Responsive Zeolitic Imidazole Framework-90 as a General Platform for Cytosolic Protein Delivery and Genome Editing. *J. Am. Chem. Soc.* **2019,** 141 (9), 3782– 3786. https://doi.org/10.1021/jacs.8b11996.
38. Kida, K.; Okita, M.; Fujita, K.; Tanaka, S.; Miyake, Y. Formation of High Crystalline ZIF-8 in an Aqueous Solution. *Cryst. Eng. Comm.* **2013,** *15* (9), 1794–1801. https://doi.org/10.1039/c2ce26847g.
39. Cravillon, J.; Nayuk, R.; Springer, S.; Feldhoff, A.; Huber, K.; Wiebcke, M. Controlling Zeolitic Imidazolate Framework Nano- and Microcrystal Formation: Insight into Crystal Growth by Time-Resolved in Situ Static Light Scattering. *Chem. Mater.* **2011,** *23* (8), 2130–2141. https://doi.org/10.1021/cm103571y.
40. Nadizadeh, Z.; Naimi-Jamal, M. R.; Panahi, L. Mechanochemical Solvent-Free in Situ Synthesis of Drug Loaded {Cu2 (1,4-Bdc)2 (Dabco)}n MOFs for Controlled Drug Delivery. *J. Solid State Chem.* **2018,** *259,* 35–42. https://doi.org/10.1016/j.jssc.2017.12.027.
41. Iacomi, P.; Maurin, G. ResponZIF Structures: Zeolitic Imidazolate Frameworks as Stimuli-Responsive Materials. *ACS Appl. Mater. Interfaces.* **2021,** *13* (43), 50602–50642. https://doi.org/10.1021/acsami.1c12403.
42. Su, H.; Sun, F.; Jia, J.; He, H.; Wang, A.; Zhu, G. A Highly Porous Medical Metal Organic Framework Constructed from Bioactive Curcumin. *Chem. Commun.* **2015,** *51* (26), 5774–5777. https://doi.org/10.1039/c4cc10159f.
43. Wang, Z.; Hu, S.; Yang, J.; Liang, A.; Li, Y.; Zhuang, Q.; Gu, J. Nanoscale Zr Based MOFs with Tailorable Size and Introduced Mesopore for Protein Delivery. *Adv. Funct. Mater.* **2018,** *28* (16), 1707356. https://doi.org/10.1002/adfm.201707356.
44. Bennett, T. D.; Cheetham, A. K. Amorphous Metal–Organic Frameworks. *Acc. Chem. Res.* **2014,** *47* (5), 1555–1562.
45. Li, Y.; Zhang, Y.; Tan, W.; Jin, P.; Zhang, P.; Li, K. Bioinspired Coassembly of Copper Ions and Nicotinamide Adenine Dinucleotides for Single-Site Nanozyme with Dual Catalytic Functions. *Anal. Chem.* **2023,** *95* (5), 2865–2873. https://doi.org/10.1021/acs.analchem.2c04389
46. Xiang, T.; Yan, H.; Peng, F.; Ke, W.; Faheem, A.; Li, M.; Hu, Y. Microorganisms@aMIL-125 (Ti), An Amorphous Metal–Organic Framework Induced by Microorganisms

and Their Applications. *ACS Omega* **2023,** *8* (2), 2164–2172. https://doi.org/10.1021/acsomega.2c06329.

47. Liu, M.; Slavney, A. H.; Tao, S.; McGillicuddy, R. D.; Lee, C. C.; Wenny, M. B.; Billinge, S. L.; Mason, J. A. Designing Glass and Crystalline Phases of Metal–Bis (acetamide) Networks to Promote High Optical Contrast. *J. Am. Chem. Soc.* **2022,** *144* (48), 22262–22271. https://doi.org/10.1021/jacs.2c10449.
48. Castel, N.; Coudert, F.-C. Atomistic Models of Amorphous Metal–Organic Frameworks. *J. Physic. Chem. C* **2022,** *126* (16), 6905–6914. https://doi.org/10.1021/acs.jpcc.2c01091
49. Orellana-Tavra, C.; Baxter, E. F.; Tian, R.; Bennett, T. D.; Slater, N. K. H.; Cheetham, A. K.; Fairen-Jimenez, D. Amorphous Metal-Organic Frameworks for Drug Delivery. *Chem. Commun.* **2015,** *51*, 13878–13881.
50. Polk, D. E. Structural Model for Amorphous Silicon and Germanium. *J. Non Cryst. Solids* **1971,** *5*, 365–376.
51. Bennett, T. D.; Andrew L. Goodwin, Martin T. Dove, David A. Keen, et al. Structure and Properties of an Amorphous Metal-Organic Framework. *Phys. Rev. Lett.* **2010,** *104* (11), 115503.
52. Yang, Y.; Shin, Y. K.; Li, S.; Bennett, T. D.; van Duin, A. C. T.; Mauro, J. C. Enabling Computational Design of ZIFs Using ReaxFF. *J. Phys. Chem. B* **2018,** *122*, 9616–9624.
53. Thyagarajan, R.; Sholl, D. S. A Database of Porous Rigid Amorphous Materials. *Chem. Mater.* **2020,** *32*, 8020–8033.
54. Horcajada, P.; Serre, C.; Vallet-Regí, M.; Sebban, M.; Taulelle, F.; Férey, G. Metal-Organic Frameworks as Efficient Materials for Drug Delivery. *Angew. Chemie—Int. Ed.* **2006,** *45* (36), 5974–5978. https://doi.org/10.1002/anie.200601878.
55. He, S.; Wu, L.; Li, X.; Sun, H.; Xiong, T.; Liu, J.; Huang, C.; Xu, H.; Sun, H.; Chen, W. and Gref, R. Metalorganic Frameworks for Advanced Drug Delivery. *Acta Pharm. Sinica B* **2021,** *11* (8), 2362–2395. https://doi.org/10.1016/j.apsb.2021.03.019.
56. Fonseca, J.; Choi, S. Synthesis of a Novel Amorphous Metal Organic Framework with Hierarchical Porosity for Adsorptive Gas Separation. *Microporous Mesoporous Mater.* **2021,** *310*, 110600. https://doi.org/10.1016/j.micromeso.2020.110600.
57. Zhang, X.; Fang, L.; Jiang, K.; He, H.; Yang, Y.; Cui, Y.; Li, B. Nanoscale Fluorescent Metal–Organic Framework Composites as a Logic Platform for Potential Diagnosis of Asthma. *Biosens. Bioelectron.* **2019,** *130*, 65–72. https://doi.org/10.1016/j.bios.2019.01.011.
58. Millward, A. R.; Yaghi, O. M. Metal−Organic Frameworks with Exceptionally High Capacity for Storage of Carbon Dioxide at Room Temperature. *J. Am. Chem. Soc.* **2005,** *127* (51), 17998–17999, pubs.acs.org/doi/abs/10.1021/ja0570032.
59. Ma, W.; Jiang, Q.; Yu, P.; Yang, L.; Mao, L. Zeolitic Imidazolate Framework-Based Electrochemical Biosensor for in Vivo Electrochemical Measurements. *Anal. Chem.* **2013,** *85* (15), 7550–7557. https://doi.org/10.1021/ac401576u.
60. Shi, Z.; Chu, C.; Zhang, Y.; Su, Z.; Lin, H.; Pang, X.; Wang, X.; Liu, G.; Li, W. Self-Assembled Metal-Organic Nanoparticles for Multimodal Imaging-Guided Photothermal Therapy of Hepatocellular Carcinoma. *J. Biomed. Nanotechn.* **2018,** *14* (11), 1934–1943. https://doi.org/10.1166/jbn.2018.2636.
61. Kundu, T.; Mitra, S.; Díaz Díaz, D.; Banerjee, R. Gadolinium (III)-Based Porous Luminescent Metal-Organic Frameworks for Bimodal Imaging. *ChemPlusChem.* **2016,** *81* (8), 728–32.

62. Zhang, J.; Hao-Tian, Z.; Du, Z.-Y.; Xueqing, W.; Yu, S.-H.; Jiang, H.-L. Water-Stable Metal–Organic Frameworks with Intrinsic Peroxidase-Like Catalytic Activity as a Colorimetric Biosensing Platform. *Chem. Commun.* **2014,** *50* (9), 1092–1094. https://doi.org/10.1039/c3cc48398c.
63. Osman, D. I.; El-Sheikh, S. M.; Sheta, S. M.; Ali, O. I.; Salem, A. M.; Shousha, W. G.; Shawky, S. M. Nucleic Acids Biosensors Based on Metal-Organic Framework (MOF), Paving the Way to Clinical Laboratory Diagnosis. *Biosens. Bioelectron.* **2019,** 111451. https://doi.org/10.1016/j.bios.2019.111451
64. Zhao, Y.; Jiang, X.; Liu, X.; Liu, X.; Liu, Z.; Liu, X. Application of Photo-Responsive Metal-Organic Framework in Cancer Therapy and Bioimaging. *Front. Bioeng. Biotechnol.* **2022,** *10*, 1031986. https://doi.org/10.3389/fbioe.2022.1031986.
65. Saeb, M. R.; Rabiee, N.; Mozafari, M.; Verpoort, F.; Voskressensky, L. G.; Luque, R. Metal-Organic Frameworks (MOFs) for Cancer Therapy. *Materials* **2021,** *14* (23), 7277. https://doi.org/10.3390/ma14237277.
66. Tamames-Tabar, C.; Imbuluzqueta, E.; Guillou, N.; Serre, C.; Miller, S. R.; Elkaïm, E.; Blanco-Prieto, M. J. A Zn Azelate MOF: Combining Antibacterial Effect. *CrystEngComm* **2015,** *17* (2), 456–462. https://doi.org/10.1039/c4ce00885e
67. Bhardwaj, N.; Pandey, S. K.; Mehta, J.; Bhardwaj, S. K.; Kim, K. H.; Deep, A. Bioactive Nano Metal-Organic Frameworks as Antimicrobials Against Gram-Positive and Gram-Negative Bacteria. *Toxicol. Res.* **2018,** *7* (5), 931–941. https://doi.org/10.1039/c8tx00087e.
68. Masschalck, B.; Van Houdt, R.; Van Haver, E. G.; Michiels, C. W. Inactivation of Gram-Negative Bacteria by Lysozyme, Denatured Lysozyme, and Lysozyme-Derived Peptides Under High Hydrostatic Pressure. *Appl. Environ. Microbiol.* **2001,** *67* (1), 339–344. https://doi.org/10.1128/AEM.67.1.339–344.2001.
69. Bouson, S.; Krittayavathananon, A.; Phattharasupakun, N.; Siwayaprahm, P.; Sawangphruk, M. Antifungal Activity of Water-Stable Copper-Containing Metal Organic Frameworks. *R. Soc. Open Sci.* **2017,** *4* (10), 170654. https://doi.org/10.1098/rsos.170654

CHAPTER 6

Metal–Organic Framework in Bioimaging and Biosensing Application

REET MINHAS, HONISHA SHAH, MITAL PATEL, GSN KOTESWARA RAO, and RAJASEKHAR REDDY ALAVALA

Shobhaben Pratapbhai Patel School of Pharmacy & Technology Management, SVKM's NMIMS, Vile Parle, Mumbai, India

ABSTRACT

The metal-organic framework (MOF) is a type of porous material composed of metal ions or clusters coordinated to organic ligands. It has gained attention in biosensing and bioimaging due to its high surface area, tunable pore size, and excellent stability. It can be functionalized with specific ligands which selectively bind to target biomolecules, resulting in a change in the optical, electrical, or magnetic properties of the MOF. This change can then be measured and used to quantify the concentration of the target biomolecule in a sample. This compilation provides insight into MOF, their types, use in biosensing and bioimaging including advancement in the field.

6.1 INTRODUCTION

Biosensing is a mechanism that has evolved through the compartmentalization of the eukaryotic cell, which helps optimize and facilitate various metabolic pathways. These metabolic pathways involve a series of chemical reactions between proteins, which may or may not be catalyzed by enzymes. The pathways can also be modulated by messenger molecules or drugs, making intracellular biosensing a valuable tool for drug development phases and in disease diagnosis.[1–3] In the past, various assay techniques have been used to quantify biomolecules within cells. However, the discovery

Metals in Medicine, Volume 1: Metals for Tissue Engineering and Pharmaceutical Applications.
Sonali Sundram, Rishabha Malviya, and GSN Koteswara Rao

of metal–organic framework (MOFs) has revolutionized diagnosis by offering noninvasive, efficient, and rapid techniques. These innovations are transforming the field of diagnostic medicine.[4] The visualization of visceral organs allows the rapid and accurate diagnosis of tumors or physiological changes in tissues and is thus central to the process of diagnosis of various severe diseases. Bioimaging, the process of visualizing probable disease in tissues or organs is made part of the diagnosis more often than not in order to have a reliable and accurate source of medical information of a patient. Bioimaging too has evolved over the years and is facing its own set of limitations and developments as the world strives to be healthier and more technology-savvy (Fig. 6.1).

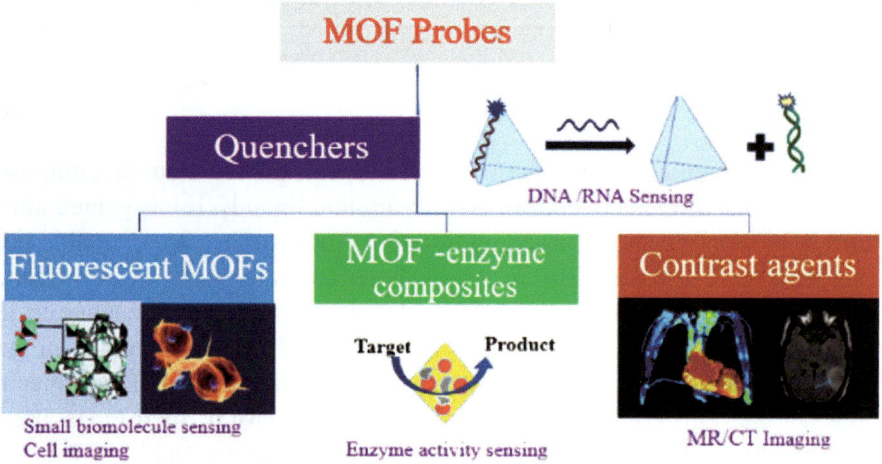

FIGURE 6.1 MOFs for biosensing and bioimaging applications.

Source: Reprinted with permission from Ref. [2]. Copyright 2017. Elsevier.

Since their inception in 1989 by Robson et al. as polymeric frameworks consisting of 3D-linked rod-like segments, MOFs have gained significant attention as a type of coordination polymer.[5] In 1995, Yaghi et al.[6] introduced the term MOF, after reporting the synthesis of a 2D-coordination compound using a Rigid Organic Ligand, Trimesic acid, and a Transition metal (Co). This marked the formal proposal of the concept of MOFs, and over the last two decades, MOFs have emerged as an independent branch of coordination chemistry with the development of numerous MOF families. Recently, MOFs have found diverse applications in fields such as material storage,[7] separations,[8–10] purification,[11] catalysis,[12–17] sensing,[18–23] bioimaging,[24,25] energy storage,[26–30] and drug delivery.[31,32] MOFs have shown great potential as biomedical candidates for biological sensing and imaging due to their luminescence properties and the ability to quench.[33,34]

6.2 USE OF MOFS IN BIOSENSING

MOFs have been the subject of significant research as innovative imaging probes in the area of biological sensing. MOF-based biosensing mainly involves two methods: (1) Designing MOFs with fluorescence or luminescence properties that can sensitively respond to their local environment or visiting species[35]; and (2) Using MOFs as fluorescence quenchers for analyte fluorophores through fluorescence resonance energy transfer (FRET), photo-induced electron transfer (PET),[36,37] or charge transfer.[38] This compilation discusses the biosensing applications of MOFs, including their use as fluorescent probes, fluorescent quenching platforms, and catalyzers. Furthermore, MOFs can be employed as biosensors for genomic biomolecules, such as DNA/RNA, small and large biomolecules, such as enzymes and dopamine, depending on their pore size and channel structure.

6.2.1 DETECTION OF NUCLEIC ACID (DNA AND RNA)

The nucleic acids detection using the fluorescence concept can be performed conventionally using platforms, such as graphene oxide (GO), single-walled carbon nanotubes, carbon nanoparticles, gold nanoparticles, and other such "quenchers." MOFs have fluorescence quenching properties and demonstrate preferential binding to single-stranded DNA (ss-DNA) compared with double-stranded DNA (ds-DNA). Chen et al. have proven the effectiveness and reliability of Cu(H2DTOA) MOF (Table 6.1) for detecting HIV-1 DNA sequences and thrombin in 2013.[39] Additionally, biosensing of virus DNA or RNA has been studied using different MOFs [Cu_3(Cmdcp)2(dps)4(H2O)4(SO4)], and the ligands H3Cmd-cpBr, H3CbdcpBr, and H2dcbbBr, [Cu(dcbb)2], [Zn(HCbdcp)2]DPSnd [Dy(Cmdcp)(H2O)3] (NO_3) $2H_2$On (Table 6.1).[37] The formed matrices can interact with two distinct carboxy fluorescein (FAM) labeled ss-DNA (single-stranded) probes in three different ways: electrostatic, p-stacking, and hydrogen-bonding interactions. The MOF has the ability to absorb M by utilizing a process called photo-induced electron transfer (PET). When the target DNA is available, the resulting ds-DNA detach from the MOF

TABLE 6.1 MOFs Application in Biosensing.

Ligand structure	Ligand abbreviation	Cation (Metal)	Metal–organic frame work formula	Surface Area (m2/g)	Pore size	Sensing Target	MOFs role	References
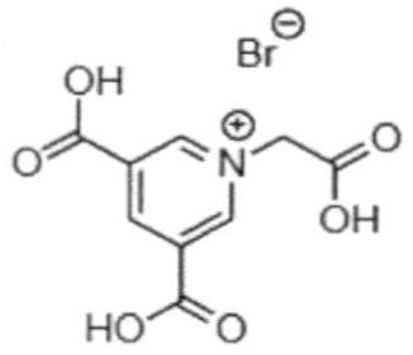	H3Cmdcp	Cu2+	[Cu3(Cmdcp)2(dps)4 (H2O)4(SO4)]n	348m2/g	9.7 16.6	HIV DNA and SUDV RNA	Fluorescence Quenching platform	[37, 40, 40]
		Dy3+	{[Dy(Cmdcp) (H2O)3] (NO3).2H2O}n	–	–			
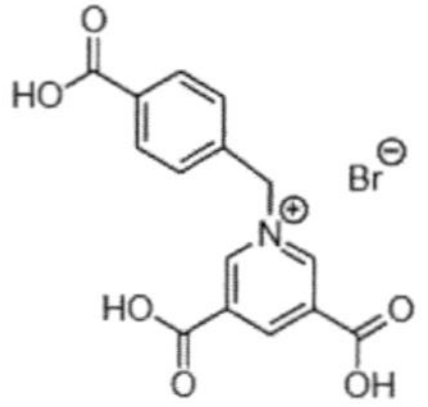	H3CbdcpBr	Zn2+	{[Zn(HCbdcp)2].H2O} n	–	–	HIV DNA	Fluorescence Quenching platform	[40]
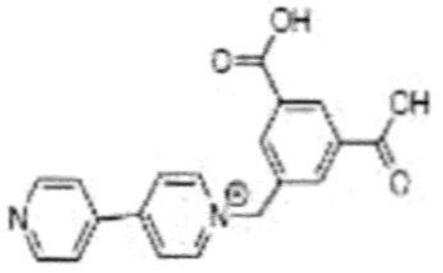	H2dcbbBr	Cu2+	[Cu(dcbb)2] n	–	–	HIV DNA	Fluorescence Quenching platform	[41]

TABLE 6.1 *(Continued)*

Ligand structure	Ligand abbreviation	Cation (Metal)	Metal–organic frame work formula	Surface Area (m2/g)	Pore size	Sensing Target	MOFs role	References
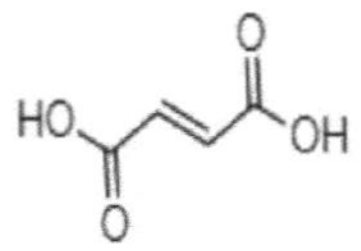	FA	Fe3+	[Fe3O(FA)3Clz.3H2O]n (MIL-88A)	347348m2/g	5–7	DNA	Fluorescence Quenching platform	[36, 42, 43]
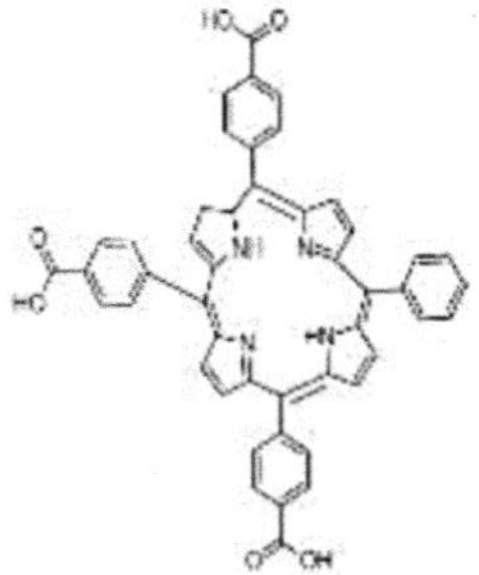	TCPP	Zr4+	[Zr6(μ3-OH)8-(TCPP)2]n (PCN-222)	2217348m2/g 32	13	Phosphoprotein	Catalyzer	[43]

surface and permits the restoration of the fluorescence intensity of FAM. These innovative platforms have proven to be effective for detecting Sudan virus RNA (SUDV RNA) and human immunodeficiency virus 1 ds-DNA (HIV ds-DNA) with detection thresholds of 196 and 73 pM, respectively, using fluorescent sensing.[40]

The platforms that have previously been used to identify DNA/RNA include GO and MoS2.[44] However, recent studies have shown that some MOFs such as MIL-101,[45] MIL—88A,[36,46] UiO-66-NH2 are highly sensitive and are able to react distinctly to changes in luminescence caused by both matched and non-complementary target sequences of DNA/RNA. MOFs often show different mechanisms of action than conventional luminescence sensing platforms, such as GNPs. For example, some MOFs exhibit peroxidase enzyme-like activity in the presence of H_2O_2 (hydrogen peroxide) and others, such as $\{[La_2(TDA)_3]_2H_2O\}n$, coated with dyes or silica, show luminescence sensing due to f–f electron transitions from dyes to the La+ during DNA/RNA sensing.[47] The positively and negatively charged segments of DNA/RNA follow different processes. These MOFs exhibit exciting and versatile sensing properties that make them highly suitable, faster, and more efficient options for biosensing of aptamers.

Aptamers, which are oligonucleotides used as an alternative to antibiotics, can be improved for biosensing purposes by immobilizing MOFs on them to enhance biocompatibility as shown in Figure 6.2. Recent examples of this application include nanoscale MOFs for the detection of DNA. To make a covalent cross-link, the MOF surface is modified with sulfosuccinimidyl 4-(N-mal-aminomethyl) cyclohexane-1-carboxylate (Sulfo-SMCC), which attaches the DNA to the MOF surface.[48] A fluorescent MOF immobilized sensor for chlorpyrifos (CPF) detection based on terbium (III) metal–organic framework (Tb–MOFs), and PDDA-aggregated-AuNPs was fabricated by Feng et al.[49] In the past, DNA biosensing, especially for the detection of gene mutation during prenatal studies, has been carried out through laborious, extensive, and complex instrumentation requiring methods such as electrophoretic separations and radioisotopic detection. The use of MOFs in highly sensitive electrochemical sensors for aptameric mutation detection is a novel area that has arisen due to the exceptional electrocatalytic properties of MOF composites. Jing et al. have presented studies on the use of MOF composites as electrochemical sensors for highly sensitive aptameric mutation detection.[50,51]

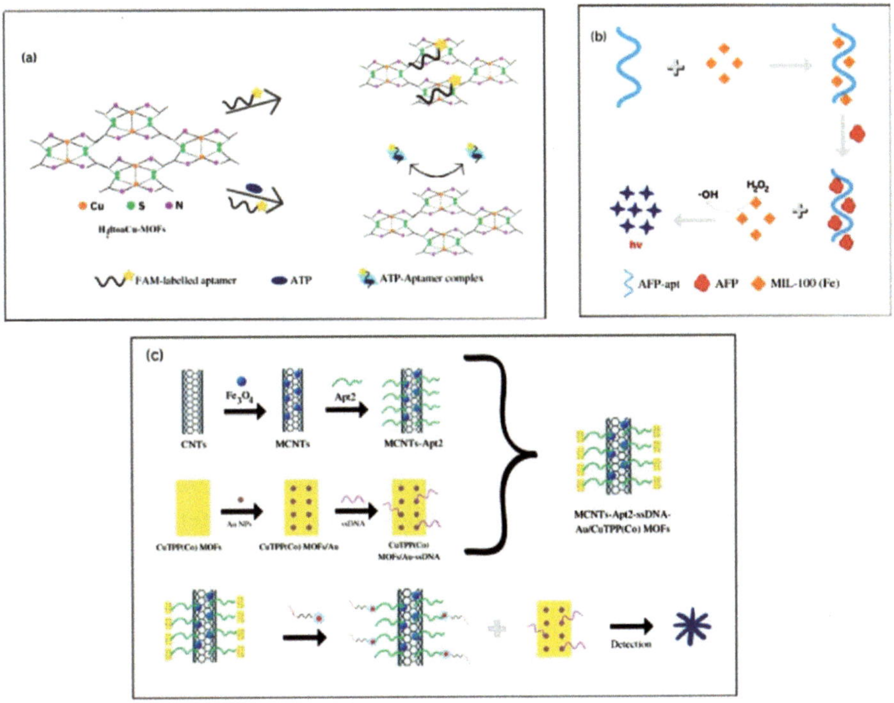

FIGURE 6.2 MOFs-based sensors. (a) A fluorescence aptasensor on H_2dtoaCu to detect ATP, (b) A chemiluminescent on the luminol–H_2O_2–MOF, (c) Cu–TCPP (Co) MOFs-based CL-Aptasensors.

Source: Reprinted with permission from Ref. [49]. Copyright 2021. Elsevier

In recent times, new technologies have revealed the potential of nMOFs for biosensing, diagnosis, and controlling SARS-CoV-2 pandemic. For instance, Li et al. developed unique sandwich Immunosensor utilizing Au-NPs@Cu(II)-HKUST-1@Tb and CoFe@N-GCT for identifying C-reactive protein test (CRP) as a critical follow-up test in COVID-19 patients (Fig. 6.3).[52] Meanwhile, Rabiee et al. created MOF nanomaterial masks for real-time COVID-19 virus diagnosis via surface-enhanced Raman scattering (SERS) mechanism, where visual color changes were observed upon adsorption of different viruses on the surface doped with Au-NPs@nMOF.[53]

MOFs are increasingly utilized for nucleic acid (DNA/RNA) sensing through fluorescence, electrochemical, and colorimetric methods. To make reliable and reproducible biosensors using MOFs, certain challenges must be overcome, such as maintaining the uniformly ordered macro and micro-pore structures of MOFs and ensuring their stability and large-scale clinical testing of real clinical targets before employing them for Biosensing and imaging nucleic acids at the population level. These techniques can potentially replace conventional and laborious methods.[54]

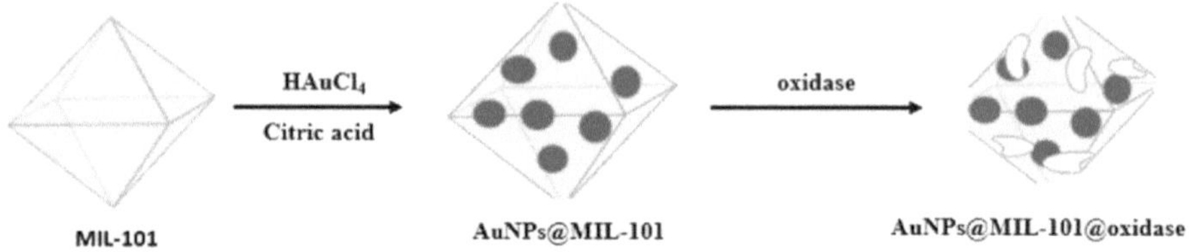

FIGURE 6.3 Schematic illustration of AuNPs@MIL-101@oxidases synthetic approach.

6.2.2 MONITORING ENZYME ACTIVITY

Proteins and enzymes are challenging to detect and visualize. However, new possibilities in biological macromolecule sensing have emerged with the use of coprecipitation, temperature-sensitivity, and electrochemical mechanisms in various MOF composites[55,56] Zang and colleagues developed a phosphoprotein sensor based on photoelectrochemical activity with Zr-based PCN-222 as given in Table 6.1. The modified electrode achieves label-free detection of α-casein by creating steric hindrance due to phosphate group coordination in the protein and ZrAO clusters, which inhibits interface electron transfer between PCN-222, O_2 media, and dopamine. The photocurrent signals are inversely proportional to the concentration of α casein because as the amount of α casein is increased, steric hindrance is also increased. This work is important because it shows that MOFs can be used for sensing biological macromolecules.

New techniques have been developed for sensing enzyme activity, such as oxidases, using Quantum dots composites (QDs) and MOFs to form core-shell nanocomposites (CSNCPs).[50,57] Lin et al. demonstrated gelatinase-A biosensor, a member of the matrix metalloproteinase, based on fluorescence resonance energy transfer (FRET) between poly(9,9-dioctyl-fluorenyl-2,7-diyl) dots and the MOF [Cu(H_2DTOA)] n, which were linked together.[57] The fluorescence was generated by semiconducting polymer nanoparticles (Pdots), which were quenched with polypeptide linker (COOH-GHHYYG-PLGVRGCNH2) through the FRET process. The MMP-2 (Substrate), is present on this polypeptide chain, so if its concentration increases, it releases Pdots and reverses the fluorescence quenching.

MOFs are used as quenching platforms for enzyme activity sensing, as certain MOFs have been found to exhibit luminance quenching abilities for dye-labeled ss-DNA.[58] Wang and colleagues developed a bio-probe for the enzyme deoxyribonuclease-I using the MOF [Ba2(L)(H_2O)].(DMF)0.5(H_2O)$_3$ (H_4L = Bis-(3,5- Dicarboxy- Phenyl) Terephthalamide), and an FAM-labeled ss-DNA-Probe (FAM-P). The biosensing is achieved through the prevention of fluorescence quenching by the enzyme deoxyribonuclease-I, which curtails the long ss-DNA chain of the probe. Biosensing is achieved by the mechanism of prevention of fluorescence quenching by the enzyme deoxyribonuclease-I, which curtails the long ss-DNA chain of the probe. Recently, simple enzyme/MOF biocomposites have also been studied for their ability to prevent enzyme degradation in unsuitable temperature/pH conditions due to the porous structure, metal-based nodes, and organic linkers of MOFs.[59]

Yang and his colleagues have developed a MOFs-in-nanochannels electrochemical device by combining TiO_2 with the nMOF ZIF-8. The device specifically affects the enzymatic activity of the entrapped CytC, which can be detected by monitoring the alterations in the flow of ions during the process of ABTS oxidation. Typically, this configuration positively affects or increases enzyme activity, and it serves as a label-free device for recording entrapped enzyme activity.[60] On the other hand, Hou and his colleagues have demonstrated that HP-PCN-224(Fe) can be used for uric acid detection, with 1.8 μM detection limit. This was achieved by immobilizing Uricase on HP-PCN-224(Fe).[61]

6.2.3 SENSING SMALL BIOMOLECULES

MOFs possess both micro and macro pore sizes, which enable them to capture small and large biomolecules as guest molecules. This property has been utilized in biosensing applications.[62] Hou and colleagues developed a MOF–enzyme composite consisting of glucose oxidase (GOx) in a zeolite imidazole framework 8 (Mzif-8) for colorimetric detection of glucose.[63] The composite demonstrated peroxidase-like activity, where GOx catalyzed glucose oxidation to produce H_2O_2. The zeolite imidazole framework (Mzif-8) then facilitated the oxidation of O-Phenylenediamine (OPD) by H_2O_2 for the production of an orange-colored compound. The technique was effectively employed to quantify glucose levels in urine samples, aiding in the diagnosis of glucosuria. Another example of MOF–enzyme composite utilizing peroxidase activity for detecting small biomolecules is the study conducted by Wei and colleagues.[64] The team measured glucose and lactate levels in living tissues to diagnose ischemic stroke, which affects glucose and lactate levels in the brain. They developed nanozymes using MOF MIL-101, graphene nanoplateletes (GNPs), and GOx/LOx (lactate oxidase), which oxidized glucose and lactate. The process involved the oxidation of leucomalachite green (LMG) into Raman active malachite green (MG) through the use of graphene nanoplateletes (GNPs), which were produced through the reaction of H_2O_2. The resulting malachite green emitted surface-enhanced Raman scattering signals that were employed to determine its activity level.[63]

6.2.4 OTHER BIOSENSING APPLICATIONS

The varying pore size and pore walls of MOFs are arguably their most beneficial characteristic in the field of biosensing and imaging because they can be suitably exploited for sensing not only genetic material (DNA/RNA), small and large biomolecules (protein, enzymes) but also other molecules such as reactive oxygen species (ROS) (O_2-, OH, RO, H_2O_2). For example, Lu et al. detected a MOF containing methyl viologen cations used for the detection of pure O_2. The detection is based on a color change in the MOF after X-ray diffraction.[65] Wang and co-workers devised a luminescent MOF of type Eu(III)-MOF for the detection of H_2O_2. The principle is based on a visible color change that occurs when in the presence of H_2O_2, Fe_2+ is oxidized to Fe_3+ via the Fenton reaction, causing fluorescence quenching of Eu-MOF.[66] All reactive oxygen species exhibit high oxidative activity which is utilized in their sensing (fluorescence quenching or electrochemical method).[67,68] Xia and co-workers demonstrated the sensing of ROS in environmental and biological samples by showing their fluorescence quenching ability of sulfur tagged $[Eu_2(TDA)_3]_2H_2O\}n$. The mode of operation involves the conversion of the thioether of TDA into sulfoxide, causing a shift in the coordination environment of Eu_3+ to a more polar state. The reduction in fluorescence intensity is a result of the transfer of charges from the oxidized sulfoxide to Eu_3+. Furthermore, a range of hybrid composites consisting of protein/enzyme-MOF have been employed in detecting H_2O_2 in biological samples using either electrochemical or colorimetric methods.[69,70] Chen and co-workers presented a biosensor that could be used in the detection of the release of the same from living cells and can further be used to identify cellular damage at inappropriate levels. The biosensor, which was developed using Boronic acid functionalized MIL-100(Cr) immobilized with horseradish peroxidase (HRP), exhibited a swift response time of under 4 seconds and a linear range spanning from 0.5 to 3000 μM.[70]

The most recent use of MOFs is seen in the sensing of possible drug pollutants from the environment as shown in Figure 6.4. For example, Artetxe and co-workers showed the capturing and biosensing of common water and environment pollutants, ibuprofen, and naproxen in varying concentrations with the help of a heptameric supramolecular MOF ($CuCr_6$) which is able to trap these drugs either by supramolecular heptameric hydrogen bonding or π-π interactions.[71] Dutta and co-workers fabricated an efficient chemosensor, UiO-66@butyne (isoreticular with UiO-66), for the detection of hg_2+, one of the most hazardous pollutants. The principle of action involved an oxymercuration reaction-based chemodosimetric pathway which proved to be highly sensitive (LOD = 10.9 nm).[72] Gu, Liu, and co-workers reported a Zn-based MOF, NH_2–Zn-MOF; $[Zn_2(TPOM)(NH_2–BDC)_2]·4\ H_2O$ for the sensing of Cr_3+ ions. The limit of detection was 4.95 μm.[73]

Tang and co-workers worked on the detection of the radioactive element, uranium from industrial effluents and seawater by employing faulty manufactured or "defected" MOFs. The concept of photocatalytic reduction activity was employed on the Zr–MOF for the capturing. This was achieved by missing linker defects and node metal substitution CytC@ZIF-8 has excellent peroxidase activity on TiO_2M which shows its potential application in the detection of H_2O_2.[74]

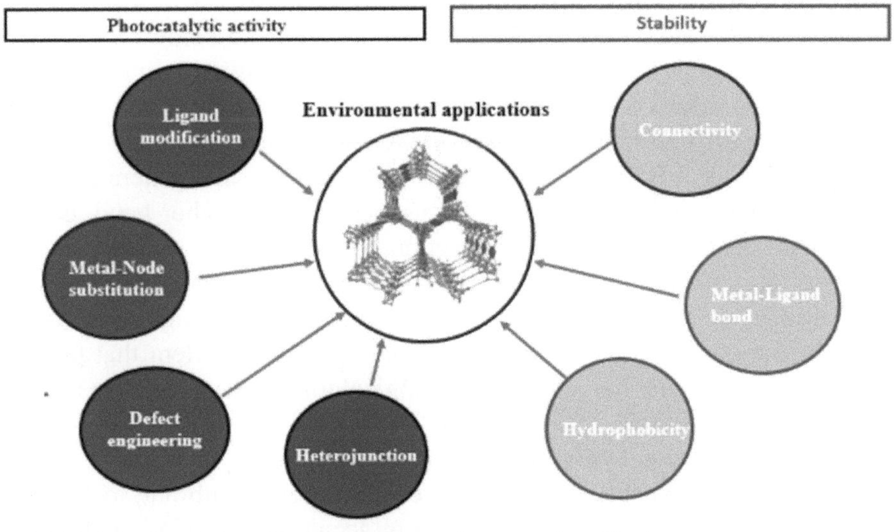

FIGURE 6.4 Properties of MOFs used in environmental applications.

6.3 APPLICATION OF MOFS IN BIOIMAGING

The failure in the delivery of proteins across cellular membranes due to the sensitivity and size of proteins, and in the endocytosis of MOFs posed the need for the scaling of MOFs down to a few nanometers. Ultrasonic exfoliation, solvothermal, and isothermal methods, for example, allow the synthesis of NMOFs while retaining the physicochemical properties of their corresponding MOFs.[75,76] NMOFs were known to have poor physiological stability in phosphate media and have been modified to include a polymer wrapping that protects the NMOF from being attacked by phosphate ions or acids.[77,78]

6.3.1 INTRACELLULAR IMAGING

Biosensing is the evaluation of the intracellular environment and/or composition in order to accurately diagnose the diseased condition in a patient. A specific, previously identified biological response is first converted into an electrochemical, electrical, optical, gravimetric, or acoustic signal (via transduction) and biosensors are designed to amplify the same to make visualization possible.[77]

Biosensors are made of nanomaterials that can penetrate into a cell and facilitate the transduction process at the site of metabolism. Biosensors typically consist of an analyte, a bioreceptor, a transducer, the amplifier or processing units, and the display as shown in Figure 6.5 below. The analyte, as shown below, is the moiety that is desired to be identified. In the determination of blood glucose concentration, glucose molecules would be treated as the analyte. The bioreceptor serves as a biological component such as enzymes, DNA or RNA, and antibodies that recognize and generate a signal upon interacting with the analyte. Transducers, on the other hand, convert the signal generated from the interaction between the bioreceptor and the analyte into another form of energy. Amplifying and processing units are responsible for enhancing the signal received and preparing it for display. Finally, the display unit includes a user interpretation system that presents the output in a numerical, tabular, or graphical format depending on the end-user's requirements.[77]

Biosensors have evolved from having the ability to detect analyte molecules that advanced to the surface of the cell membrane to have the ability to detect not only the intracellular molecules but also intracellular pH.

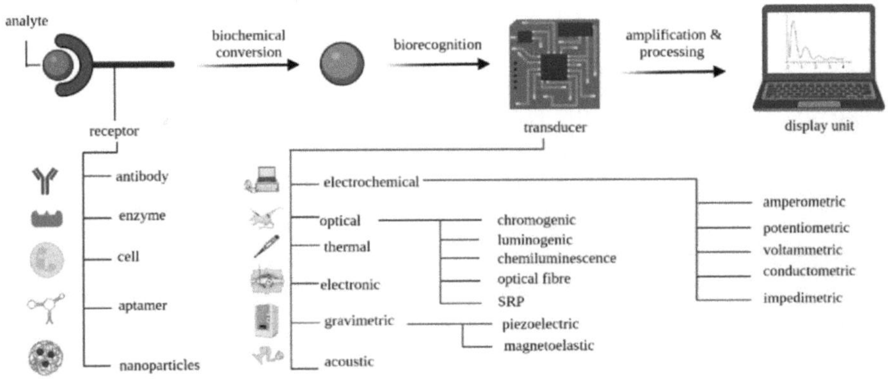

FIGURE 6.5 The composition of a biosensor and its function.

Source: Adapted from Ref. [77]

The evolution of biosensors has indeed rendered nanoparticles redundant since nanometal-organic frameworks (NMOFs) facilitate the direct interaction of enzymes with the electrode and thereby reduce the cost of the biosensor and allow multiple repeats of the diagnostic test.

NMOFs can be used to quantify and/or characterize.[77]

1. the DNA and RNA present in healthy or diseased/ cancerous cells,
2. small biomolecules such as the highly-reactive oxygen species,
3. the pH in and around a cell and its organelles.

Diseased conditions often alter the regulation or composition of microRNAs—single-stranded, non-coding length of nucleotides that regulate gene expression by cleaving or repressing mRNA. While some diseased conditions result in the up-regulation of miRNAs, some result in down-regulation of the same.

DNA or RNA probes contain known sequences of nucleotides that bind to their complementary segments in the endogenous DNA or miRNA. Conjugating these probes with fluorophore groups enables the inference of the composition of the endogenous DNA or RNA on the basis of the fluorescence observed in the sample (under UV light). An ideal fluorophore-containing biosensor must have distinct excitation and emission wavelengths, accurate target recognition, and good biocompatibility including but not limited to cell permeability and photostability.[79] Fluorophore-labeled DNA probes are used in conjugation with nickel-isoreticular metal-organic frameworks (Ni-IRMOF). This technique is known as fluorescence quenching. The NMOF coats the fluorophore-labeled probes to repress the intensity of their fluorescence properties. On combination with its complimentary segment in the miRNA, the probes are expelled out of the NMOFs and elicit their fluorescence property. The hybridized double-stranded RNA is more stable than the miRNA by itself. Hence, the reaction equilibrium is toward the hybridized RNA and the fluorescence property is observable under the light of a particular wavelength as shown in Figure 6.6 below.[80]

Fluorescence quenching can also be achieved with the usage of gold nanoparticles, graphene oxide or carbon nanotubes. The monitoring of oxygen releasing reactions (ORR) has been extensively carried out using platinum and carbon metals. Mao et al. developed a strategy to replace the expensive metal—platinum, that easily corroded carbon and formed aggregates, with Cu-based MOFs. Graphene oxide, hereby increased the conductivity of the biosensor.60 Graphene oxide is used as a signal amplifier in fluorescence probe based biosensing. In the detection of the human immunodeficiency virus (HIV) Rev peptide, for example, GO acts as an amplifier to attain the combination of the fluorophore-containing probes with the antagonists of the HIV-Rev peptide.[81] Chen et al. developed three-dimensional structures of carbon nanotubes on carbon nanoplates that have shown excellent electromagnetic wave absorption (EMWA) properties. EMWA properties protect one from the electromagnetic radiation from electronic devices.[82]

NMOFS, however, have intrinsic fluorescence quenching properties due to the presence of central metal ligands, a large surface area due to their high porosity, and the resilience to design-related modifications to their chemical properties. NMOFs are now known to be the more advantageous biosensors.[80]

Fluorophore-labeled TAMRA (trimethylrhodamine) and FAM (fluorescein amidite) probes were used in conjugation with lanthanide-based nanosheets to sense the presence of the corresponding DNA segments in cells. The hybridization of the endogenous DNA with the ss-DNA conjugated in the Ln-based nanosheets decreased the affinity of the ss-DNA to the Ln-based nanosheets eventually expelling the latter out of the framework, able to elicit its fluorescence properties. The recovery of fluorescence of the quenched TAMRA and FAM probes yielded unexpected results and led to the hypothesis for another successful discovery discussed hereafter. The TAMRA-labeled probes experienced a "turn-up" fluorescence, that is, an enhancement in its fluorescence properties while the FAM-labeled probes experienced a "turn-down" fluorescence, that is, repression of its fluorescence properties on quenching and recovery of the fluorescence properties.[47]

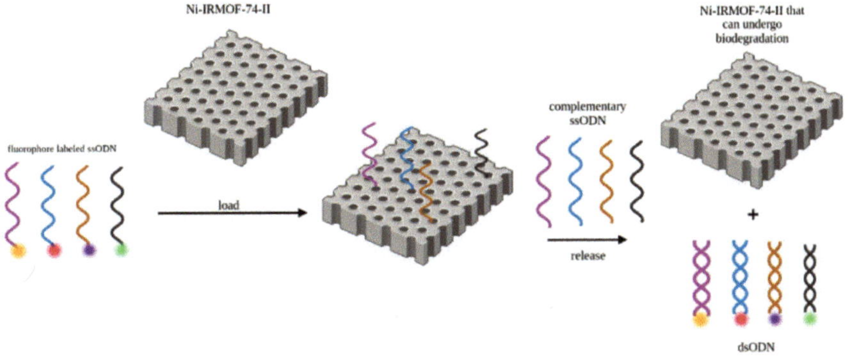

FIGURE 6.6 An illustration of the working of Ni-RMOF-74-II frameworks in conjugation with fluorophore-labeled ssODN.

Source: Adapted from Ref. [80]

These findings were applied to develop methods to sense the ATP activity that is often altered in diseased conditions in cells. A combination of TAMRA and FAM labeled probes provided high-contrast images of a cell containing ATP. The green, fluorophore-labeled probes would appear orange on hybridization with their corresponding endogenous ATP molecules. The difference in the turn-up and turn-down tendencies of the two probes made the diagnosis more sensitive and thus ideal for diagnosis.[47]

The zeolithic imidazalate framework—8 (ZIF-8) possesses excellent biocompatibility and is easy to manufacture. ZIF-8; however, displays poor fluorescence properties and thus insufficient quenching in the diagnosis of DNA. To overcome its limitations and be able to benefit off of its advantageous properties, ZIF-8 is doped with a Ln_3+ on its surface. The use of a Ln_3+ core-shell increased the fluorescence properties by about 8 times and made the synthesis of the CS-ZIF-8-La biosensor more economical and functional.[83]

An important breakthrough in the journey of NMOFs is that of the detection of the extracellular presence of H_2S in case of diseases, such as the Alzheimer's disease, Down's syndrome, etc. H_2S is a poisonous gas that is a product of the cystathionine β-synthase (CBS) catalyzed metabolic reactions. The observation of a significant decrease in the levels of H_2S, the third most important biomolecule after NO and CO, in the brains of the patients of the Alzheimer's disease[83,84] and the up-regulation of the cystathionine β-synthase to produce elevated levels of H_2S in cancer patients correctly identified the analyte used in the diagnosis of the aforementioned diseases.[85]

Conventional techniques of H_2S quantification demanded complex instruments, and skilled manpower and could also damage healthy tissues.

The reactivity and diffusion properties of H_2S made gas chromatography, colorimetric or electrochemical quantification of H_2S difficult. H_2S is known to participate in characteristic nucleophilic addition, precipitation, or thiolysis types of reactions but the variation in response times, detection limits, and the presence of toxic organic solvents make this kind of H_2S sensing inaccurate and unreliable.[86]

The consequent hunt for miniaturized, highly sensitive probes for H_2S detection culminated in the development of NMOF-based biosensors that could be visualized by luminescent, cataluminescent, capacitance-based, or other methods of sensing.[87]

Cu_{2+} ions are used as central metal ligands, that H_2S can bind to in NMOFs. The porosity of the NMOFs imparts high selectivity and surface area over which binding can take place. [Cu(TCPP)(AlOH)2]n frameworks show an enhancement in the fluorescence of the probes on incubation with NO donors. UiO-66-N_3, on the other hand, is used to monitor the mediation of the diazotization (of amide to azide) by H_2S. The turn-up in fluorescence is similar to that observed in the CD-MONT-2 (NMOF based on b-cyclodextrin) also used to detect intracellular H_2S.

Since, proteins are sensitive to pH and must maintain their structural integrity to maintain their function, intracellular and extracellular pH is stringently regulated. Intracellular pH imaging finds numerous applications in diagnosis since diseased conditions either alter the composition of proteins in a cell or repress the production of function of the same. Intracellular pH can be measured using proton-permeable electrodes, NMR, absorption spectroscopy, and fluorescence imaging. Fluorescence imaging is particularly the most sought-after technique of intracellular pH measurement owing to its high sensitivity and resolution.

Fluorescein isothiocyanate (FITC) can be conjugated with the UiO framework in order to detect fluorescence as a function of the intracellular pH. F-UiO, however, is known to escape a cell rapidly and can thus lead to discrepancies in the obtained results. F-UiO frameworks can detect pH from 5.0 to 7.0 on rapid and efficient endocytosis into a cell.[88] UiO frameworks can also be conjugated with RITC (rhodamine-β-isothiocyanate) in order to sense O_2 in living cells. O_2 is a vital component in the respiration of living cells and is used as a biomarker in the case of vascular, pulmonary or tumor-causing diseases. Once again, fluorescence-based techniques provide higher specificity and resolution than the conventional techniques of positron emission tomography, immunohistological staining or O_2 needle electrodes[88] O_2 sensing is effectively performed using ratiometric sensing which involves the use of an O_2 insensitive probe and an O_2—sensitive probe. This technique allows the measurement of the emission ratios at different wavelengths and can thereby give an accurate estimate of the O_2 concentrations in a cell. R-UiO NMOFs have been validated as accurate sensors of intracellular O_2 levels using confocal laser scanning microscopy (CLSM) methods on mouse colon carcinoma cells. The use of such frameworks is advantageous especially because the rhodamine dyes are known to not leach into the cells and provide the most stable O_2—sensing technique discovered so far.[88]

Recent advancements in the glutathione stabilization of gold nanoclusters have enhanced the fluorescence properties of hROS by as much as 10 times. Owing to their intrinsic biodegradability, the enhancement of fluorescence properties is rapidly reversed in the metabolism of the NMOFs used in the detection of hROS.

6.3.2 *MAGNETIC RESONANCE IMAGING (MRI)*

Bioimaging is the noninvasive visualization of the biological activity in a cell or tissue in a specified period of time. It is an important branch of diagnostics and is developing with the knowledge of MOFs since MOFs can help enhance the contrast between various components observed by probes. Bioimaging finds application in the detection of tumor-forming units in the body among many others.[95] Bioimaging either provides information about the internal structures as in MRI, CT, and ultrasound scans, or functional information about molecules in the target cell as in PET, SPECT, or magnetic resonance spectroscopy.

Magnetic resonance imaging (MRI) is a commonly used diagnostic procedure that enables the visualization of internal organs within the body. This is achieved through the measurement of the nuclear spin reorientations of atoms, such as hydrogen, in a magnetic field.[96,97] To enhance the contrast between two areas of interest in an MRI scan, a combination of two agents is used. A positive contrast agent reduces the longitudinal relaxation time (T1) of the water molecule protons, while a negative contrast agent shortens the transverse relaxation time (T2) of the protons in the body. This approach is widely employed in MRI to improve the clarity of images.[98,99] Positive contrast agents typically involve the use of transitional metal ions, such as Gd3+ or Mn^{2+}, that are chelated with MOFs or other components to mitigate their adverse effects. On the other hand, negative contrast agents generally consist of superparamagnetic iron oxides (SPIOs) that cause a reduction in image intensity or negative image enhancement. This approach is widely employed in order to enhance the clarity of images while minimizing potential side effects.[100]

TABLE 6.2 MOFs Application in Bioimaging.

Ligand structures	Ligand abbreviation	Metal	MOF formula	Preparation approach	MOF particle size	Imaging applications	References
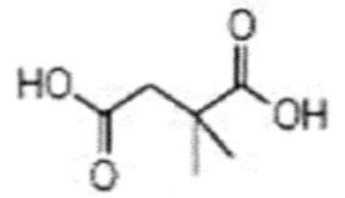	$C_6H_{10}O_4$	Mn^{2+}	$[Mn(C_6H_8O_4)(H_2O)]n$ (MnDMS)	Ultrasonic Exfoliation	~200 nm	DNA & RNA	[89]
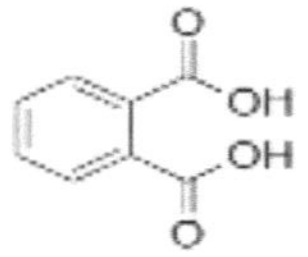	BDC	Zr^{4+}	$[Zr_6O_4(OH)_4(BDC)6]n$ (UiO-66)	Solvothermal method	125 nm	RNA	[90]
			$[Gd(BDC)_{1.5}(H_2O)_2]n$	Reverse Microemulsion Process	155 ± 30 nm	MRI and CT	[91]
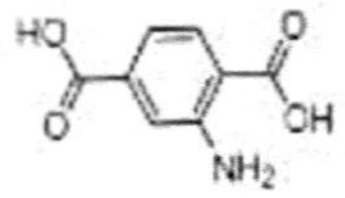	NH2-BDC		$[Zn_4O(H_2\text{-BDC})_3]n$ IRMOF$_{-3}$	Surface modification	250 nm	MRI	[92]
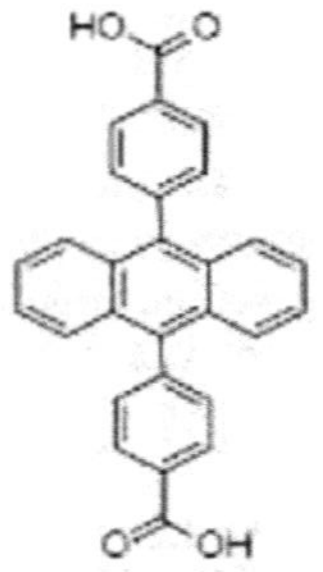	H_2L	Hf+4	Hf- UiO	Solvothermal method	50–200 nm	CT	[93]
		Zr+4	Zr- UiO	Solvothermal method	50–200 nm	CT	[94]

6.3.3 DUAL-MODE IMAGING WITH MRI AND CT

Computer tomography (CT) scan is one of the most cost-effective methods that can provide tomographical information about internal anatomy. A CT scan basically involves the irradiation of the patient's body with X-rays from a source that is a hollow cylinder in shape (commonly called a gantry), can accommodate the patient in itself, and can rotate 360°. The sensors on the gantry detect the intensity of the reflected rays from the patient and thus characterize the condition of tissues present in the detected part of the patient's body.[81] MOFs have shown useful applications in enhancing the contrast between tissues of similar densities and are thus integral to the concept of computer tomography. Zhang et al. reported a type of iodine–boron–dipyrromethene containing NMOF (BODIPY), UiO-PDT to be useful contrasting agents in CT scans. The UiO-PDT nanocrystals, that are about 70 nm wide, accumulate at sites of tumors. The UiO-PDT nanocrystals show higher X-ray attenuation than healthy cells and thus guarantee accurate and sensitive detection of tumor sites in the body.[100,101]

Nanoscale coordination polymers (NCPs) are utilized together with Gd3+ and Ru[4,4′-(COOH)2 bipyridyl(bpy)]32+ (LRu) due to their strong ability to enhance the longitudinal relaxation rate and their ability to emit red fluorescence, respectively. NCPs have desirable physicochemical properties like that of low toxicity, high-contrast imaging efficiency, and simple manufacturing techniques. Hence, NCPs and their application in MRI practices have been studied in the past on HepG2 cells, zebrafish, and tumor-bearing mice as models.[97] Mn^{2+}-based nanoparticles have also been used more often as a result of their low cytotoxicity and efficient T1-weighted contrast enhancement.[102] Overexposure of free Mn^{2+} ions is, however, known to cause neurodegenerative diseases and the manufacture and design of chelation thus becomes imperative.[103]

A typical example of the T2 contrasting agents is that of Fe_3O_4 nanoparticles coated with NMOFs. It also makes for an example of a theranostic molecule that is involved in the therapeutic as well as diagnostic processes of a disease. The Fe_3O_4 nanoparticles serve as a T2 contrasting agent in MRI while the UiO-66 core traps the drug molecule in the framework it builds on the Fe_3O_4 nanoparticles. As a result, this framework provides sustained release of the drug, enhanced contrast in MRI, effective chemotherapeutic activity, and high drug loading capacity all while ensuring good biocompatibility and degradability.[102]

Fe_3O_4@IRMOF-3,[104,105] Fe_3O_4@ZIF8 and Fe_3O_4@ZIF-90 frameworks are pH and glutathione-responsive T1 and T2 MRI contrasting agents and are overexpressed in the GSH tumor microenvironments. Disassembly of this framework expels the contrasting effect of these agents and enables high-contrast MRI. Fortunately, the Fe_3O_4-ZIF-8 frameworks have been studied to be non-toxic to HeLa and NIH3T3 cells and can be further studied to improve its applications.[106] Tian et al. were the first to combine the utilities of CT and MRI scans while simultaneously overcoming each of their limitations. CT scans, for example, have poor resolution in soft tissues and MRI scans have poorer sensitivity than CT scans. Tian et al. hence designed the GdMOF-PAA-Au hybrid system to enhance contrast in scans obtained on dual imaging and take bioimaging to newer heights.[100] The in vivo imaging on the detection of brain cancer has also been made possible via gold nanorod composites with Fe in the form of MIL-88, MIL-100, and MIL-101. The possibility of dual imaging.[107–109]

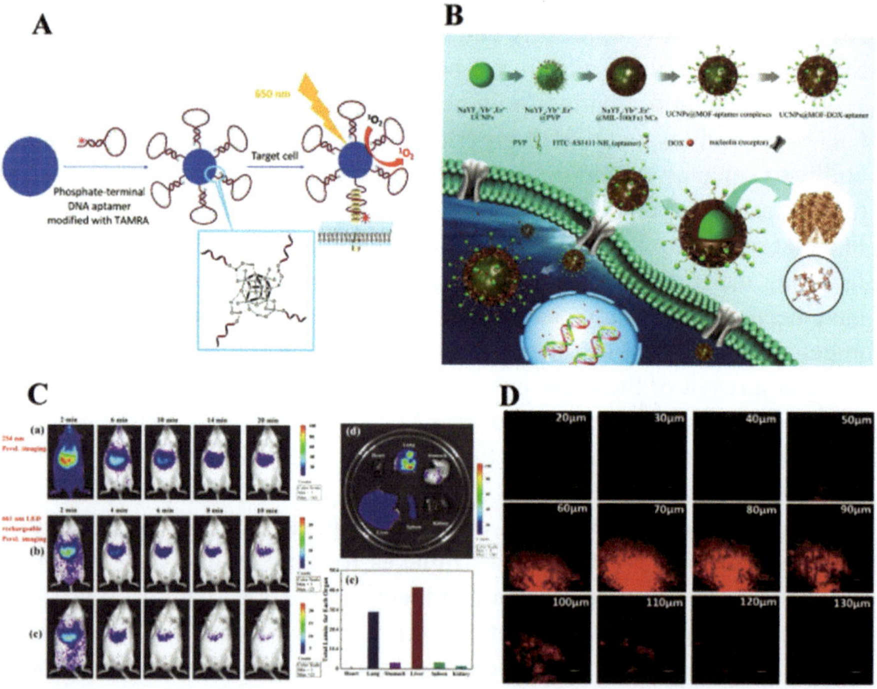

FIGURE 6.7 (a) phosphate-terminal DNA aptamer to a Zr–MOF nanoparticle quencher can be used for imaging and photodynamic therapy; (b) targeted UCNPs@MOF core-shell NCs, loading them with drugs, and using receptor-mediated endocytosis; (c) In vivo NIR PersL imaging; (d) Ex vivo NIR PersL imaging.

Source: Reprinted with permission from Ref. [100]. https://creativecommons.org/licenses/by/4.0/

Liu et al. made incredible use of the Zr-based MOF by designing a nanoparticle quencher that not only provides target-based bioimaging but also photodynamic therapy. The Zr–MOF, as seen in Figure 6.7a. conjugates with the DNA aptamer in order to undergo a structural change. This binding and change in structure causes the fluorescence quenching of TAMRA (tetramethylrhodamine) dyes and provides target-based imaging (Fig. 6.7c and d).

6.4 SUMMARY

MOFs are currently being actively researched for their potential use in diagnosis. To increase their efficiency and uptake, these frameworks are being scaled down to nanometer units. In addition to their diagnostic applications, nanoscale MOFs (NMOFs) are being used to detect contaminants in water and other everyday settings. MOFs have also been used as transducers to detect biological molecules, such as enzymes, antibodies, and DNA due to their high surface area and porosity, which allows for high loading of these biomolecules and enables highly sensitive and specific detection of target analytes. MOFs can be engineered to have specific optical or magnetic properties, making them ideal for targeted imaging of specific tissues or cells in bioimaging applications, such as contrast agents for magnetic resonance imaging (MRI) and fluorescent and photoacoustic imaging. MOFs' biocompatibility and biodegradability make them promising candidates for use in vivo. The future perspective for MOF application in biosensors and bioimaging is optimistic, with continued research and development likely leading to enhanced sensitivity and specificity of biosensors and improved imaging capabilities in vivo. Nevertheless, MOFs' stability, biocompatibility, and biodegradability require further optimization for clinical applications.

KEYWORDS

- **metal-organic framework (MOF)**
- **biosensing**
- **bioimaging**
- **aptamer**
- **nanocomposite**

REFERENCES

1. Liu, Y.; Jiang, T.; Liu, Z. Metal-Organic Frameworks for Bioimaging: Strategies and Challenges. *Nanotheranostics* **2022,** *6* (2), 143–160. https://doi.org/10.7150/ntno.63458.
2. Wang, H. S. Metal–Organic Frameworks for Biosensing and Bioimaging Applications. *Coord. Chem. Rev.* **2017,** *349*, 139–155. https://doi.org/10.1016/J.CCR.2017.08.015.
3. Munawar, J.; Khan, M. S.; Zehra Syeda, S. E.; Nawaz, S.; Janjhi, F. A.; Ul Haq, H.; Rashid, E. U.; Jesionowski, T.; Bilal, M. Metal-Organic Framework-Based Smart Nanoplatforms for Biosensing, Drug Delivery, and Cancer Theranostics. *Inorg. Chem. Commun.* **2023,** *147* (October 2022), 110145. https://doi.org/10.1016/j.inoche.2022.110145.
4. Casey, J. R.; Grinstein, S.; Orlowski, J. Sensors and Regulators of Intracellular PH. *Nat. Rev. Mol. Cell Biol.* **2009,** *11* (1), 50–61. https://doi.org/10.1038/nrm2820.
5. Hoskins, B. F.; Robson, R. Infinite Polymeric Frameworks Consisting of Three Dimensionally Linked Rod-like Segments. *J. Am. Chem. Soc.* **1989,** *111* (15), 5962–5964. https://doi.org/10.1021/JA00197A079/SUPPL_FILE/JA00197A079_SI_001.PDF.
6. Yaghi, O. M.; Li, G.; Li, H. Selective Binding and Removal of Guests in a Microporous Metal–Organic Framework. *Nature* **1995,** *378* (6558), 703–706. https://doi.org/10.1038/378703a0.
7. Liang, C. C.; Shi, Z. L.; He, C. T.; Tan, J.; Zhou, H. D.; Zhou, H. L.; Lee, Y.; Zhang, Y. B. Engineering of Pore Geometry for Ultrahigh Capacity Methane Storage in Mesoporous Metal-Organic Frameworks. *J. Am. Chem. Soc.* **2017,** *139* (38), 13300–13303. https://doi.org/10.1021/JACS.7B08347/SUPPL_FILE/JA7B08347_SI_005.CIF.
8. Zhang, X.; Chuah, C. Y.; Dong, P.; Cha, Y. H.; Bae, T. H.; Song, M. K. Hierarchically Porous Co-MOF-74 Hollow Nanorods for Enhanced Dynamic CO 2 Separation. *ACS Appl. Mater. Interfaces* **2018,** *10* (50), 43316–43322. https://doi.org/10.1021/ACSAMI.8B17180/SUPPL_FILE/AM8B17180_SI_001.PDF.
9. Prasetya, N.; Ladewig, B. P. New Azo-DMOF-1 MOF as a Photoresponsive Low-Energy CO2 Adsorbent and Its Exceptional CO2/N2 Separation Performance in Mixed Matrix Membranes. *ACS Appl. Mater. Interfaces* **2018,** *10* (40), 34291–34301. https://doi.org/10.1021/ACSAMI.8B12261.
10. Marti, A. M.; Venna, S. R.; Roth, E. A.; Culp, J. T.; Hopkinson, D. P. Simple Fabrication Method for Mixed Matrix Membranes with in Situ MOF Growth for Gas Separation. *ACS Appl. Mater. Interfaces* **2018,** *10* (29), 24784–24790. https://doi.org/10.1021/ACSAMI.8B06592.
11. Wang, L.; Zhu, H.; Shi, Y.; Ge, Y.; Feng, X.; Liu, R.; Li, Y.; Ma, Y.; Wang, L. Novel Catalytic Micromotor of Porous Zeolitic Imidazolate Framework-67 for Precise Drug Delivery. *Nanoscale* **2018,** *10* (24), 11384–11391. https://doi.org/10.1039/C8NR02493F.
12. Liu, X.; Qi, W.; Wang, Y.; Lin, D.; Yang, X.; Su, R.; He, Z. Rational Design of Mimic Multienzyme Systems in Hierarchically Porous Biomimetic Metal–Organic Frameworks. *ACS Appl. Mater. Interfaces* **2018.** https://doi.org/10.1021/ACSAMI.8B09388.
13. Salgaonkar, M.; Nadar, S. S.; Rathod, V. K. Combi-Metal Organic Framework (Combi-MOF) of α-Amylase and Glucoamylase for One Pot Starch Hydrolysis. *Int. J. Biol. Macromol.* **2018,** *113*, 464–475. https://doi.org/10.1016/J.IJBIOMAC.2018.02.092.
14. Yang, J. C.; Shang, Y.; Li, Y. H.; Cui, Y.; Yin, X. B. An “All-in-One” Antitumor and Anti-Recurrence/Metastasis Nanomedicine with Multi-Drug Co-Loading and Burst Drug Release for Multi-Modality Therapy. *Chem. Sci.* **2018,** *9* (36), 7210. https://doi.org/10.1039/C8SC02305K.

15. Zhao, W.; Wan, G.; Peng, C.; Sheng, H.; Wen, J.; Chen, H. Key Single-Atom Electrocatalysis in Metal-Organic Framework (MOF)-Derived Bifunctional Catalysts. *ChemSusChem* **2018,** *11* (19), 3473–3479. https://doi.org/10.1002/CSSC.201801473.
16. Zou, M. Z.; Liu, W. L.; Li, C. X.; Zheng, D. W.; Zeng, J. Y.; Gao, F.; Ye, J. J.; Zhang, X. Z. A Multifunctional Biomimetic Nanoplatform for Relieving Hypoxia to Enhance Chemotherapy and Inhibit the PD-1/PD-L1 Axis. *Small* **2018,** *14* (28). https://doi.org/10.1002/SMLL.201801120.
17. Han, S. Y.; Pan, D. L.; Chen, H.; Bu, X. B.; Gao, Y. X.; Gao, H.; Tian, Y.; Li, G. S.; Wang, G.; Cao, S. L.; et al. A Methylthio-Functionalized-MOF Photocatalyst with High Performance for Visible-Light-Driven H2 Evolution. *Angew. Chem. Int. Ed. Engl.* **2018,** *57* (31), 9864–9869. https://doi.org/10.1002/ANIE.201806077.
18. Qu, F.; Li, X.; Lv, X.; You, J.; Han, W. Highly Selective Metal–Organic Framework-Based Sensor for Protamine through Photoinduced Electron Transfer. *J. Mater. Sci.* **2019,** *54* (4), 3144–3155. https://doi.org/10.1007/S10853-018-3041-6.
19. Qin, J.; Cho, M.; Lee, Y. Ferrocene-Encapsulated Zn Zeolitic Imidazole Framework (ZIF-8) for Optical and Electrochemical Sensing of Amyloid-β Oligomers and for the Early Diagnosis of Alzheimer's Disease. *ACS Appl. Mater. Interfaces* **2019,** *11* (12), 11743–11748. https://doi.org/10.1021/ACSAMI.8B21425/SUPPL_FILE/AM8B21425_SI_001.PDF.
20. Masih, D.; Chernikova, V.; Shekhah, O.; Eddaoudi, M.; Mohammed, O. F. Zeolite-like Metal-Organic Framework (MOF) Encaged Pt(II)-Porphyrin for Anion-Selective Sensing. *ACS Appl. Mater. Interfaces* **2018,** *10* (14), 11399–11405. https://doi.org/10.1021/ACSAMI.7B19282.
21. Lei, B.; Wang, M.; Jiang, Z.; Qi, W.; Su, R.; He, Z. Constructing Redox-Responsive Metal-Organic Framework Nanocarriers for Anticancer Drug Delivery. *ACS Appl. Mater. Interfaces* **2018,** *10* (19), 16698–16706. https://doi.org/10.1021/ACSAMI.7B19693.
22. Liu, L. L.; Yu, Y. Z.; Zhao, X. J.; Wang, Y. R.; Cheng, F. Y.; Zhang, M. K.; Shu, J. J.; Liu, L. A Robust Zn(II)/Na(I)-MOF Decorated with [(OAc)2(H2O)2]N2n− Anions for the Luminescence Sensing of Copper Ions Based on the Inner Filter Effect. *Dalt. Trans.* **2018,** *47* (23), 7787–7794. https://doi.org/10.1039/C8DT00908B.
23. Yang, X.; Yu, Y. Q.; Peng, L. Z.; Lei, Y. M.; Chai, Y. Q.; Yuan, R.; Zhuo, Y. Strong Electrochemiluminescence from MOF Accelerator Enriched Quantum Dots for Enhanced Sensing of Trace CTnI. *Anal. Chem.* **2018,** *90* (6), 3995–4002. https://doi.org/10.1021/ACS.ANALCHEM.7B05137.
24. Zhang, H.; Shang, Y.; Li, Y. H.; Sun, S. K.; Yin, X. B. Smart Metal-Organic Framework-Based Nanoplatforms for Imaging-Guided Precise Chemotherapy. *ACS Appl. Mater. Interfaces* **2019,** *11* (2), 1886–1895. https://doi.org/10.1021/ACSAMI.8B19048.
25. Robison, L.; Zhang, L.; Drout, R. J.; Li, P.; Haney, C. R.; Brikha, A.; Noh, H.; Mehdi, B. L.; Browning, N. D.; Dravid, V. P.; et al. A Bismuth Metal-Organic Framework as a Contrast Agent for X-Ray Computed Tomography. *ACS Appl. bio Mater.* **2019,** *2* (3), 1197–1203. https://doi.org/10.1021/ACSABM.8B00778.
26. Yang, Z. L.; Tian, W.; Wang, Q.; Zhao, Y.; Zhang, Y. L.; Tian, Y.; Tang, Y. X.; Wang, S. J.; Liu, Y.; Ni, Q. Q.; et al. Oxygen-Evolving Mesoporous Organosilica Coated Prussian Blue Nanoplatform for Highly Efficient Photodynamic Therapy of Tumors. *Adv. Sci.* **2018,** *5* (5). https://doi.org/10.1002/ADVS.201700847.

27. Zhang, Y.; Wang, F.; Liu, C.; Wang, Z.; Kang, L.; Huang, Y.; Dong, K.; Ren, J.; Qu, X. Nanozyme Decorated Metal-Organic Frameworks for Enhanced Photodynamic Therapy. *ACS Nano*, **2018,** *12* (1), 651–661. https://doi.org/10.1021/ACSNANO.7B07746.
28. Hong, X. J.; Tang, X. Y.; Wei, Q.; Song, C. L.; Wang, S. Y.; Dong, R. F.; Cai, Y. P.; Si, L. P. Efficient Encapsulation of Small S2-4 Molecules in MOF-Derived Flowerlike Nitrogen-Doped Microporous Carbon Nanosheets for High-Performance Li-S Batteries. *ACS Appl. Mater. Interfaces* **2018,** *10* (11), 9435–9443. https://doi.org/10.1021/ACSAMI.7B19609.
29. Zou, G.; Hou, H.; Ge, P.; Huang, Z.; Zhao, G.; Yin, D.; Ji, X. Metal-Organic Framework-Derived Materials for Sodium Energy Storage. *Small* **2018,** *14* (3). https://doi.org/10.1002/SMLL.201702648.
30. Qu, C.; Liang, Z.; Jiao, Y.; Zhao, B.; Zhu, B.; Dang, D.; Dai, S.; Chen, Y.; Zou, R.; Liu, M. "One-for-All" Strategy in Fast Energy Storage: Production of Pillared MOF Nanorod-Templated Positive/Negative Electrodes for the Application of High-Performance Hybrid Supercapacitor. *Small* **2018,** *14* (23), 1800285. https://doi.org/10.1002/SMLL.201800285.
31. Wang, S.; Chen, Y.; Wang, S.; Li, P.; Mirkin, C. A.; Farha, O. K. DNA-Functionalized Metal-Organic Framework Nanoparticles for Intracellular Delivery of Proteins. *J. Am. Chem. Soc.* **2019,** *141* (6), 2215–2219. https://doi.org/10.1021/JACS.8B12705/ASSET/IMAGES/LARGE/JA-2018-12705W_0003.JPEG.
32. Zhao, H.; Hou, S.; Zhao, X.; Liu, D. Adsorption and PH-Responsive Release of Tinidazole on Metal-Organic Framework CAU-1. *J. Chem. Eng. Data* **2019,** *64* (4), 1851–1858. https://doi.org/10.1021/ACS.JCED.9B00106/SUPPL_FILE/JE9B00106_SI_001.PDF.
33. Mukoyoshi, M.; Kitagawa, H. Nanoparticle/Metal–Organic Framework Hybrid Catalysts: Elucidating the Role of the MOF. *Chem. Commun.* **2022,** *58* (77), 10757–10767. https://doi.org/10.1039/D2CC03233C.
34. Yang, P.; Men, Y.; Tian, Y.; Cao, Y.; Zhang, L.; Yao, X.; Yang, W. Metal-Organic Framework Nanoparticles with Near-Infrared Dye for Multimodal Imaging and Guided Phototherapy. *ACS Appl. Mater. Interfaces* **2019,** *11* (12), 11209–11219. https://doi.org/10.1021/ACSAMI.9B01286.
35. Zheng, H. Q.; Liu, C. Y.; Zeng, X. Y.; Chen, J.; Lü, J.; Lin, R. G.; Cao, R.; Lin, Z. J.; Su, J. W. MOF-808: A Metal-Organic Framework with Intrinsic Peroxidase-Like Catalytic Activity at Neutral PH for Colorimetric Biosensing. *Inorg. Chem.* **2018,** *57* (15), 9096–9104. https://doi.org/10.1021/ACS.INORGCHEM.8B01097.
36. Tan, H.; Tang, G.; Wang, Z.; Li, Q.; Gao, J.; Wu, S. Magnetic Porous Carbon Nanocomposites Derived from Metal-Organic Frameworks as a Sensing Platform for DNA Fluorescent Detection. *Anal. Chim. Acta* **2016,** *940*, 136–142. https://doi.org/10.1016/J.ACA.2016.08.024.
37. Yang, S. P.; Chen, S. R.; Liu, S. W.; Tang, X. Y.; Qin, L.; Qiu, G. H.; Chen, J. X.; Chen, W. H. Platforms Formed from a Three-Dimensional Cu-Based Zwitterionic Metal-Organic Framework and Probe Ss-DNA: Selective Fluorescent Biosensors for Human Immunodeficiency Virus 1 Ds-DNA and Sudan Virus RNA Sequences. *Anal. Chem.* **2015,** *87* (24), 12206–12214. https://doi.org/10.1021/ACS.ANALCHEM.5B03084/SUPPL_FILE/AC5B03084_SI_003.CIF.
38. Miller, S. E.; Teplensky, M. H.; Moghadam, P. Z.; Fairen-Jimenez, D. Metal-Organic Frameworks as Biosensors for Luminescence-Based Detection and Imaging. *Interface Focus* **2016,** *6* (4). https://doi.org/10.1098/RSFS.2016.0027.

39. Zhu, X.; Zheng, H.; Wei, X.; Lin, Z.; Guo, L.; Qiu, B.; Chen, G. Metal–Organic Framework (MOF): A Novel Sensing Platform for Biomolecules. *Chem. Commun.* **2013,** *49* (13), 1276–1278. https://doi.org/10.1039/C2CC36661D.
40. Qin, L.; Lin, L. X.; Fang, Z. P.; Yang, S. P.; Qiu, G. H.; Chen, J. X.; Chen, W. H. A Water-Stable Metal–Organic Framework of a Zwitterionic Carboxylate with Dysprosium: A Sensing Platform for Ebolavirus RNA Sequences. *Chem. Commun.* **2015,** *52* (1), 132–135. https://doi.org/10.1039/C5CC06697B.
41. Zhao, H. Q.; Qiu, G. H.; Liang, Z.; Li, M. M.; Sun, B.; Qin, L.; Yang, S. P.; Chen, W. H.; Chen, J. X. A Zinc(II)-Based Two-Dimensional MOF for Sensitive and Selective Sensing of HIV-1 Ds-DNA Sequences. *Anal. Chim. Acta* **2016,** *922*, 55–63. https://doi.org/10.1016/J.ACA.2016.03.054.
42. Férey, C.; Mellot-Draznieks, C.; Serre, C.; Millange, F.; Dutour, J.; Surblé, S.; Margiolaki, I. A Chromium Terephthalate-Based Solid with Unusually Large Pore Volumes and Surface Area. *Science* **2005,** *309* (5743), 2040–2042. https://doi.org/10.1126/SCIENCE.1116275.
43. Zhang, G. Y.; Zhuang, Y. H.; Shan, D.; Su, G. F.; Cosnier, S.; Zhang, X. J. Zirconium-Based Porphyrinic Metal-Organic Framework (PCN-222): Enhanced Photoelectrochemical Response and Its Application for Label-Free Phosphoprotein Detection. *Anal. Chem.* **2016,** *88* (22), 11207–11212. https://doi.org/10.1021/ACS.ANALCHEM.6B03484.
44. Zhu, C.; Zeng, Z.; Li, H.; Li, F.; Fan, C.; Zhang, H. Single-Layer MoS2-Based Nanoprobes for Homogeneous Detection of Biomolecules. *J. Am. Chem. Soc.* **2013,** *135* (16), 5998–6001. https://doi.org/10.1021/JA4019572.
45. Zhao, S. N.; Wu, L. L.; Feng, J.; Song, S. Y.; Zhang, H. J. An Ideal Detector Composed of a 3D Gd-Based Coordination Polymer for DNA and Hg2+ Ion. *Inorg. Chem. Front.* **2016,** *3* (3), 376–380. https://doi.org/10.1039/C5QI00252D.
46. Serre, C.; Mellot-Draznieks, C.; Surblé, S.; Audebrand, N.; Filinchuk, Y.; Férey, G. Role of Solvent-Host Interactions That Lead to Very Large Swelling of Hybrid Frameworks. *Science* **2007,** *315* (5820), 1828–1831. https://doi.org/10.1126/SCIENCE.1137975.
47. Wang, H. S.; Li, J.; Li, J. Y.; Wang, K.; Ding, Y.; Xia, X. H. Lanthanide-Based Metal-Organic Framework Nanosheets with Unique Fluorescence Quenching Properties for Two-Color Intracellular Adenosine Imaging in Living Cells. *NPG Asia Mater.* **2017,** *9* (3), e354–e354. https://doi.org/10.1038/am.2017.7.
48. Zhang, X.; Yan, T.; Wu, T.; Feng, Y.; Sun, M.; Yan, L.; Du, B.; Wei, Q. Fabrication of Hierarchical MIL-68(In)-NH2/MWCNT/CdS Composites for Constructing Label-Free Photoelectrochemical Tetracycline Aptasensor Platform. *Biosens. Bioelectron.* **2019,** *135*, 88–94. https://doi.org/10.1016/J.BIOS.2019.03.062.
49. Lv, M.; Zhou, W.; Tavakoli, H.; Bautista, C.; Xia, J.; Wang, Z.; Li, X. J. Aptamer-Functionalized Metal-Organic Frameworks (MOFs) for Biosensing. *Biosens. Bioelectron.* **2021,** *176*. https://doi.org/10.1016/J.BIOS.2020.112947.
50. Wang, K.; Li, N.; Zhang, J.; Zhang, Z.; Dang, F. Size-Selective QD@MOF Core-Shell Nanocomposites for the Highly Sensitive Monitoring of Oxidase Activities. *Biosens. Bioelectron.* **2017,** *87*, 339–344. https://doi.org/10.1016/J.BIOS.2016.08.026.
51. Ling, P.; Lei, J.; Zhang, L.; Ju, H. Porphyrin-Encapsulated Metal-Organic Frameworks as Mimetic Catalysts for Electrochemical DNA Sensing via Allosteric Switch of Hairpin DNA. *Anal. Chem.* **2015,** *87* (7), 3957–3963. https://doi.org/10.1021/ACS.ANALCHEM.5B00001.

52. Sheta, S. M.; El-Sheikh, S. M. Nanomaterials and Metal-Organic Frameworks for Biosensing Applications of Mutations of the Emerging Viruses. *Anal. Biochem.* **2022,** *648*. https://doi.org/10.1016/J.AB.2022.114680.
53. Rabiee, N.; Bagherzadeh, M.; Ghasemi, A.; Zare, H.; Ahmadi, S.; Fatahi, Y.; Dinarvand, R.; Rabiee, M.; Ramakrishna, S.; Shokouhimehr, M.; et al. Point-of-Use Rapid Detection of SARS-CoV-2: Nanotechnology-Enabled Solutions for the COVID-19 Pandemic. *Int. J. Mol. Sci.* **2020,** *21* (14), 5126. https://doi.org/10.3390/IJMS21145126.
54. Osman, D. I.; El-Sheikh, S. M.; Sheta, S. M.; Ali, O. I.; Salem, A. M.; Shousha, W. G.; EL-Khamisy, S. F.; Shawky, S. M. Nucleic Acids Biosensors Based on Metal-Organic Framework (MOF): Paving the Way to Clinical Laboratory Diagnosis. *Biosens. Bioelectron.* **2019,** *141*. https://doi.org/10.1016/J.BIOS.2019.111451.
55. Guo, T.; Deng, Q.; Fang, G.; Gu, D.; Yang, Y.; Wang, S. Upconversion Fluorescence Metal-Organic Frameworks Thermo-Sensitive Imprinted Polymer for Enrichment and Sensing Protein. *Biosens. Bioelectron.* **2016,** *79*, 341–346. https://doi.org/10.1016/J.BIOS.2015.12.040.
56. Lyu, F.; Zhang, Y.; Zare, R. N.; Ge, J.; Liu, Z. One-Pot Synthesis of Protein-Embedded Metal-Organic Frameworks with Enhanced Biological Activities. *Nano Lett.* **2014,** *14* (10), 5761–5765. https://doi.org/10.1021/NL5026419.
57. Zhang, G. Y.; Zhuang, Y. H.; Shan, D.; Su, G. F.; Cosnier, S.; Zhang, X. J. Zirconium-Based Porphyrinic Metal-Organic Framework (PCN-222): Enhanced Photoelectrochemical Response and Its Application for Label-Free Phosphoprotein Detection. *Anal. Chem.* **2016,** *88* (22), 11207–11212. https://doi.org/10.1021/ACS.ANALCHEM.6B03484/SUPPL_FILE/AC6B03484_SI_001.PDF.
58. Yi, F. Y.; Chen, D.; Wu, M. K.; Han, L.; Jiang, H. L. Chemical Sensors Based on Metal–Organic Frameworks. *Chempluschem* **2016,** *81* (8), 675–690. https://doi.org/10.1002/CPLU.201600137.
59. Liang, W.; Wied, P.; Carraro, F.; Sumby, C. J.; Nidetzky, B.; Tsung, C. K.; Falcaro, P.; Doonan, C. J. Metal-Organic Framework-Based Enzyme Biocomposites. *Chem. Rev.* **2021,** *121* (3), 1077–1129. https://doi.org/10.1021/ACS.CHEMREV.0C01029/SUPPL_FILE/CR0C01029_SI_008.MP4.
60. Guo, J.; Yang, L.; Gao, Z.; Zhao, C.; Mei, Y.; Song, Y. Y. Insight of MOF Environment-Dependent Enzyme Activity via MOFs-in-Nanochannels Configuration. *ACS Catal.* **2020,** *10* (10), 5949–5958. https://doi.org/10.1021/ACSCATAL.0C00591/SUPPL_FILE/CS0C00591_SI_001.PDF.
61. Xia, H.; Li, N.; Zhong, X.; Jiang, Y. Metal-Organic Frameworks: A Potential Platform for Enzyme Immobilization and Related Applications. *Front. Bioeng. Biotechnol.* **2020,** *8*, 695. https://doi.org/10.3389/FBIOE.2020.00695/BIBTEX.
62. Lyu, F.; Zhang, Y.; Zare, R. N.; Ge, J.; Liu, Z. One-Pot Synthesis of Protein-Embedded Metal-Organic Frameworks with Enhanced Biological Activities. *Nano Lett.* **2014,** *14* (10), 5761–5765. https://doi.org/10.1021/NL5026419/SUPPL_FILE/NL5026419_SI_001.PDF.
63. Hou, C.; Wang, Y.; Ding, Q.; Jiang, L.; Li, M.; Zhu, W.; Pan, D.; Zhu, H.; Liu, M. Facile Synthesis of Enzyme-Embedded Magnetic Metal–Organic Frameworks as a Reusable Mimic Multi-Enzyme System: Mimetic Peroxidase Properties and Colorimetric Sensor. *Nanoscale* **2015,** *7* (44), 18770–18779. https://doi.org/10.1039/C5NR04994F.
64. Hu, Y.; Cheng, H.; Zhao, X.; Wu, J.; Muhammad, F.; Lin, S.; He, J.; Zhou, L.; Zhang, C.; Deng, Y.; et al. Surface-Enhanced Raman Scattering Active Gold Nanoparticles with

Enzyme-Mimicking Activities for Measuring Glucose and Lactate in Living Tissues. *ACS Nano* **2017,** *11* (6), 5558–5566. https://doi.org/10.1021/ACSNANO.7B00905/SUPPL_FILE/NN7B00905_SI_001.PDF.
65. Li, H. Y.; Zhao, S. N.; Zang, S. Q.; Li, J. Functional Metal–Organic Frameworks as Effective Sensors of Gases and Volatile Compounds. *Chem. Soc. Rev.* **2020,** *49* (17), 6364–6401. https://doi.org/10.1039/C9CS00778D.
66. Mao, X.; Liu, S.; Su, B.; Wang, D.; Huang, Z.; Li, J.; Zhang, Y. Luminescent Europium(III)-Organic Framework for Visual and on-Site Detection of Hydrogen Peroxide via a Tablet Computer. *Microchim. Acta* **2020,** *187* (7), 1–11. https://doi.org/10.1007/S00604-020-04379-4/METRICS.
67. Zhang, S. Y.; Shi, W.; Cheng, P.; Zaworotko, M. J. A Mixed-Crystal Lanthanide Zeolite-like Metal-Organic Framework as a Fluorescent Indicator for Lysophosphatidic Acid, a Cancer Biomarker. *J. Am. Chem. Soc.* **2015,** *137* (38), 12203–12206. https://doi.org/10.1021/JACS.5B06929/SUPPL_FILE/JA5B06929_SI_002.CIF.
68. Wang, H. S.; Bao, W. J.; Ren, S. Bin; Chen, M.; Wang, K.; Xia, X. H. Fluorescent Sulfur-Tagged Europium(III) Coordination Polymers for Monitoring Reactive Oxygen Species. *Anal. Chem.* **2015,** *87* (13), 6828–6833. https://doi.org/10.1021/ACS.ANALCHEM.5B01104/SUPPL_FILE/AC5B01104_SI_001.PDF.
69. Wang, Q.; Yang, Y.; Gao, F.; Ni, J.; Zhang, Y.; Lin, Z. Graphene Oxide Directed One-Step Synthesis of Flowerlike Graphene@HKUST-1 for Enzyme-Free Detection of Hydrogen Peroxide in Biological Samples. *ACS Appl. Mater. Interfaces* **2016,** *8* (47), 32477–32487. https://doi.org/10.1021/ACSAMI.6B11965/SUPPL_FILE/AM6B11965_SI_001.PDF.
70. Dai, H.; Lü, W.; Zuo, X.; Zhu, Q.; Pan, C.; Niu, X.; Liu, J.; Chen, H. L.; Chen, X. A Novel Biosensor Based on Boronic Acid Functionalized Metal-Organic Frameworks for the Determination of Hydrogen Peroxide Released from Living Cells. *Biosens. Bioelectron.* **2017,** *95*, 131–137. https://doi.org/10.1016/J.BIOS.2017.04.021.
71. Pérez-Aguirre, R.; Artetxe, B.; Beobide, G.; Castillo, O.; de Pedro, I.; Luque, A.; Pérez-Yáñez, S.; Wuttke, S. Ferromagnetic Supramolecular Metal-Organic Frameworks for Active Capture and Magnetic Sensing of Emerging Drug Pollutants. *Cell Reports Phys. Sci.* **2021,** *2* (5). https://doi.org/10.1016/j.xcrp.2021.100421.
72. Samanta, P.; Desai, A. V.; Sharma, S.; Chandra, P.; Ghosh, S. K. Selective Recognition of Hg2+ Ion in Water by a Functionalized Metal-Organic Framework (MOF) Based Chemodosimeter. *Inorg. Chem.* **2018,** *57* (5), 2360–2364. https://doi.org/10.1021/ACS.INORGCHEM.7B02426/SUPPL_FILE/IC7B02426_SI_001.PDF.
73. Lv, R.; Wang, J.; Zhang, Y.; Li, H.; Yang, L.; Liao, S.; Gu, W.; Liu, X. An Amino-Decorated Dual-Functional Metal–Organic Framework for Highly Selective Sensing of Cr(III) and Cr(VI) Ions and Detection of Nitroaromatic Explosives. *J. Mater. Chem. A* **2016,** *4* (40), 15494–15500. https://doi.org/10.1039/C6TA05965A.
74. Guo, J.; Yang, L.; Gao, Z.; Zhao, C.; Mei, Y.; Song, Y. Y. Insight of MOF Environment-Dependent Enzyme Activity via MOFs-in-Nanochannels Configuration. *ACS Catal.* **2020,** *10* (10), 5949–5958. https://doi.org/10.1021/ACSCATAL.0C00591/SUPPL_FILE/CS0C00591_SI_001.PDF.
75. Della Rocca, J.; Liu, D.; Lin, W. Nanoscale Metal-Organic Frameworks for Biomedical Imaging and Drug Delivery. *Acc. Chem. Res.* **2011,** *44* (10), 957–968. https://doi.org/10.1021/AR200028A/ASSET/IMAGES/MEDIUM/AR-2011-00028A_0013.GIF.

76. Awasthi, G.; Shivgotra, S.; Nikhar, S.; Sundarrajan, S.; Ramakrishna, S.; Kumar, P. Progressive Trends on the Biomedical Applications of Metal Organic Frameworks. *Polymers (Basel).* **2022,** *14* (21), 1–28. https://doi.org/10.3390/polym14214710.
77. Naresh, V.; Lee, N. A Review on Biosensors and Recent Development of Nanostructured Materials-Enabled Biosensors. *Sensors* **2021,** *21* (4), 1109. https://doi.org/10.3390/S21041109.
78. Wang, S.; Chen, Y.; Wang, S.; Li, P.; Mirkin, C. A.; Farha, O. K. DNA-Functionalized Metal-Organic Framework Nanoparticles for Intracellular Delivery of Proteins. *J. Am. Chem. Soc.* **2019,** *141* (6), 2215–2219. https://doi.org/10.1021/JACS.8B12705.
79. Lin, Y.; Huang, Y.; Chen, X. Recent Advances in Metal-Organic Frameworks for Biomacromolecule Sensing. *Chemosens.* **2022,** *10* (10), 412. https://doi.org/10.3390/CHEMOSENSORS10100412.
80. Peng, S.; Liu, M.; Bie, B.; Zhang, Y.; Tang, H.; Sun, Y.; Zhou, X. Multiplexed MicroRNA Detection Using Metal-Organic Framework for Signal Output. *ACS Appl. Bio Mater.* **2020,** *3* (5), 2604–2609. https://doi.org/10.1021/ACSABM.9B01189.
81. Zhang, Y.; Tang, H.; Chen, W.; Zhang, J. Nanomaterials Used in Fluorescence Polarization Based Biosensors. *Int. J. Mol. Sci.* **2022,** *23* (15), 8625. https://doi.org/10.3390/IJMS23158625.
82. Wang, Q.; Astruc, D. State of the Art and Prospects in Metal-Organic Framework (MOF)-Based and MOF-Derived Nanocatalysis. *Chem. Rev.* **2020,** *120* (2), 1438–1511. https://doi.org/10.1021/ACS.CHEMREV.9B00223/ASSET/IMAGES/MEDIUM/CR-2019-00223Z_0061.GIF.
83. Hao, Y. B.; Shao, Z. S.; Cheng, C.; Xie, X. Y.; Zhang, J.; Song, W. J.; Wang, H. S. Regulating Fluorescent Aptamer-Sensing Behavior of Zeolitic Imidazolate Framework (ZIF-8) Platform via Lanthanide Ion Doping. *ACS Appl. Mater. Interfaces* **2019,** *11* (35), 31755–31762. https://doi.org/10.1021/ACSAMI.9B12253/SUPPL_FILE/AM9B12253_SI_001.PDF.
84. Eto, K.; Asada, T.; Arima, K.; Makifuchi, T.; Kimura, H. Brain Hydrogen Sulfide Is Severely Decreased in Alzheimer's Disease. *Biochem. Biophys. Res. Commun.* **2002,** *293* (5), 1485–1488. https://doi.org/10.1016/S0006-291X(02)00422-9.
85. Szabo, C.; Coletta, C.; Chao, C.; Módis, K.; Szczesny, B.; Papapetropoulos, A.; Hellmich, M. R. Tumor-Derived Hydrogen Sulfide, Produced by Cystathionine-β-Synthase, Stimulates Bioenergetics, Cell Proliferation, and Angiogenesis in Colon Cancer. *Proc. Natl. Acad. Sci. USA* **2013,** *110* (30), 12474–12479. https://doi.org/10.1073/PNAS.1306241110.
86. Ma, Y.; Su, H.; Kuang, X.; Li, X.; Zhang, T.; Tang, B. Heterogeneous Nano Metal-Organic Framework Fluorescence Probe for Highly Selective and Sensitive Detection of Hydrogen Sulfide in Living Cells. *Anal. Chem.* **2014,** *86* (22), 11459–11463. https://doi.org/10.1021/AC503622N/SUPPL_FILE/AC503622N_SI_001.PDF.
87. Vikrant, K.; Kumar, V.; Ok, Y. S.; Kim, K. H.; Deep, A. Metal-Organic Framework (MOF)-Based Advanced Sensing Platforms for the Detection of Hydrogen Sulfide. *TrAC Trends Anal. Chem.* **2018,** *105*, 263–281. https://doi.org/10.1016/J.TRAC.2018.05.013.
88. He, C.; Lu, K.; Lin, W. Nanoscale Metal-Organic Frameworks for Real-Time Intracellular PH Sensing in Live Cells. *J. Am. Chem. Soc.* **2014,** *136* (35), 12253–12256. https://doi.org/10.1021/JA507333C/SUPPL_FILE/JA507333C_SI_003.AVI.
89. Tan, J. C.; Saines, P. J.; Bithell, E. G.; Cheetham, A. K. Hybrid Nanosheets of an Inorganic-Organic Framework Material: Facile Synthesis, Structure, and Elastic

Properties. *ACS Nano* **2012,** *6* (1), 615–621. https://doi.org/10.1021/NN204054K/SUPPL_FILE/NN204054K_SI_002.CIF.

90. Furukawa, H.; Gándara, F.; Zhang, Y. B.; Jiang, J.; Queen, W. L.; Hudson, M. R.; Yaghi, O. M. Water Adsorption in Porous Metal-Organic Frameworks and Related Materials. *J. Am. Chem. Soc.* **2014,** *136* (11), 4369–4381. https://doi.org/10.1021/JA500330A/SUPPL_FILE/JA500330A_SI_010.PDF.
91. Rieter, W. J.; Taylor, K. M. L.; An, H.; Lin, W.; Lin, W. Nanoscale Metal-Organic Frameworks as Potential Multimodal Contrast Enhancing Agents. *J. Am. Chem. Soc.* **2006,** *128* (28), 9024–9025. https://doi.org/10.1021/JA0627444/SUPPL_FILE/JA0627444SI20060606_103648.PDF.
92. Isobe, T.; Arai, Y.; Yanagida, S.; Matsushita, S.; Nakajima, A. Solvothermal Preparation and Gas Permeability of an IRMOF-3 Membrane. *Microporous Mesoporous Mater.* **2017,** *241*, 218–225. https://doi.org/10.1016/J.MICROMESO.2016.12.031.
93. Wang, C.; Volotskova, O.; Lu, K.; Ahmad, M.; Sun, C.; Xing, L.; Lin, W. Synergistic Assembly of Heavy Metal Clusters and Luminescent Organic Bridging Ligands in Metal-Organic Frameworks for Highly Efficient X-Ray Scintillation. *J. Am. Chem. Soc.* **2014,** *136* (17), 6171–6174. https://doi.org/10.1021/JA500671H.
94. Dekrafft, K. E.; Boyle, W. S.; Burk, L. M.; Zhou, O. Z.; Lin, W. Zr- and Hf-Based Nanoscale Metal–Organic Frameworks as Contrast Agents for Computed Tomography. *J. Mater. Chem.* **2012,** *22* (35), 18139–18144. https://doi.org/10.1039/C2JM32299D.
95. Wang, Y. M.; Liu, W.; Yin, X. B. Self-Limiting Growth Nanoscale Coordination Polymers for Fluorescence and Magnetic Resonance Dual-Modality Imaging. *Adv. Funct. Mater.* **2016,** *26* (46), 8463–8470. https://doi.org/10.1002/ADFM.201602925.
96. Fox, M. D.; Raichle, M. E. Spontaneous Fluctuations in Brain Activity Observed with Functional Magnetic Resonance Imaging. *Nat. Rev. Neurosci.* **2007,** *8* (9), 700–711. https://doi.org/10.1038/nrn2201.
97. Sereno, M. I.; Dale, A. M.; Reppas, J. B.; Kwong, K. K.; Belliveau, J. W.; Brady, T. J.; Rosen, B. R.; Tootell, R. B. H. Borders of Multiple Visual Areas in Humans Revealed by Functional Magnetic Resonance Imaging. *Science* **1995,** *268* (5212), 889–893. https://doi.org/10.1126/SCIENCE.7754376.
98. Chowdhury, M. A. Metal-Organic-Frameworks for Biomedical Applications in Drug Delivery, and as MRI Contrast Agents. *J. Biomed. Mater. Res. A* **2017,** *105* (4), 1184–1194. https://doi.org/10.1002/JBM.A.35995.
99. Rocca, J. Della; Lin, W. Nanoscale Metal–Organic Frameworks: Magnetic Resonance Imaging Contrast Agents and Beyond. *Eur. J. Inorg. Chem.* **2010,** *2010* (24), 3725–3734. https://doi.org/10.1002/EJIC.201000496.
100. Liu, Y.; Jiang, T.; Liu, Z. Metal-Organic Frameworks for Bioimaging: Strategies and Challenges. *Nanotheranostics* **2022,** *6* (2), 143–160. https://doi.org/10.7150/NTNO.63458.
101. Liu, D.; He, C.; Poon, C.; Lin, W. Theranostic Nanoscale Coordination Polymers for Magnetic Resonance Imaging and Bisphosphonate Delivery. *J. Mater. Chem. B* **2014,** *2* (46), 8249–8255. https://doi.org/10.1039/C4TB00751D.
102. Zhao, H. X.; Zou, Q.; Sun, S. K.; Yu, C.; Zhang, X.; Li, R. J.; Fu, Y. Y. Theranostic Metal–Organic Framework Core–Shell Composites for Magnetic Resonance Imaging and Drug Delivery. *Chem. Sci.* **2016,** *7* (8), 5294–5301. https://doi.org/10.1039/C6SC01359G.

103. Pan, D.; Schmieder, A. H.; Wickline, S. A.; Lanza, G. M. Manganese-Based MRI Contrast Agents: Past, Present and Future. *Tetrahedron* **2011,** *67* (44), 8431–8444. https://doi.org/10.1016/J.TET.2011.07.076.
104. Chowdhuri, A. R.; Singh, T.; Ghosh, S. K.; Sahu, S. K. Carbon Dots Embedded Magnetic Nanoparticles @Chitosan @Metal Organic Framework as a Nanoprobe for PH Sensitive Targeted Anticancer Drug Delivery. *ACS Appl. Mater. Interfaces* **2016,** *8* (26), 16573–16583. https://doi.org/10.1021/ACSAMI.6B03988/SUPPL_FILE/AM6B03988_SI_001.PDF.
105. Ray Chowdhuri, A.; Bhattacharya, D.; Sahu, S. K. Magnetic Nanoscale Metal Organic Frameworks for Potential Targeted Anticancer Drug Delivery, Imaging and as an MRI Contrast Agent. *Dalt. Trans.* **2016,** *45* (7), 2963–2973. https://doi.org/10.1039/C5DT03736K.
106. Sun, W.; Li, S.; Tang, G.; Luo, Y.; Ma, S.; Sun, S.; Ren, J.; Gong, Y.; Xie, C. Recent Progress of Nanoscale Metal-Organic Frameworks in Cancer Theranostics and the Challenges of Their Clinical Application. *Int. J. Nanomed.* **2019,** *14*, 10195. https://doi.org/10.2147/IJN.S230524.
107. Zimpel, A.; Preiß, T.; Röder, R.; Engelke, H.; Ingrisch, M.; Peller, M.; Rädler, J. O.; Wagner, E.; Bein, T.; Lächelt, U.; et al. Imparting Functionality to MOF Nanoparticles by External Surface Selective Covalent Attachment of Polymers. *Chem. Mater.* **2016,** *28* (10), 3318–3326. https://doi.org/10.1021/ACS.CHEMMATER.6B00180/SUPPL_FILE/CM6B00180_SI_001.PDF.
108. Wang, D.; Zhou, J.; Chen, R.; Shi, R.; Zhao, G.; Xia, G.; Li, R.; Liu, Z.; Tian, J.; Wang, H.; et al. Controllable Synthesis of Dual-MOFs Nanostructures for PH-Responsive Artemisinin Delivery, Magnetic Resonance and Optical Dual-Model Imaging-Guided Chemo/Photothermal Combinational Cancer Therapy. *Biomaterials* **2016,** *100*, 27–40. https://doi.org/10.1016/J.BIOMATERIALS.2016.05.027.
109. Chen, X.; Zhang, M.; Li, S.; Li, L.; Zhang, L.; Wang, T.; Yu, M.; Mou, Z.; Wang, C. Facile Synthesis of Polypyrrole@metal–Organic Framework Core–Shell Nanocomposites for Dual-Mode Imaging and Synergistic Chemo-Photothermal Therapy of Cancer Cells. *J. Mater. Chem. B* **2017,** *5* (9), 1772–1778. https://doi.org/10.1039/C6TB03218D.

CHAPTER 7

Synthesis, Properties, and Biomedical Application of Platinum and Palladium-based Nanoparticles

MAHESH V. KAMBLE, SACHIN V. OTARI, and KIRAN D. PAWAR

School of Nanoscience and Biotechnology, Shivaji University, Kolhapur, Maharashtra, India

ABSTRACT

Metals have been utilized in medicine for a very long time, since different processed metals, such as gold, silver, mercury lead, copper, etc., were used to treat various disease conditions. In antiquity, both platinum (Pt) and palladium (Pd) also been used to cure a number of diseases. Recently, Pt and Pd considered as a crucial ingredient in many medications, especially those that are used to treat cancer. For instance, chemotherapy for cancer included the use of substances containing Pt, such as cisplatin, oxaliplatin, and carboplatin. Similarly, Pd has an indispensable role in the treatment of cancer and other disorders. Pt and Pd are utilized in the medical industry for a wide range of purposes, namely, construction of medical implants and devices, due to their remarkable qualities, including biocompatibility, inertness within the body, durability, electroconductivity, high corrosion resistance, oxidation resistance, fine machinability, radiopaque properties, and radiopacity. Moreover, Pt and Pd have special qualities that make them the ideal materials for building compact, durable structures that can resist extreme stress without breaking or deforming. Therefore, research is increasingly concentrating on creating novel PtNPs and PdNPs with distinctive optical, electronic, and biomedical properties that can be used in various biomedical applications.

Metals in Medicine, Volume 1: Metals for Tissue Engineering and Pharmaceutical Applications.
Sonali Sundram, Rishabha Malviya, and GSN Koteswara Rao

7.1 INTRODUCTION

From ancient time, various processed metals were used in the preparation of medicines to treat various illness conditions, namely, mercury, gold, silver, lead, zinc, copper, etc. Before being utilized in medicine, these metals underwent incredibly complex manufacturing procedures that were documented in Ayurvedic texts, particularly Rasashastra.[1] At that time, the use of various metals in pharmaceutical formulations to treat a range of illness problems was referred to as "metals in medicine" in its broadest sense. For instance, one of the earliest written accounts of the use of metals in medicine found in Egyptian book written by Ebers papyrus in 1500 BCE describes the treatments which include the application of topical iron-rich meat to wounds and the use of copper for headaches.[2] Platinum (Pt) and palladium (Pd)-based materials have been utilized for a very long time and a variety of applications in biomedical research, dating back to antiquity. However, in the modern era, the use of Pt and Pd in biomedical applications started late compared to other metals. However, with the advancement of knowledge regarding Pt and Pd, both the metals are currently being used in various fields and technologies at all research scales, from macro to nano to discover and develop new formulations and technologies. After that, it is now widely accepted as a result of the development of nanoscience that metal in its nano form has many advantages over its macro form.

The efficacy of Pt and Pd can be improved by creating metal nanoparticles (NPs) of respective metals.[3] For instance, platinum nanoparticles (PtNPs) and Pt nanoparticles (PdNPs) have several advantages over large metal molecules in applications, such as the capacity to create materials that are more robust, lightweight, and durable. Additionally, the utility and effectiveness of metals are increased when nanomaterial composed of different metals is used as alloy. Such NP-based alloys material are excellent materials can be used in engineering as ideal materials for a variety of uses. Many PtNPs and PdNPs with various special features have currently been created by researchers. Researchers are working hard to create combinations of PtNPs and PdNPs and also with other metal NPs to get benefit from the special qualities of both PtNPs and PdNPs metals as well as other metals.[4] Currently, a variety of metal alloys are employed for biomedical purposes, including stainless steel, cobalt–chromium alloys, amalgam, titanium-based alloys, etc. As a result, PtNPs and PdNPs are investigated by the medical sector as a potential next-generation biomaterial for use in therapeutic and diagnostic purposes.

Numerous PtNPs and PdNPs have also been found to possess therapeutic benefits, including antioxidant, antibacterial, and anticancer activities, making them appropriate for use as metallodrugs in the treatment of several illnesses.[5–7] Researchers are actively striving to synthesize different combinations of metal and metal oxides NPs with the intention of taking advantage of the rare possibility of gaining the properties of all the metals involved.[4]

Many PtNPs and PdNPs have also been discovered to have therapeutic advantages, such as antioxidant, antibacterial, and anticancer activity, making them appropriate for use as metallodrugs in the treatment of a range of ailments.[5–7]

Recently, Pt and Pd and their alloys attracted growing interest because of their distinctive physicochemical features such as chemical permanence, high magnetization, curie temperature, and X-ray absorption, which make them useful in functional applications such as nanocarriers, nanozymes, and nanosensors. Moreover, PtNPs and PdNPs are known for demonstrating a variety of biomedical applications, including photoablation treatment, targeted medication delivery, hyperthermia, antibacterial agents, and bioimaging and biosensing, among others. Furthermore, PtNPs and PdNPs both display excellent constancy, solubility, controlled release, amassing, and specific targeting, and neither pose any toxicological hazards to people. Utilizing PtNPs and PdNPs may allow great expansion of therapeutic and theranostic platforms to simplifying, speeding up, and reducing the invasiveness of the diagnostic processes. PtNPs and PdNPs may also be used more effectively in biomedicine as nanotheranostic entities as novel nanocomposites with multifunctional modalities are created.[8]

In this chapter, we briefly discussed biomedical applications of PtNPs and PdNPs, along with this we discussed various methods of PtNPs and PdNPs synthesis. We also discussed their biological applications, toxicological implications, and utilization in combination therapy.

7.2 METHODS OF SYNTHESIS OF PTNPS AND PDNPs

The synthesis methods are essential to obtain NPs with desideratum features. In general, for the synthesis of PtNPs and PdNPs, top–down and bottom–up methods are used (Fig 7.1). Top–down approaches involves the production of NPs from the large metal through mechanical breakdown using physical or mechanochemical methods. Here, the processes involved in this approach are time-consuming and require of sophisticated infrastructure. The main benefit of this strategy is we can control the size and shape of NPs during the synthesis process. Several physical methods such as laser ablation, photolithography, electroexplosion, sputtering, electrolithography, motorized milling techniques, and plasma etching follow the top–down approach in the formation of NP. In bottom–up approaches, molecules are assembled to form nanomaterials. This approach includes methods such as chemical precipitation, oxidation–reduction, sol–gel techniques, polymerization, chemical vapor deposition (CVD), thermolysis, flame spraying synthesis, and biogenic synthesis. Currently, various physical, chemical, and biological methods are utilized for the formation of PtNPs and PdNPs.

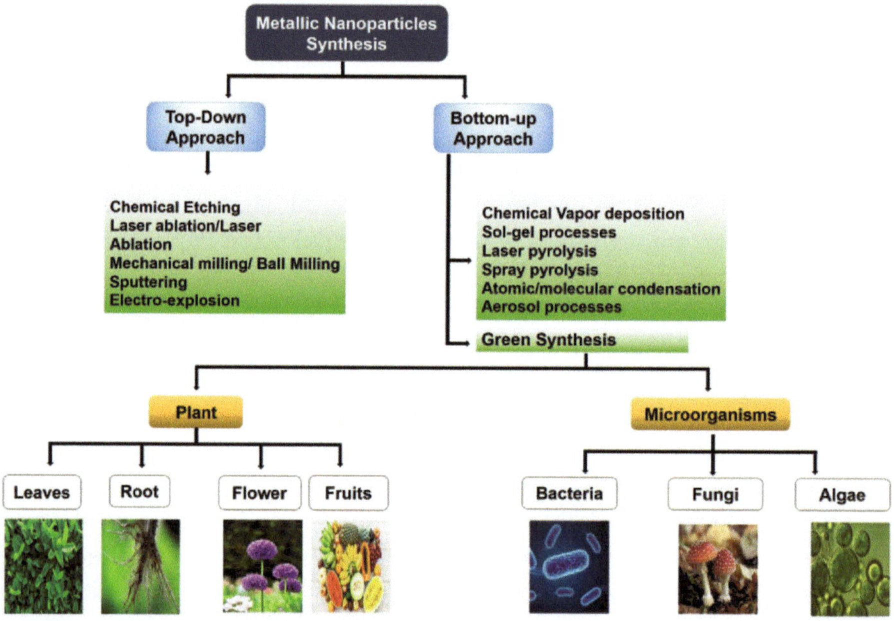

FIGURE 7.1 Methods of metal NP synthesis.

Source: Adapted from Ref. [9]

7.2.1 PHYSICAL METHODS

The physical methods are being used by industrial-scale production of the PtNPs and PdNPs which, in general, require sophisticated and expensive instrumental infrastructures that require high electricity, heat, and pressure. The less or no use of deadly chemicals is the major advantage of the physical methods. Physical processes such as melt mixing, ball milling, sputter deposition, laser ablation, microwave irradiation, arc discharge, sonochemical reduction vapor deposition, and flame pyrolysis are all available. Over the past two decades, laser bombardment of metal solid surfaces technique has been popular for the synthesis of a wide variety of metal NPs for producing NPs in solvents.[10] several attempts have been made to synthesize PtNPs and PdNPs in water using a laser ablation process where the stable, colloidal, and uniformed size NPs are produced using solid Pt and Pd metal surfaces.[11,12] plasma sputtering is another physical method employed for the synthesis of PtNPs and PdNPs where a pulsed power supply is used to create plasma applying special waveforms of voltage and current. Also, synthesis of both metal NPs was performed on the solid surface or NPs thin films as well as in the solvents.[13–18] The physical synthesis of organic and inorganic NPs from bulk materials to smaller ones has long been done using the milling method.[19] The inert gas condensation (ICG) method is also implied for the synthesis of metal NPs where the inert gas-filled vacuum chamber is utilized for the evaporation of metals involving the inter collision of gas atoms and evaporated metal atoms leads to the formation of crystals of the metal ions due to loss of kinetic energy in the liquid energy. There are very studies involved in the formation of PtNPs, PdNPs, and alloys of both NPs using the ICG method as the method involves sophisticated instrumentation and critical expertise for large-scale production.[20]

7.2.2 CHEMICAL SYNTHESIS

The chemical synthesis of PtNPs and PdNPs has been the most common and followed synthesis route to get the desired forms and size of NPs. Aside from the cost of the metal precursors and reducing agents, this method has several advantages, including ease of functionalization, high stability, and reduced polydispersity. It can also be done at room temperature and pressure with only a few sophisticated infrastructures. The most common chemical NPs synthesis methods are the sol–gel technique, pyrolysis, microemulsion, hydrothermal, and CVD. The nucleation reaction occurring during the reduction of the metal precursor led to the formation of thermodynamically stable nanostructures. The uncontrolled chemical reaction often forms aggregated nanostructures. The surfactants or capping agents are used in the chemical reduction process along with reducing agents to avoid the assemblage of NPs. The appropriate ratio of the capping agent, reducing agent and precursors can form NPs of uniform shapes and sizes. The most often used chemical process for producing PtNPs and PdNPs is chemical reduction, which involves reducing agents such as hydrazine hydrate,[21,22] Sodium borohydride,[23,24] trisodium citrate,[25,26] formic acid,[27,28] and potassium bitartrate.[29] Other chemical methods, such as solvothermal,[30,31] emulsion process,[32,33] chemical vapor accumulation,[34,35] sonochemical,[36,37] electrochemical deposition process[38] photochemical process,[39,40] coprecipitation,[41] etc. The abovementioned synthesis processes have been demonstrated for the creation of alloys of Pd and PtNPs. Although chemical synthesis is economical compared to physical one, the use and generation of toxic chemicals or gases are the major disadvantages that encourage investigators to follow the green chemistry approach for PtNPs and PdNPs synthesis.

7.2.3 BIOLOGICAL SYNTHESIS

Biological-mediated synthesis has gained remarkable attention over the past few decades which has proved to follow a green chemistry approach with no use or release of toxic chemicals during and after the synthesis process. The nontoxic, simple, economic, rapid, and facile nature of the biological route of synthesis is the major advantage compared to physical and chemical methods. Several biomaterials including plant part extracts, microorganisms, proteins, enzymes, and peptides have been demonstrated which can be useful in the biosynthesis of PtNPs and PdNPs. Li et al. reported the synthesis of PtNPs with varying sizes ranging from 1.73 to 3.54 nm using selected peptides where the structural features of the nanocrystals can be controlled through peptide selection.[42] The PdNPs synthesis on peptide synthesized using arginine as a building block is also documented.[43] One report demonstrated the regulation of PtNP synthesis with the regulation of protein expression in *Escherichia coli* forming 2–3 nm sized, uniform PtNPs.

Among the various biomaterials, synthesis using plant extracts is the most explored biosynthesis method for various metal and metal oxide NPs due to the ease of method, abundance availability of biomaterials, and requirement of ambient temperature and pressure. Several plant component extracts, including those from fruits, leaves, seeds, and other plant parts, have been used to synthesize PtNPs from diverse plant species.[44,45] For the synthesis of PdNPs, the leaf extract of plant species, for example, *Sapium sebiferum*,[46] *Gymnema sylvestre*,[47] *Glycine max* (Soybean), *Filicium decipiens*,[48] and for the synthesis of PtNPs, *Diopyros kaki*,[49] *Bacopa monnieri*,[50] *Combretum erythrophyllum*,[51] *Tragia involucrate*,[52] and other plant species have been utilized successfully. Similarly, aqueous seed extracts of plant species,

Peganum harmala L.,[53] *Phyllanthus emblica*,[54] *Annona squamosa*,[55] *Nigella sativa L.*, and *Coffea arabica*[56] (Bogireddy et al., 2021) are shown to have potential to synthesize PtNPs and PdNPs which are further utilized for the biomedical applications. In some studies, fruit extracts are also demonstrated for the synthesis of PtNPs and PdNPs.[57–59] The composites and bimetallic NPs of PtNPs and PdNPs are also synthesized using plant materials with Fe_3O_4, CuO, TiO_2, Au NPs, etc.[60,61] The biomolecules such as flavonoids, alkaloids, terpenoids, proteins, peptides, enzymes, and carbohydrates in various plant part extracts not only have been shown to possess reducing abilities but also act as functionalizing and stabilizing agents forming stable and uniform structured nanostructures.

Microbial synthesis is another biological synthesis method employed under the green chemistry approach where microorganisms (bacteria, algae, and fungi) and their cell-free extracts are used as reducing agents of metal ions.[62] Bloch and coauthors have collected the information in form review for intra- and extracellular synthesis of PtNPs where various microbial species such as *Acinetobacter*, *Acetobacter*, *Desulfovibrio*, *Escherichia*, *Plectonema*, *Calothrix*, *Pseudomonas*, *Shewanella*, *Streptomyces*, *Vibrio*, *Sporosarcina*, *Kocuria*, sulfate reducing bacteria.[16] Similarly, extracellular synthesis PdNPs is also demonstrated using a wide range of microbial species, for example, *Shewanella loihica*,[63] *Shewanella oneidensis*,[64] *Geobacter sulfurreducens*,[65] *Bacillus thuringiensis*,[66] *Citrobacter*,[67] *Chlorella vulgaris*,[68] *Agaricus bisporus*,[69] *Desulfovibriode sulfuricans*, and *Bacillus benzeovorans* are also shown to synthesize PdNPs intracellularly where the electron microscopy studies revealed cytoplasmic accumulation of PdNPs.[70] The metal ions reduction by bacterial cell membrane proteins, cytochrome, and cytoplasmic enzymes (hydrogenase) to create PtNPs and PdNPs has been explained by a number of different methods.[9]

7.3 STRUCTURAL AND OPTICAL PROPERTIES OF PTNPs AND PDNPs

It is crucial to have a deeper understanding of the nature, fate, and behavior of NPs, because, it affects the structural, physical, chemical, and optical properties of metal nanomaterials. Every industry, including the biomedical one, has a wide range of practical uses for NPs of various forms, sizes, and characteristics. The structural features of NPs' size, shape, crystallinity, surface topography, specific surface area, size distribution, aggregation state, and other factors are only a few of the ones that are now being examined more extensively.[71] Moreover, it is reported that metal has unique size-dependent properties at the nanoscale, and nanotechnology offers the chance to regulate the production of NPs with preferred sizes and properties using physical, chemical, and biological processes discussed in detail in the aforementioned sections. Therefore, efforts were done to give information regarding structural and optical features of PtNPs and PdNPs and their applications.

7.3.1 STRUCTURAL PROPERTIES

It is now well accepted that all of the optical, electrical, catalytic, and thermal properties of NPs largely depend on their size, shape, and composition.[72] Studies also suggest that the size and structural characteristics of NP affect its surface characteristics, which are crucial for drug delivery.[73] Also, the manufacturing processes and reducing agents used to produce them have a considerable impact on their structural properties and composition. At present, multiple methods and factors were identified, which can affect size and shape of PtNPs and PdNPs. In general, many geometrical shapes, including spheres, tetrahedrons, cubes, octahedrons, decahedrons, dodecahedrons, truncated octahedrons, cuboctahedrons, and icosahedrons, are displayed by PtNPs and PdNPs.[74] Different geometrical shapes have different atomic arrangements leads to variation in properties toward the same application. It is also widely recognized that dwindle in the interatomic Pt–Pt distance, improves the dissociative chemisorption of oxygen atoms, which has a positive influence on the catalytic activity in oxygen reduction reactions. In 2009, Z. Bayindir examined the effects of PtNP's surface and size on its electrical behavior.[75] Additionally, it is feasible to alter the electrical characteristics of PtNPs and PdNPs by altering their surface shape, particle size, and alloying content.

When considering metallic catalysts, Pt is a frequent component.[76] Pd also has specific qualities that are typically essential as catalysts.[77] Both metals are more expensive than gold, though. Consequently, using an alloy of Pt and Pd with another metal is one feasible technique to lower the cost of products. Additionally, nanoalloy displays peculiar physicochemical characteristics that differ from those of the bulk substance or each of its component's parts. PtNPs are an excellent example; they are stable and useful for catalysis, and their catalytic reactions heavily depend on the surface structure. By controlling, the way how the elements combine together helps to precisely tune its physicochemical properties.

7.3.2 OPTICAL PROPERTIES

NPs' optical properties, such as absorption, transmission, reflection, and light emission, can be used for a variety of purposes, such as biosensing, solar cells, photocatalysis, imaging, and light emission and detection.[78] By adjusting its shape, size, and surface functionality, a variety of optical effects can be created. Also, the type, size, or form of them might affect the color they generate.[79] For instance, 25 nm diameter spherical gold NPs appear green, while those between 100 and 200 nm appear orange. E. Gharibshahi in 2017 made size-controlled PtNPs using the gamma radiolytic synthesis technique to examine the effects of size variation on optical properties.[80] Also, it is well known that the optical features of nanomaterials are influenced by their intrinsic electrical structure. And, the surface plasma resonance effect is responsible for the color seen in nanomaterials, and the relationship between color and particle size may be depicted mathematically.[81] Optical properties such as emission and adsorption occur when an electron switches between two states. Additionally, this change in the dimension of the electronic structure of NPs caused the electron to transition between the two states.

Moreover, the quantum effect property of PtNPs and PdNPs made them suitable to use as semiconducting materials, because they provide zero-dimensional advanced materials due to their extremely diminutive size and can be used in various optical devices and computing applications. Y Chen in 2022, used *Bacillus megaterium* to create PdNPs, which were then examined for their optical characteristics and their effect on other applications.[66] They found that the antibacterial capabilities of the PdNPs were greatly enhanced by the high photothermal conversion of particles under NIR irradiation. Metal NPs' optical properties are also employed in dye remediation, where dye degradation is facilitated by the photodegradation activity of NPs. In 2022, Wei Zhang created PdNPs embedded in nutshells, utilized them as visible-light-responsive photocatalysts, and researched the removal of nitrogen oxide (NO) from the same.[82] It was discovered that nutshells with PdNPs implanted in them exhibited the highest photocatalytic activity with reduced NO elimination of up to 58%, making them suitable for usage as semiconductor material.

7.4 BIOMEDICAL APPLICATION OF PTNPs AND PDNPs

PtNPs and PdNPs are being used in the medical field for a variety of applications (Fig. 7.2), each of which has been discussed in detail in the following.

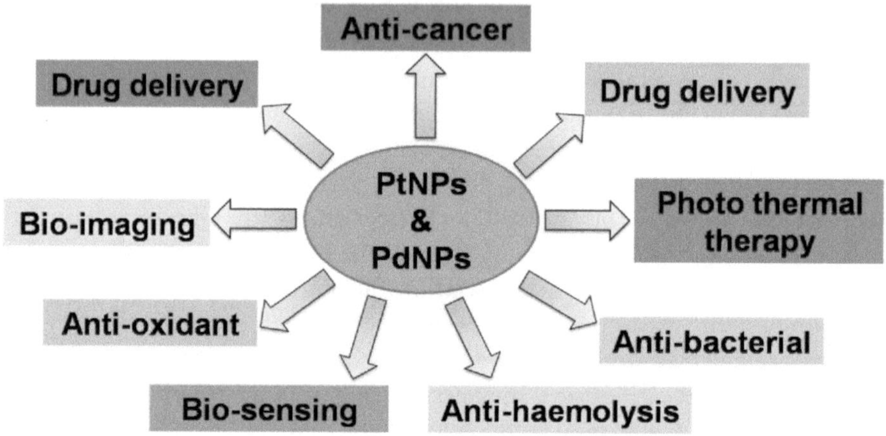

FIGURE 7.2 Various applications of PtNPs and PdNPs in the medical field.

7.4.1 *IN BIOIMAGING*

Bioimaging is an important process of visualizing organs, tissue, subcellular structures, entire cell, and their activity at the molecular and cellular levels during various biological and pathological processes in a real-time.[83] Bioimaging is central to medical treatment since it provides a noninvasive diagnosis of diseases and other disorders without being intrusive and allows medical professionals to assess the human body and organs through noninvasive means. Presently, various bioimaging techniques are used in medical diagnosis such as X-rays, computer tomography (CT scan), thermal imaging, hyperspectral imaging, magnetic resonance imaging (MRI), ultrasounds, endoscopies, tactile imaging, etc. All of the imaging systems operate on the same core premise: the body or body part to be diagnosed is passed through a wave beam that transmits or reflects radiation, and a detector records this change in radiation pattern to produce an interpretable pattern. The sources used in all bioimaging methods include light, electrons, ultrasound, fluorescence, X-rays, and magnetic resonance. In addition to that, several fluorescent probes such as organic dyes, quantum dots, fluorescent proteins, carbon dots, lanthanides, etc. are important parts of effective bioimaging. For the past few decades, number of metal particles have been used as a probe in bioimaging for successful bioimaging because of having unique fluorophore properties. For instance, in the early 20th century, patients receiving X-rays were given barium sulfate orally.[84]

Recently, the use of noble metals such as Pt and Pd attracted the huge interest of researchers for bioimaging due to their optical, catalytic, and thermal properties.[85] In addition, it possesses several physiochemical qualities, including high solubility, stability, and flexibility. Also, PtNPs and PdNPs showed strong relationship with electronic and structural characteristics which make them the ideal fluorophores for imaging.[86] At present, several PtNPs and PdNPs with different sizes and properties have been synthesized by numerous researchers using various methods.

In terms of bioimaging, Pt and its NPs are currently utilized mostly as fluorescent probes. Different fluorescent PtNPs are already being used for bioimaging of cell lines, and some findings suggest that PtNPs have lower cytotoxicity than conventional probes.[87] For instance, Chen in 2015 synthesized PtNPs with fluorescent properties which used in vivo fluorescence imaging for precise monitoring of tumor cells helps in early detection.[88] Also, Pasha et al., in 2016 synthesized water-soluble Pt complexes which give strong green luminescence in solution and can be employed in bioimaging.[89] This Pt complex also demonstrated cell membrane penetration in both cancer cells and normal cells. In 2016, Pasha et al. developed water-soluble Pt composites that exhibit potent green fluorescence in solution and can be used for bioimaging. Additionally, they noticed that produced Pt complex penetrated cell membranes in both normal and cancerous cells and cell membrane penetration of Pt complex's is more in cancerous cells than normal cells and can be used in bioimaging to study cancerous cell. Additionally, PtNPs, are simple to utilize in protein marking experiments by using functionalize PtNPs with antibodies, which strengthens the electron signal when paired with diaminobenzindine (DAB) and osmium tetroxide. Also, fluorophore PtNPs probes can be utilized in Correlative light and electron microscopy (CLEM) bioimaging. However, conventional Pt fluorophores used for bioimaging have some drawbacks such as they are frequently hampered by low photostability, quick photobleaching, and high plasma protein binding rates, making them unsuitable for long-term bioimaging. Also, the radiopaque properties of PtNPs and PdNPs assist in obtaining clearly visible X-ray images, enabling medical professionals to track the location of the device inside the body while administering treatment.[90]

Similar to Pt, Pd is getting a lot of attention from researchers who are interested in bioimaging because of its important characteristics, which include excellent physicochemical properties, namely, catalytic, electrical, physical, mechanical, and optical capabilities.[91,92] Additionally, PdNp-based materials exhibit substantial near-infrared (NIR) absorption, which have excellent photothermal stability and photothermal conversion ability, which make them a crucial component of bioimaging.[93] PdNp-based materials have emerged as leading contenders for bioimaging by taking advantage of their specific characteristics. PdNPs have, however, been employed in very few studies compared to other metals for usage in the biomedical field, and of those, they are mostly used in bioimaging as fluorophore probes.

Recently, by using the intrinsic optical feature of PdNPs and PdNPs-based photoacoustic agent were developed and studied for early tumor diagnostics, revealing PdNPs as potential photoacoustic agents for bioimaging.[94] Nie et al. PdNPs' use in cancer PA imaging was first established by Nie et al. in 2014.[95] Also, PdNPs are generally promising candidates for bioimaging of cell lines because their optical absorption, which varies with size but is mostly centered in the NIR range, is size dependent.

7.4.2 IN THERAPEUTICS

Numerous NP-based therapeutic treatments are now being developed for various diseases and medical disorders for the prevention, treatment, or mitigation of a disease condition in humans. Recently, the usage of PtNPs and PdNPs in the development of different medicinal formulations has been steadily rising. PtNPs and PdNPs-based materials are reported to have good therapeutic applications, such as anti-tumor, antioxidant, and antibacterial agents. Also, their unique photothermal properties can be employed in the treatment of cancer as photothermal agent. PtNPs and PdNPs are innovative classes of chemotherapeutics that have just recently been used in a few studies to diagnose and treat various malignancies. Furthermore, PtNPs and PdNPs showed certain physicochemical characteristics that allow the medicine to enter the systemic circulation and target a specific organ or tissue in the body. This allows for the avoidance of side effects by limiting drug exposure to nontarget sites, making PtNPs and PdNPs ideal drug-delivery agents. Additionally, cisplatin drug-loaded PtNPs and PdNPs had excellent therapeutic benefits and were successful in overcoming cisplatin resistance.[96] However, because of the lack of comprehensive understanding and the necessity for additional research, PdNPs and PdNPs have not yet been used effectively in therapeutic fields. Therefore, it is important to know how cells react to NPs and by what mechanism since certain physicochemical characteristics of nanomaterials may offer potential dangers to human health.

Due to the ability of Pt ions to bind with DNA and hinder replication, PtNPs have a more potent cytotoxic impact and may be employed in cancer therapy.[97] The surface functionalization characteristics of nanotherapeutics, which boost solubility, biocompatibility, and the potential for precise targeting, have been shown in several investigations to result in higher desired effects than those of traditional medications. Bioactive substances such as antibodies, biocompatible polymers, peptides, and other biomolecules can be used to fictionalize PtNPs. Researchers recently demonstrated that functionalized PtNPs selectively affect cancer cells via particular routes.[98] Due to their concentration at the site of the tumor, they can also enhance radiation. Moreover, illness diagnosis has been done with PtNPs. When compared to other metals employed in therapy, PdNPs have superior photostability and a better capacity for light sensitization; as a result, they require less laser power density. Additionally, they are capable of converting light into heat. Researchers hypothesized that PdNPs would be helpful in the treatment of cancer after discovering that they could stop the cell death caused by laser irradiation. PdNPs can also act as a platform for combination therapy with follow-up response monitoring, and they have a significant impact on the development of new strategies for drug delivery in the fight against cancer. For instance, Pd nanoparticles coated with doxorubicin (DOX) are suggested as a potential cancer treatment.[99]

To develop nanotherapeutics using green methods, Q Ma et al., 2018 conducted experiments and obtained PtNPs with dynamic light scattering properties which can be used in various treatments.[100] PdNPs are a viable option for photothermal therapy. PdNPs have not, however, yet been effectively used in therapeutic sectors. PdNPs are a viable option for photothermal therapy. S. D. Brown et al., 2010 were able to create Pt NPs with dynamic light-scattering capabilities that may be used in a variety of treatments to create nanotherapies utilizing environmentally friendly techniques.[101] Photothermal properties are also observed in PtNPs and PdNPs which can be used in photothermal therapy.[102] However, PdNPs still have not been practically exploited in the therapeutic fields but can be used in the future after further research.

7.4.3 DRUG-DELIVERY APPLICATIONS

In recent years, engineered NPs attracting interest as a potential therapeutic agent to overcome the limitations of conventional pharmacological treatments due to their controlled drug delivery and intracellular trafficking, target specificity or cell/tissue-specific targeting, and organelle-specific transport, less toxicity.[103,104] Nonetheless, as a nanoscale delivery vehicle, NPs promise higher stability and solubility of encapsulated drugs and their release across the biomembrane with effective circulation times.[105] Currently, gold, silver, and iron nanostructures are currently the subject of much research in the biomedical sector; several of these studies have advanced them into clinical application.[106] To deal with the variety of patients and their disease states, this aids in the construction of customized or personalized NPs-mediated drug-delivery systems. Recent research has revealed that PdNPs and PdNPs offer superior physicochemical features to those of other materials, including strong thermal and chemical stability, outstanding photocatalytic activity, electrical properties, and optical qualities.[107] PtNPs and PdNPs also have the benefit of having a large variety of shapes and sizes that can be coated with various biopolymers to produce NPs with a variety of properties.[107,108]

Recent research has examined the usefulness of PtNPs as a chemotherapeutic delivery mechanism, particularly for solid malignancies including bone marrow, bladder, and testicular cancer.[109,110] PtNPs conjugated with cisplatin (*cis*-diamminedichlo-Pt, CDDP) was the first permitted for chemotherapy[111] that inhibits DNA transcription and replication of delivered cells, which leads to cellular apoptosis. However, due to its higher side effects, scientists are now looking for a better version of PtNPs-based drug-delivery system with less cellular toxicity such as carboplatin, oxaliplatin, nedaplatin, lobaplatin, and heptaplatin which have very much similar mechanisms to cisplatin.[112] These nanoconjugates frequently leave the body quickly after being introduced. Doxorubicin, which induces the death of cancer cells, was used by Mukherjee et al. in 2020 to create a PtNPs-based drug-delivery system (PtNPs–DOX) that was approved by the FDA.[113] To increase blood flow and retention period while lowering rapid clearance and nonspecific interactions with serum proteins, they additionally combined PtNPs with polyethylene glycol (PEG). In a similar effort, Ruiz et al., 2021 group developed a poly(lactic-co-glycolic acid) (PLGA) encapsulated PtNP drug-delivery system to increase circulation time, target specificity, and increased accumulation at the target site.[114] Several PtNP-based drug-delivery systems have entered clinical phase trials. Soon, these studies will provide efficient PtNP-based clinical chemotherapy practices to deliver important drugs more efficiently.

To date, only a few numbers of studies reported the applicability of PdNPs in drug delivery, gene therapy, and a wide range of biomedical fields, photoacoustic agents, and drug carriers. The high porosity of PdNPs helps greatly with the loading and delivery of drugs and in gene therapy. In a recent comparison study, porous PdNPs outperformed porous gold (AuNPs) and PtNPs in terms of gene loading and delivery.[115] To silence the HCV NS3 gene, the author used fluorescein-labeled thiolated DNAzymes (FAM-Dz) that were supplied using AuNPs, PtNPs, and PdNPs. Their results demonstrated that porous PdNPs performed remarkably well in photothermal conversion, therapeutic gene loading/releasing, cytotoxicity, and in vitro cancer treatment across the board. Due to their excellent thermal tolerance, PdNPs appear to have a variety of potential functions for the treatment of cancer. In the presence of photothermal and chemo treatments, studies revealed that mesoporous silica NPs embellished with Pd nanosheets loaded with DOX showed a substantial synergistic effect. Also, reports showed the efficiency of PdNPs synthesized from chaga mushroom to carry the cancer drug DOX and its site-specific release within 6 hours in a neutral condition. It is also shown that a slightly acidic condition (pH 5.7) helps release more than 92% of DOX release to tumor cells compared to neutral conditions. PdNPs conjugated with therapeutic drugs through linking molecules were also found to be equally effective for target-specific drug delivery. A pH-responsive releasing profile was observed while DOX was linked with PEGylated PdNPs and targeted in human cervical cancer cells (HeLa).[116] Another study also reported a higher permeation and retention rate in the breast cancer microenvironment and fewer side effects or cellular toxicity effects of the anticancer drug Paclitaxel when delivered through PdNPs conjugated with phthalocyanine. PdNP conjugated tubastatin A found to be extraordinarily successful against the inhibition of breast cancer cells compared to traditional methods. Recently, PdNP-based drug-delivery systems have gained attention among scientists due to their stability and lesser toxicity.[117] In a recent study, it has been proved that PdNPs-based systems can be used as transition metal complexes for higher drug stability with controlled interaction between ligands and drug molecules with increased drug delivery at specific sites.[118] These findings promise a more efficient gene or drug-delivery system based on PtNPs and PdNPs in the near future.

7.4.4 IN BIOSENSING

Currently, a number of biomedical sensors are used for the detection of physical and chemical changes occurring in the human body due to various disease conditions increasing day by day for early detection of disease.[119] The development of sensors mainly focused on detecting various forms of energy sources, including thermal, electrical, magnetic, radiant, and chemical energy.[120] Presently, several sensing techniques are being used for sensing purposes, namely, cyclic voltammetry (CV), differential pulse voltammetry (DPV), electrochemilumeinescence (ECL), photoelectron–chemical chemistry (PEC), square wave voltammetry (SWV), and electrochemical impedance spectroscopy (EIS). However, sensitivity, selectivity, stability, response time, linear range, distortion, minimum detectable signal, and reproducibility of above sensing techniques are mainly depends on the sensing material. Sensing techniques involved number of chemical elements having moderate to good sensing properties including metals. Metals are far ahead in this race because of their unique properties. Due to their useful and fascinating properties, such as their high catalytic activity and large surface–volume ratio, research is currently focusing on exploiting NPs of various metals that offer further benefits in biosensing.[121]

Noble metals and their NPs are essential for creating more effective electrodes for sensors because of their better optical, surface electrical, and catalytic capabilities, all of which are required to produce sensors for biosensing applications. And, the development of biosensors with improved electrodes leads to increased response performance, which is the current focus of biosensor research. PtNPs and PdNPs are the noble metals recently coming forward as preferred sensing materials and have great potential as sensing material to detect various chemical and physical changes due to their excellent electrical and thermal conductivity, chemical stability, and more specific surface area along with good biocompatibility.[122] Therefore, researchers trying to develop methodologies that can incorporate PtNPs and PdNPs into polymer material for the production of modified electrodes. Presently, PtNPs have been widely employed in the biosensing of bioactive substances such as glucose, glutamic acid, and hormones. Similarly, PdNPs are being used as a sensing material in biosensing of glucose, hydrogen peroxide, and electrochemical DNA biosensing, etc.[123–125] PtNPs and PtNPs both exhibit several specific size-dependent phenomena, including the quantum size effect, volume effects, surface effects, and many more. To measure the amount of glucose in human serum, Zhong Ping Li created a glucose biosensor with success.[123] They experimented with employing n-alkylamine-stabilized PdNPs for immobilizing GOx (H_2O_2) in glucose biosensing, which is based on the enzymatic oxidation of glucose to produce hydrogen peroxide.

Today's cutting-edge research centers on the hybridization of NPs made of different metals and other chemicals to create composite nanomaterials that can be used to create the best possible sensors. In 2012, Qiu, JianDing, et al. created hybrid Pt polyaniline-modified graphene nanosheets (Pt/PANI/GNs), which can be employed as an appealing and cutting-edge electrode material to create biosensors and electrochemical sensors.[126] Similar to this, Harley-Trochimczyk (2015) built functionalized low-power consuming polysilicon microheaters using PtNP catalyst loaded in a graphene aerogel substrate which can be used as low-power catalytic hydrogen biosensors.[127] The developed hydrogen sensor can detect hydrogen at 65 ppm, with a recovery time of up to 0.72 s, and also these catalytic hydrogen sensors have a low power requirement.

7.4.5 IN ANTIBACTERIAL THERAPY

NPs can target bacteria and can become new nonantibiotic antibacterial/antimicrobials.[128] The antibacterial/antimicrobial properties of different NPs depend upon varied factors such as their ionic states, biosynthesis, shape, size, and their conjugation with different active compounds. Recent studies demonstrated that metallic NPs synthesized from Au, Ag, Fe, Zn, Cu, and Pt exhibit high antimicrobial activity due to their negative zeta potential. Several studies showed the antimicrobial properties of PtNPs is dose-dependent and exhibit additional negative zeta potential which causes serious oxidative damage to cells.[129] The antimicrobial capabilities of PtNPs are also influenced by their size; smaller sizes can more easily move inside the cell wall of *Staphylococcus aureus*, which may produce more reactive oxygen species (ROS), which improves antibacterial activity.[130] PtNPs with an NP size of less than 5 nm were found to have an antibacterial action by Hashimoto et al. in 2017.[131] PdNPs have very similar properties to PtNPs.

Similar to this, Adams et al. (2014) discovered that at concentrations as low as 2.5 nM, PdNPs (size 2 nm) had more antibacterial effects against Gram-positive *S. aureus* than against Gram-negative *E. coli*.[132] Also, few reports suggest that PtNPs and PdNPs can both inhibit a variety of food-borne pathogens, including *Salmonella*, *Staphylococcus*, *E. coli*, and *Listeria* up to a range of 55.2–99 and 83.8–99%, respectively, with increasing concentrations PdNPs from 22.25–44.5 to 50.5–101 mg/L.

According to this, NPs can be highly helpful for creating effective medication, vaccines, and peptide delivery systems against microbiological infections. Rajendran S. et al. demonstrated in 2020 that synthetic AuNPs and PtNPs coated with the pyrimidine-based ligand 2-4,6-dimethoxypyrimidine-2-yl, methyleneenamino-6-methoxyphenol (DPMM) can interact with DNA and possess antimicrobial properties against a variety of bacteria, including *E. coli*, *Klebsiella pneumonia*, Pseudomonas fluor.[133,134] Lopes et al. proved that Pt-bound polysaccharides such as porphyrins NPs are highly potent agents to control biofilm due to their high microbial photodynamic inactivation and thus can inhibit multi-drug resistant bacteria, namely, *S. aureus*.[135] Similarly, studies proved that PtNPs and PdNPs coated with pharmacologically active compounds showed a higher degree of antimicrobial activity than conventional drugs. Tetracycline-coated PdNPs were discovered to be sixteen times more efficient than uncoated PdNPs against the tetracycline-resistant *E. coli* strain HB101/pBR32. Thiosemicarbazone-conjugated Pt (II) and Pd (II) NPs were discovered to be extremely deadly against Mycobacterium TB. Plant-based synthesis of PdNPs also shows antibacterial activity for *Bacillus substilis* and *Pseudomonas aeruginosa*.[136] PdNPs conjugated with polyamide S-containing sulfones showed high antifungal and antibacterial properties against *Aspergillum flavus* and *Candida albicans*, respectively.

The antibacterial properties of various nitrogen, sulfur, and oxygen-based Schiff base complexes are also well recognized.[137] As a result, researchers worldwide are working to create brand-new antimicrobial medications based on PtNPs and PdNPs. The biological activity of chitosans has been improved by recently developed PtNPs and PdNPs-based complexes with salicylaldehyde amphiphilic Schiff bases, which have higher antibacterial efficacy against *Pseudomonas syringaea* and antifungal activity against *Fusarium graminearum* fungi.[138] PdNPs were also recorded for antibacterial and antibiofilm properties against multidrug-resistant clinical microorganisms.[139]

Another important scientific study is developing new nanomaterial-based antimicrobial therapy to overcome multidrug resistance to conventional therapy. One such recent method is photothermal therapy that generates high heat with higher biocompatibility to kill pathogenic microbes within host cells. In this method, bacteria are killed by converting NIR light to heat using a photothermal transducer. Recently, Pd nanostructures have become a new contender for photothermal transducers. Moreover, PdNPs with varying sizes and shapes display exceptional photothermal stability and excellent optical extinction coefficients when compared to other metallic NPs. Chen et al., in 2010 successfully demonstrated 99.99% disinfection of both *S.*

aureus and *E. coli* within less than 10 min with a low dosage of PdNPs (20 mg/L).[139] This innovative approach to antimicrobial medication therapy claims to be environmentally friendly, with the potential to shorten treatment times and, most significantly, to prevent the formation of multidrug-resistant microorganisms.

7.4.6 IN BIOMEDICAL IMPLANTS AND DEVICES CONSTRUCTION

In general, medical implants are used for monitoring and replacing damaged human organs and other organs and tissues, as well as for diagnostic and therapeutic purposes.[140] In modern era, metals have been used to make implants since more than 100 years ago when Lane in 1895 developed metal implants for bone fracture fixation. Furthermore, since the early 1970s, Pt started to construct variety of medical devices. According to "Medical Equipment Global Market Report 2022," the global market for medical accessories is anticipated to increase from US$574.46 billion in 2021 to US$640.25 billion in 2022 at an annual growth rate of 11.5%. Also, the business is estimated to grow up to US$939.98 billion in 2026 at an annual growth rate of 10.1%.[141]

Overall, there are many different shapes, sizes, and levels of sophistication in biomedical tools and equipment. Safety is a key factor in selecting materials for biomedical device development and manufacturing; these materials must also not interact negatively with or harm exposed biological tissues. The corrosive nature of naturally occurring fluids in the body must be considered while researching a material's resistance to corrosion, as the chemical composition and concentration of the human body are not constant and fluctuate depending on a number of circumstances. Currently, medical implants and gadgets are made mostly from body tissues, ceramics, metals, and polymers.[142] However, metals, and their alloys remain the material of choice because of their qualities such as great mechanical strength, high ductility, high density, toughness, durability, high resistance to corrosion, and biocompatibility. At present, metals make up over 80% of implantable medical devices. Base metals, such as steel, titanium, copper, and nickel are used to develop a number of biomedical tools and devices such as surgical equipment, orthopedic devices, dentistry supplies, cardiovascular devices, diabetes care devices, etc. However, uses of these metals have a number of drawbacks and limitations. Identifying a more suitable metal is necessary since, for instance, copper and nickel can affect bodily tissue, generating intoxication effects that may cause a bad impact on human health.[143] However, there are several drawbacks and limitations to the usage of these metals. As metals such as copper and nickel can corrode and react with biological tissue, causing intoxication can harm human health therefore finding a more acceptable metal is crucial.

For more than 40 years, Pt and Pt alloys have been widely used in the medical industry for a range of purposes. Due to its strong corrosion resistance and resilience to changes in chemical conditions within the body, Pt is considered an important material for constructing biomedical devices and implants. Additionally, because of its strong biocompatibility, inherent corrosion resistance, and radiopacity properties, Pt is perfect for a range of biomedical applications. Also, the mechanical characteristics and ductility of Pt make it suitable for fabricating small, complex, and strong structures that can tolerate high stress without deforming or splitting. Furthermore, the biocompatibility features of structures made by Ptmake them an ideal implantable material for long-term use. Presently Pt and Pd are used in medical treatments including stenting, angioplasty, and balloon angioplasty frequently use Pt.[144] because of its many physical features, including sterility, durability, high melting point, fine machinability, and X-ray visibility. In addition, Pt's strong electrical conductivity is utilized to create electrodes for the majority of biomedical equipment. Pt has also been used in the creation of implanted hearing aids to assist with hearing restoration in a more discrete way (cochlear implants).

As a result of the recent advancements in nanotechnology, it is now possible to produce PtNPs and PdNPs NPs of various sizes and qualities to enhance the functionality of biomedical equipment and devices. Currently, a number of tools and devices built of PtNPs, PdNPs, and their alloys are employed in the medical field, including bone grafts, coronary stents, and Pt wires for the treatment of brain aneurysms.[145] Use of PtNPs and PdNPs in medical implants and devices as an electrode will increase effectiveness and durability. Various types of medical implants and devices are shown in Figure 7.3.

7.5 TOXICITY RELEVANCE OF PTNPs AND PDNPs

Metal toxicity, often known as metal poisoning, is the toxic impact of specific metals on the human body when exposed to certain concentrations. The severity of metal toxicity depends upon, the amount of metal ingested, the way it was exposed, and how long it was exposed and may affect a whole body, or an organ. In general, the toxic effects of any toxin are dose-dependent; even a drug that is necessary can cause intoxication when taken in excess, and even

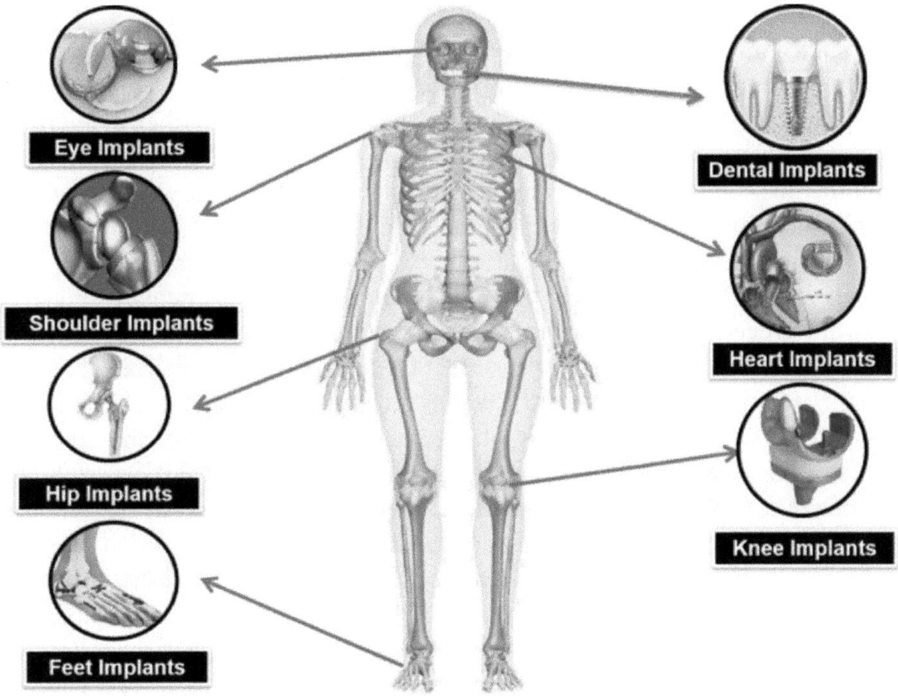

FIGURE 7.3 Types of medical implants and devices.

Source: Reprinted with permission from Ref. [146]. Copyright 2022. Elsevier

a substance that is extremely toxic, such as snake venom, has a minimum dose below which no toxic impact is detectable. Presently, numerous equipment, tools, and devices made up of various metals and metal alloys are employed in the medical industry for several applications and researchers are still working very hard to develop and identify new metals and metal alloys suitable for different biomedical applications with excellent qualities. Therefore, it is absolutely important to do a preclinical toxicity assessment of each implant on different biological systems including humans before use. Toxicity tests help to investigate various adverse effects on the human body such as cancer, different allergies, cardio-toxicity, nausea, skin/eye irritation, etc.[147] Importantly, toxicity testing helps to determine no observed adverse effect level (NOAEL) quantity which is necessary for clinical studies.[148]

There are several factors to take into account, but metal corrosion is one of the crucial factors for toxicity studies.[149] This is because implants made of more corrosive materials result in metal debris inside the body due to surface corrosion, which can release metal ions inside the body. The uptake of such ions by cells by means of endocytotic processes leads to cytotoxicity, chromosomal damage, and oxidative stress.[150] Moreover, metal ions that have been released into the body can combine with other elements to generate hazardous compounds that could have negative effects. Hence, all biomedical equipment and implants must be created in a way that allows them to withstand substantial changes in the chemical environment they are utilized in without losing stability.[151] Additionally, metal ions that have been released into the body can combine with other elements to generate hazardous compounds that could have negative effects. To maintain stability, biomedical implants, and devices must be designed with materials that have ability to withstand substantial changes happening inside the human body.

PtNPs and PdNPs, provide a better option as material for the manufacture of biomedical implants and devices. Both PtNPs and PdNPs are highly resistant to corrosion. Which releases very less or no metal debris and ions inside the human body. Aseptic loosening and osteolysis, which are typically brought on by free ions released by corrosive implants, are less likely to develop in the body when implants composed of PtNPs and PdNPs are used. Orthopedic metals typically result in immunological reactions that support a cell-mediated hypersensitive response, according to experimental research. PtNPs and PdNPs implants, on the other hand, showed good tissue biocompatibility and are safe for human use. Because of its biocompatibility, Pt is used in a number of treatments since it is perfect for both temporary and long-term implantation in the body.[152] It has several significant qualities that are not shared by base metals and may be formed into small, intricate shapes when used as a metal. Unlike inert metals such as nickel and copper, which can occasionally trigger allergic reactions, it does not corrode inside the body since it is inert. Many Pt alloys have also been extensively employed in procedures for treating coronary artery disease such as balloon angioplasty and stenting because of their inertness and good X-ray visibility. At present, devices which usually put inside the human body such as neuromodulation and cardiac rhythm disorders have taken advantage of these special properties of PtNPs and PdNPs such as inertness, durability, and electrical conductivity as ideal electrode material.

7.6 CONCLUSION AND FUTURE PERSPECTIVES

The extensive investigations have made metal and metal oxide nanomaterials applicable for various applications due to their inherent physical, chemical, electrical, and optical properties. Noble metal NPs are good examples of nanomaterials that have been part of human day-to-day life from ancient time. Together with AuNPs and AgNPs, PtNPs and PdNPs are becoming more popular among noble metal nanomaterials. PtNPs and PdNPs have been commercialized in several industrial processes thanks to research into their catalytic efficacy for industrial applications. For few decades, the biomedical applications of PtNPs and PdNPs have been reported with in vivo experimental demonstrations. The following chapter gives a summary of the synthesis processes, as well as the structural, biological, chemical, and physical characteristics of PtNPs and PdNPs. The chapter primarily focused on the biomedical application of PtNPs and PdNPs. The antimicrobial, therapeutic, drug delivery, biosensing, bioimaging, medical implants, and device construction applications are discussed with commercial aspects in the field of healthcare industries.

The advancement in technologies has facilitated the use of nanomaterials in biomedical applications. Though several nanostructures are part of the therapeutic and diagnostic formulations, toxicity and biocompatibility are still the major concerns in the applicability of nanomaterials due to the lack of extensive toxicology study data. Compared to other metal NPs, PtNPs, and PdNPs have very significantly low toxicity. Ayurveda has shown the medicinal efficacy of PtNPs at very low concentrations. Thus, the toxicity studies of these nanomaterials at different concentrations are crucial for future uses. The technological barrier has to be minimized for convincing usage of PtNPs and PdNPs. Also, the economics involved in the application of these metal NPs is too high to get them to be reached to common people which can be controlled or minimized by using bimetallic or composites of PtNPs and PdNPs. So, comprehensive and insightful investigations are inevitable for commercial healthcare applications.

ACKNOWLEDGMENT

The authors are thankful to the Department of Biotechnology, Government of India, India for providing funds for the research through the DBT-BUILDER SUK programme.

KEYWORDS

- **platinum nanoparticles**
- **palladium nanoparticles**
- **biomedical applications**
- **structural properties**
- **biocompatible**

REFERENCES

1. Barve, M.; Mashru, M.; Jagtap, C.; Patgiri, B. J.; Prajapati, P. K. Therapeutic Potentials of Metals in Ancient India: A Review Through Charaka Samhita. *J. Ayurveda Integr. Med.* **2011,** *2* (2), 55.
2. Tran, A.; Desai, S.; Mraz Robinson, D. From Ancient Egypt to the Dermatologic Office: An overview of Skin Substitutes and Modern-Day Applications in Dermatologic Surgery. *Health Sci. Rep.* **2023,** *6* (1), e1067.
3. Shoeib, M. A.; Abdel-Gawad, S. A. High Performance Nano Hydroxyapatite Coating on Zinc for Biomedical Applications. *J. Mater. Sci.* **2023,** , 1–7.
4. Aygun, A.; Gulbagca, F.; Altuner, E. E.; Bekmezci, M.; Gur, T.; Karimi-Maleh, H.; Karimi, F.; Vasseghian, Y.; Sen, F. Highly Active PdPt Bimetallic Nanoparticles Synthesized by One-Step Bioreduction Method: Characterizations, Anticancer, Antibacterial Activities and Evaluation of Their Catalytic Effect for Hydrogen Generation. *Int. J. Hydrogen Energy* **2023,** *48* (17), 6666–6679.
5. Yaray, K.; Norbakhsh, A.; Rashidzadeh, H.; Mohammadi, A.; Mozafari, F.; Ghaffarlou, M.; Mousazadeh, N.; Ghaderzadeh, R.; Ghorbani, Y.; Nasehi, L.; Danafar, H. Chemoradiation Therapy of 4T1 Cancer Cells with Methotrexate Conjugated Platinum Nanoparticles Under X-ray Irradiation. *Inorg. Chem. Commun.* **2023,** , 110457.
6. Wani, R. B.; Dwivedi, D. K. Antibacterial Activity Of Platinum Nanoparticles Using Leaf Extracts Of Cinnamomum Camphora: An Eco-Friendly Approach. *J. Pharma. Negative Results* **2023,** , 7260–7269.
7. Guleria, A.; Aishwarya, J.; Kunwar, A.; Neogy, S.; Debnath, A. K.; Rath, M. C.; Adhikari, S.; Tyagi, A. K. Solvated Electron-Induced Synthesis of Cyclodextrin-Coated Pd Nanoparticles: Mechanistic, Catalytic, and Anticancer Studies. *Dalton Trans.* **2023,** *52* (4), 1036–1051.
8. Zhang, Y.; Gao, W.; Ma, Y.; Cheng, L.; Zhang, L.; Liu, Q.; Chen, J.; Zhao, Y.; Tu, K.; Zhang, M.; Liu, C. Integrating Pt Nanoparticles with Carbon Nanodots to achieve Robust Cascade Superoxide Dismutase-Catalase Nanozyme for Antioxidant Therapy. *Nano Today* **2023,** *49*, 101768.
9. Bloch, K.; Pardesi, K.; Satriano, C.; Ghosh, S. Bacteriogenic Platinum Nanoparticles for Application in Nanomedicine. *Front. Chem.* **2021,** *9*, 624344.

10. Mafuné, F.; Kohno, J. Y.; Takeda, Y.; Kondow, T. Formation of Stable Platinum Nanoparticles by Laser Ablation in Water. *J. Phys. Chem. B* **2003,** *107* (18), 4218–4223.
11. Boutinguiza, M.; Meixus, M.; Del Val, J.; Riveiro, A.; Comesaña, R.; Lusquiños, F.; Pou, J. Synthesis and Characterization of Pd Nanoparticles by Laser Ablation in Water Using Nanosecond Laser. *Phys. Procedia* **2016,** *83*, 36–45.
12. Fernández-Arias, M.; Vilas, A. M.; Boutinguiza, M.; Rodríguez, D.; Arias-González, F.; Pou-Álvarez, P.; Riveiro, A.; Gil, J.; Pou, J. Palladium Nanoparticles Synthesized by Laser Ablation in Liquids for Antimicrobial Applications. *Nanomaterials* **2022,** *12* (15), 2621.
13. Hu, X.; Takai, O.; Saito, N. Simple Synthesis of Platinum Nanoparticles by Plasma Sputtering in Water. *Jpn J. Appl. Phys.* **2013,** *52* (1S), 01AN05.
14. Dao, V. D.; Tran, C. Q.; Ko, S. H.; Choi, H. S. Dry Plasma Reduction to Synthesize Supported Platinum Nanoparticles for Flexible Dye-Sensitized Solar Cells. *J. Mater. Chem. A* **2013,** *1* (14), 4436–4443.
15. Brown, R.; Lonn, B.; Pfeiffer, R.; Frederiksen, H.; Wickman, B. Plasma-Induced Heating Effects on Platinum Nanoparticle Size During Sputter Deposition Synthesis in Polymer and Ionic Liquid Substrates. *Langmuir* **2021,** *37* (29), 8821–8828.
16. Su, N.; Hu, X.; Zhang, J.; Huang, H.; Cheng, J.; Yu, J.; Ge, C. Plasma-Induced Synthesis of Pt Nanoparticles Supported on TiO_2 Nanotubes for Enhanced Methanol Electro-Oxidation. *Appl. Surface Sci.* **2017,** *399*, 403–410.
17. Aggarwal, K. Synthesis and Characterization of Palladium Nanocomposites Prepared by Atom Beam Sputtering Technique. *AIP Conf. Proc.* **2021,** *2352* (1), 040002.
18. Lüsi, M.; Erikson, H.; Treshchalov, A.; Rähn, M.; Merisalu, M.; Kikas, A.; Kisand, V.; Sammelselg, V.; Tammeveski, K. Oxygen Reduction Reaction on Pd Nanocatalysts Prepared by Plasma-Assisted Synthesis on Different Carbon Nanomaterials. *Nanotechnology* **2020,** *32* (3), 035401.
19. Ullah, M.; Eaqub Ali, M.; Bee Abd Hamid, S. Structure-Controlled Nanomaterial Synthesis Using Surfactant-Assisted Ball Milling—A Review. *Curr. Nanosci.* **2014,** *10* (3), 344–354.
20. Valizadeh, Z.; Abbaspour, M. Surface Energy, Relative Stability, and Structural Properties of Au-Pt, Au-Rh, Au-Cu, and Au-Pd Nanoclusters Created in Inert-Gas Condensation Process Using MD Simulation. *J. Phys. Chem. Solids* **2020,** *144*, 109480.
21. Kalbasi, R. J.; Mosaddegh, N.; Abbaspourrad, A. A Novel Catalyst Containing Palladium Nanoparticles Supported on Poly (2-Hydroxyethyl Methacrylate)/CMK-1: Synthesis, Characterization and Comparison with Mesoporous Silica Nanocomposite. *Appl. Catal. A: Gen.* **2012,** *423*, 78–90.
22. Salabat, A.; Nabiyouni, G.; Far, M. R. Effect of Platinum Precursor on the Nanoparticle Size Synthesised in Microemulsion System. *J. Exp. Nanosci.* **2011,** *6* (3), 305–310.
23. Wang, Y.; Du, M.; Xu, J.; Yang, P.; Du, Y. Size-Controlled Synthesis of Palladium Nanoparticles. *J. Dispersion Sci. Technol.* **2008,** *29* (6), 891–894.
24. Imai, T.; Abe, Y.; Nishio, K.; Tamura, R.; Shibata, H.; Kineri, T.; Gunji, T. Preparation of Platinum Nanoparticles That Are Dispersible in Water Over a Wide pH Range. *Polym. J.* **2013,** *45* (5), 540–544.
25. Stavropoulou, A. P.; Theodosiou, M.; Sakellis, E.; Boukos, N.; Papanastasiou, G.; Wang, C.; Tavares, A.; Corral, C. A.; Gournis, D.; Chalmpes, N.; Gobbo, O. L. Bimetallic Gold-Platinum Nanoparticles as a Drug Delivery System Coated with a New Drug to Target Glioblastoma. *Colloids and Surfaces B: Biointerfaces* **2022,** *214*, 112463.

26. Sun, Y.; Zhang, L.; Zhou, H.; Zhu, Y.; Sutter, E.; Ji, Y.; Rafailovich, M. H.; Sokolov, J. C. Seedless and Templateless Synthesis of Rectangular Palladium Nanoparticles. *Chem. Mater.* **2007,** *19* (8), 2065–2070.
27. Wang, Q.; Wang, Y.; Guo, P.; Li, Q.; Ding, R.; Wang, B.; Li, H.; Liu, J.; Zhao, X. S. Formic Acid-Assisted Synthesis of Palladium Nanocrystals and Their Electrocatalytic Properties. *Langmuir* **2014,** *30* (1), 440–446.
28. Wang, L.; Wang, H.; Nemoto, Y.; Yamauchi, Y. Rapid and Efficient Synthesis of Platinum Nanodendrites with High Surface Area by Chemical Reduction with Formic Acid. *Chem. Mater.* **2010,** *22* (9), 2835–2841.
29. Tan, Y.; Dai, X.; Li, Y.; Zhu, D. Preparation of Gold, Platinum, Palladium and Silver Nanoparticles by the Reduction of Their Salts with a Weak Reductant–Potassium Bitartrate. *J. Mater. Chem.* **2003,** *13* (5), 1069–1075.
30. Zhang, L.; Wang, L.; Jiang, Z.; Xie, Z. Synthesis of Size-Controlled Monodisperse Pd Nanoparticles via a Non-Aqueous Seed-Mediated Growth. *Nanosc. Res. Lett.* **2012,** *7* (1), 1–6.
31. Carpenter, M. K.; Moylan, T. E.; Kukreja, R. S.; Atwan, M. H.; Tessema, M. M. Solvothermal Synthesis of Platinum Alloy Nanoparticles for Oxygen Reduction Electrocatalysis. *J. Am. Chem. Soc.* **2012,** *134* (20), 8535–8542.
32. Martínez-Rodríguez, R. A.; Vidal-Iglesias, F. J.; Solla-Gullon, J.; Cabrera, C. R.; Feliu, J. M. Synthesis of Pt Nanoparticles in Water-in-Oil Microemulsion: Effect of HCl on Their Surface Structure. *J. Am. Chem. Soc.* **2014,** *136* (4), 1280–1283.
33. Wang, C. C.; Chen, D. H.; Huang, T. C. Synthesis of Palladium Nanoparticles in Water-in-Oil Microemulsions. *Colloids Surfaces A: Physicochem. Eng. Aspects* **2001,** *189* (1–3), 145–154.
34. Liang, C.; Xia, W.; Soltani-Ahmadi, H.; Schlüter, O.; Fischer, R. A.; Muhler, M. The Two-Step Chemical Vapor Deposition of Pd (allyl) Cp as an Atom-Efficient Route to Synthesize Highly Dispersed Palladium Nanoparticles on Carbon Nanofibers. *Chem. Commun.* **2005,** *6* (2), 282–284.
35. Choi, D. S.; Robertson, A. W.; Warner, J. H.; Kim, S. O.; Kim, H. Low-Temperature Chemical Vapor Deposition Synthesis of Pt–Co Alloyed Nanoparticles with Enhanced Oxygen Reduction Reaction Catalysis. *Adv. Mater.* **2016,** *28* (33), 7115–7122.
36. Chen, W.; Cai, W.; Lei, Y.; Zhang, L. A Sonochemical Approach to the Confined Synthesis of Palladium Nanoparticles in Mesoporous Silica. *Mater. Lett.* **2001,** *50* (2–3), 53–56.
37. Hansen, H. E.; Seland, F.; Sunde, S.; Burheim, O. S.; Pollet, B. G. Two Routes for Sonochemical Synthesis of Platinum Nanoparticles with Narrow Size Distribution. *Mater. Adv.* **2021,** *2* (6), 1962–1971.
38. Guo, D. J.; Li, H. L. Electrochemical Synthesis of Pd Nanoparticles on Functional MWNT Surfaces. *Electrochem. Commun.* **2004,** *6* (10), 999–1003.
39. Mäsing, F.; Nüsse, H.; Klingauf, J.; Studer, A. Light Mediated Preparation of Palladium Nanoparticles as Catalysts for Alkyne *cis*-Semihydrogenation. *Org. Lett.* **2017,** *19* (10), 2658–2661.
40. Tjoa, V.; Chua, J.; Pramana, S. S.; Wei, J.; Mhaisalkar, S. G.; Mathews, N. Facile Photochemical Synthesis of Graphene-Pt Nanoparticle Composite for Counter Electrode in Dye Sensitized Solar Cell. *ACS Appl. Mater. Interfaces.* **2012,** *4* (7), 3447–3452.
41. Kumar, A. P.; Kumar, B. P.; Kumar, A. K.; Huy, B. T.; Lee, Y. I. Preparation of Palladium Nanoparticles on Alumina Surface by Chemical Co-Precipitation Method and Catalytic Applications. *Appl. Surface Sci.* **2013,** *265*, 500–509.

42. Li, Y.; Whyburn, G. P.; Huang, Y. Specific Peptide Regulated Synthesis of Ultrasmall Platinum Nanocrystals. *J. Am. Chem. Soc.* **2009,** *131* (44), 15998–15999.
43. Ghorbani-Choghamarani, A.; Taherinia, Z. Synthesis of Peptide Nanofibers Decorated with Palladium Nanoparticles and Its Application as an Efficient Catalyst for the Synthesis of Sulfides via Reaction of Aryl Halides with Thiourea or 2-Mercaptobenzothiazole. *RSC Adv.* **2016,** *6* (64), 59410–59421.
44. Qazi, F.; Hussain, Z.; Tahir, M. N. Advances in Biogenic Synthesis of Palladium Nanoparticles. *RSC Adv.* **2016,** *6* (65), 60277–60286.
45. Vishnukumar, P.; Vivekanandhan, S.; Muthuramkumar, S. Plant-Mediated Biogenic Synthesis of Palladium Nanoparticles: Recent Trends and Emerging Opportunities. *ChemBioEng Rev.* **2017,** *4* (1), 18–36.
46. Tahir, K.; Nazir, S.; Li, B.; Ahmad, A.; Nasir, T.; Khan, A. U.; Shah, S. A.; Khan, Z. U.; Yasin, G.; Hameed, M. U. *Sapium sebiferum* Leaf Extract Mediated Synthesis of Palladium Nanoparticles and In Vitro Investigation of Their Bacterial and Photocatalytic Activities. *J. Photochem. Photobiol. B: Biol.* **2016,** *164*, 164–173.
47. Kadam, J.; Madiwale, S.; Bashte, B.; Dindorkar, S.; Dhawal, P.; More, P. Green Mediated synthesis of Palladium Nanoparticles Using Aqueous Leaf Extract of *Gymnema sylvestre* for Catalytic Reduction of Cr (VI). *SN Appl. Sci.* **2020,** *2*, 1–3.
48. Sharmila, G.; Fathima, M. F.; Haries, S.; Geetha, S.; Kumar, N. M.; Muthukumaran, C. Green Synthesis, Characterization and Antibacterial Efficacy of Palladium Nanoparticles Synthesized Using *Filicium decipiens* Leaf Extract. *J. Mol. Struct.* **2017,** *1138*, 35–40.
49. Song, J. Y.; Kwon, E. Y.; Kim, B. S. Biological Synthesis of Platinum Nanoparticles Using *Diopyros kaki* Leaf Extract. *Bioprocess Biosyst. Eng.* **2010,** *33*, 159–164.
50. Nellore, J.; Pauline, C.; Amarnath, K. *Bacopa monnieri* Phytochemicals Mediated Synthesis of Platinum Nanoparticles and Its Neurorescue Effect on 1-Methyl 4-Phenyl 1, 2, 3, 6 Tetrahydropyridine-Induced Experimental Parkinsonism in Zebrafish. *J. Neurodegen. Dis.* **2013,** 2013.
51. Fanoro, O. T.; Parani, S.; Maluleke, R.; Lebepe, T. C.; Varghese, R. J.; Mgedle, N.; Mavumengwana, V.; Oluwafemi, O. S. Biosynthesis of Smaller-Sized Platinum Nanoparticles Using the Leaf Extract of *Combretum erythrophyllum* and Its Antibacterial Activities. *Antibiotics* **2021,** *10* (11), 1275.
52. Selvi, A. M.; Palanisamy, S.; Jeyanthi, S.; Vinosha, M.; Mohandoss, S.; Tabarsa, M.; You, S.; Kannapiran, E.; Prabhu, N. M. Synthesis of Tragia Involucrata Mediated Platinum Nanoparticles for Comprehensive Therapeutic Applications: Antioxidant, Antibacterial and Mitochondria-Associated Apoptosis in HeLa cells. Process Biochemistry. 2020 Nov 1;98:21–33.
53. Fahmy, S. A.; Fawzy, I. M.; Saleh, B. M.; Issa, M. Y.; Bakowsky, U.; Azzazy, H. M. Green Synthesis of Platinum and Palladium Nanoparticles Using *Peganum harmala*, L. Seed Alkaloids: Biological and Computational Studies. *Nanomaterials.* **2021,** *11* (4), 965.
54. Dinesh, M.; Roopan, S. M.; Selvaraj, C. I.; Arunachalam, P. *Phyllanthus emblica* Seed Extract Mediated Synthesis of PdNPs Against Antibacterial, Heamolytic and Cytotoxic Studies. *J. Photochem. Photobiol.: Biol.* **2017,** *167*, 64–71.
55. Anila, P. A.; Keerthiga, B.; Ramesh, M.; Muralisankar, T. Synthesis and Characterization of Palladium Nanoparticles by Chemical and Green Methods: A Comparative Study on Hepatic Toxicity Using Zebrafish as an Animal Model. *Compar. Biochem. Physiol. Part C: Toxicol. Pharmacol.* **2021,** *244*, 108979.

56. Bogireddy, N. K.; Pal, U.; Kumar, M. K.; Domínguez, J. M.; Gomez, L. M.; Agarwal, V. Green Fabrication of 2D Platinum Superstructures and Their High Catalytic Activity for Mitigation of Organic Pollutants. *Catalysis Today* **2021,** *360*, 185–193.
57. Al-Radadi, N. S.; Adam, S. I. Green Biosynthesis of Pt-Nanoparticles from Anbara Fruits: Toxic and Protective Effects on CCl4 Induced Hepatotoxicity in Wister Rats. *Arab. J. Chem.* **2020,** *13* (2), 4386–4403.
58. Kumar, H.; Bhardwaj, K.; Dhanjal, D. S.; Nepovimova, E.; Şen, F.; Regassa, H.; Singh, R.; Verma, R.; Kumar, V.; Kumar, D.; Bhatia, S. K. Fruit Extract Mediated Green Synthesis of Metallic Nanoparticles: A New Avenue in Pomology Applications. *Int. J. Mol. Sci.* **2020,** *21* (22), 8458.
59. Lakshmipathy, R.; Palakshi Reddy, B.; Sarada, N. C.; Chidambaram, K.; Khadeer Pasha, S. K. Watermelon Rind-Mediated Green Synthesis of Noble Palladium Nanoparticles: Catalytic Application. *Appl. Nanosci.* **2015,** *5*, 223–228.
60. Zhan, G.; Huang, J.; Du, M.; Abdul-Rauf, I.; Ma, Y.; Li, Q. Green Synthesis of Au–Pd Bimetallic Nanoparticles: Single-Step Bioreduction Method with Plant Extract. *Mater. Lett.* **2011,** *65* (19–20), 2989–2991.
61. Nasrollahzadeh, M.; Sajadi, S. M. Green Synthesis, Characterization and Catalytic Activity of the Pd/TiO_2 Nanoparticles for the Ligand-Free Suzuki–Miyaura Coupling Reaction. *J. Colloid Interface Sci.* **2016,** *465*, 121–127.
62. Ghosh, S.; Ahmad, R.; Banerjee, K.; AlAjmi, M. F.; Rahman, S. Mechanistic Aspects of Microbe-Mediated Nanoparticle Synthesis. *Front. Microbiol.* **2021,** *12*, 638068.
63. Wang, W.; Zhang, B.; Liu, Q.; Du, P.; Liu, W.; He, Z. Biosynthesis of Palladium Nanoparticles Using *Shewanella loihica* PV-4 for Excellent Catalytic Reduction of Chromium (VI). *Environ. Sci.: Nano* **2018,** *5* (3), 730–739.
64. Wu, R.; Tian, X.; Xiao, Y.; Ulstrup, J.; Christensen, H. E.; Zhao, F.; Zhang, J. Selective Electrocatalysis of Biofuel Molecular Oxidation Using Palladium Nanoparticles Generated on *Shewanella oneidensis* MR-1. *J. Mater. Chem.* A **2018,** *6* (23), 10655–10662.
65. Yates, M. D.; Cusick, R. D.; Logan, B. E. Extracellular Palladium Nanoparticle Production Using *Geobacter sulfurreducens*. *ACS Sustain. Chem. Eng.* **2013,** *1* (9), 1165–1171.
66. Chen, Y.; Chen, Y.; Wang, B.; Mao, C.; Liu, C.; Liu, R.; Yan, B. From Trash to Treasure: Microbial Conversion of Palladium Contaminants into Valuable Pd Nanoparticles by *Bacillus thuringiensis* Y9. *J. Clean. Prod.* **2022,** *366*, 132880.
67. Matsena, M. T.; Tichapondwa, S. M.; Chirwa, E. M. Synthesis of Biogenic Palladium Nanoparticles Using Citrobacter sp. for Application as Anode Electrocatalyst in a Microbial Fuel Cell. *Catalysts* **2020,** *10* (8), 838.
68. Arsiya, F.; Sayadi, M. H.; Sobhani, S. Green Synthesis of Palladium Nanoparticles Using *Chlorella vulgaris*. *Mater. Lett.* **2017,** *186*, 113–115.
69. Mohana, S.; Sumathi, S. Multi-Functional Biological Effects of Palladium Nanoparticles Synthesized Using *Agaricus bisporus*. *J. Cluster Sci.* **2020,** *31*, 391–400.
70. Omajali, J. B.; Mikheenko, I. P.; Merroun, M. L.; Wood, J.; Macaskie, L. E. Characterization of Intracellular Palladium Nanoparticles Synthesized by *Desulfovibrio desulfuricans* and *Bacillus benzeovorans*. *J. Nanopart. Res.* **2015,** *17*, 1–7.
71. Goryunov, A. S.; Borisova, A. G.; Rozhkov, S. S.; Rozhkova, N. N. Structural and Colloid Effects of Interaction between Shungite Carbon Nanoparticles and Linoleic Fatty Acid. *Curr. Nanosci.* **2023,** *19* (1), 68–75.

72. Putta, S.; Sharma, R. K.; Khandelwal, P. Metal Nanoparticles: Synthesis, Characterization, and Biomedical Applications. In: *Nanomaterials*; Springer: Singapore, 2023; pp 85–102.
73. Dristant, U.; Mukherjee, K.; Saha, S.; Maity, D. An Overview of Polymeric Nanoparticles-Based Drug Delivery System in Cancer Treatment. *Technol. Cancer Res. Treatment* **2023,** *22*, 15330338231152083.
74. Luo, X. M.; Li, Y. K.; Dong, X. Y.; Zang, S. Q. Platonic and Archimedean Solids in Discrete Metal-Containing Clusters. *Chem. Soc. Rev*. **2023**.
75. Proniewicz, E.; Gralec, B.; Ozaki, Y. Homogeneous Pt Nanostructures Surface Functionalized with Phenylboronic Acid Phosphonic Acid Derivatives as Potential Biochemical Nanosensors and Drugs: SERS and TERS Studies. *J. Biomed. Mater. Res. Part B: Appl. Biomater*. **2023**.
76. Saadi, K.; Fan, X.; Hardisty, S. S.; Pintauro, P.; Zitoun, D. Ultralow Platinum Loading for Redox-Flow Battery by Electrospinning the Electrocatalyst and the Ionomer in Core-Shell Fibers. *J. Energy Storage* **2023,** *59*, 106430.
77. Bie, Z.; Yao, Z.; Jie, S.; Hu, J.; Pei, L.; Li, B. G.; Wang, P.; Wang, Z. Activation of a Palladium-Based Catalyst by Hexafluoroisopropanol for Polyketone Synthesis via Homogeneous Solution Polymerization. *Ind. Eng. Chem. Res*. **2023**.
78. Tomar, R.; Singh, N. B.; Singh, N. P. Optical Properties of Nanocomposite Materials. In: *Nanocomposites*; Jenny Stanford Publishing, 2023; pp 155–185.
79. Janik, M.; Khachatryan, K.; Khachatryan, G.; Krystyjan, M.; Oszczęda, Z. Comparison of Physicochemical Properties of Silver and Gold Nanocomposites Based on Potato Starch in Distilled and Cold Plasma-Treated Water. *Int. J. Mol. Sci*. **2023,** *24* (3), 2200.
80. Gharibshahi, E.; Saion, E.; Ashraf, A.; Gharibshahi, L. Size-Controlled and Optical Properties of Platinum Nanoparticles by Gamma Radiolytic Synthesis. *Appl. Radiat. Isotopes* **2017,** *130*, 211–217.
81. González, L. A.; Bishop-Hurley, G.; Henry, D.; Charmley, E. Wireless Sensor Networks to Study, Monitor and Manage Cattle in Grazing Systems. *Anim. Prod. Sci*. **2014,** *54* (10), 1687–1693.
82. Zhang, W.; Zhao, J.; Allam, A. A.; Xin, Y.; Lin, J.; Gao, T.; Ajarem, J. S.; Li, X.; Wang, C.; Bahnemann, D. W. Palladium Nanoparticles Embedded Nutshell-like Bi2WO6 as an Efficient and Stable Visible-Light-Responsive Photocatalysts for NO Removal. *Energy Fuels* **2022,** *36* (22), 13852–13862.
83. Tang, L.; Zhou, L.; Yan, X.; Zhong, K.; Gao, X.; Liu, X.; Li, J. A Simple Benzothiazole-Based Mitochondrial-Targeting Fluorescent Probe for Visualizing and Monitoring Viscosity in Living Cell, Lung Organ Tissue, and Living Mice. *Dyes Pigments* **2020,** *182*, 108644.
84. Hsu, J. C.; Nieves, L. M.; Betzer, O.; Sadan, T.; Noël, P. B.; Popovtzer, R.; Cormode, D. P. Nanoparticle Contrast Agents for X-ray Imaging Applications. *Wiley Interdisc. Rev.: Nanomed. Nanobiotechnol*. **2020,** *12* (6), e1642.
85. Verma, A. K.; Yadav, N.; Singh, S. P.; Dey, K. K.; Singh, D.; Yadav, R. R. Study of Ultrasonic Attenuation and Thermal Conduction in Bimetallic Gold/Platinum Nanofluids: Effect of Thermal Conductivity on Ultrasonic Attenuation of Gold and Gold/Platinum Nanofluids. *Johnson Matthey Technol. Rev*. **2021,** *65* (4), 556–567.
86. Capek, I. Viral Nanoparticles, Noble Metal Decorated Viruses and Their Nanoconjugates. *Adv. Colloid Interface Sci*. **2015,** *222*, 119–134.
87. Pedone, D.; Moglianetti, M.; De Luca, E.; Bardi, G.; Pompa, P. P. Platinum Nanoparticles in Nanobiomedicine. *Chem. Soc. Rev*. **2017,** *46* (16), 4951–4975.

88. Chen, A.; Ostrom, C. Palladium-Based Nanomaterials: Synthesis and Electrochemical Applications. *Chem. Rev.* **2015,** *115* (21), 11999–12044.
89. Pasha, S. S.; Das, P.; Rath, N. P.; Bandyopadhyay, D.; Jana, N. R.; Laskar, I. R. Water Soluble Luminescent Cyclometalated Platinum (II) Complex—A Suitable Probe for Bio-Imaging Applications. *Inorg. Chem. Commun.* **2016,** *67*, 107–111.
90. Dong, Y. C.; Bouche, M.; Uman, S.; Burdick, J. A.; Cormode, D. P. Detecting and Monitoring Hydrogels with Medical Imaging. *ACS Biomater. Sci. Eng.* **2021,** *7* (9), 4027–4047.
91. Cheng, L.; Wang, X.; Gong, F.; Liu, T.; Liu, Z. 2D Nanomaterials for Cancer Theranostic Applications. *Adv. Mater.* **2020,** *32* (13), 1902333.
92. Yaqoob, S. B.; Adnan, R.; Rameez Khan, R. M.; Rashid, M. Gold, Silver, and Palladium Nanoparticles: A Chemical Tool for Biomedical Applications. *Front. Chem.* **2020,** *8*, 376.
93. Andoy, N. M.; Jeon, K.; Kreis, C. T.; Sullan, R. M. Multifunctional and Stimuli-Responsive Polydopamine Nanoparticle-Based Platform for Targeted Antimicrobial Applications. *Adv. Funct. Mater.* **2020,** *30* (40), 2004503.
94. Zhao, R.; Xiang, J.; Wang, B.; Chen, L.; Tan, S. Recent Advances in the Development of Noble Metal NPs for Cancer Therapy. *Bioinorg. Chem. App.* **2022,** *2022*.
95. Nie, L.; Chen, M.; Sun, X.; Rong, P.; Zheng, N.; Chen, X. Palladium Nanosheets as Highly Stable and Effective Contrast Agents for In Vivo Photoacoustic Molecular Imaging. *Nanoscale* **2014,** *6* (3), 1271–1276.
96. Jeyaraj, M.; Gurunathan, S.; Qasim, M.; Kang, M. H.; Kim, J. H. A Comprehensive Review on the Synthesis, Characterization, and Biomedical Application of Platinum Nanoparticles. *Nanomaterials* **2019,** *9* (12), 1719.
97. Nejdl, L.; Kudr, J.; Moulick, A.; Hegerova, D.; Ruttkay-Nedecky, B.; Gumulec, J.; Cihalova, K.; Smerkova, K.; Dostalova, S.; Krizkova, S.; Novotna, M. Platinum Nanoparticles Induce Damage to DNA and Inhibit DNA Replication. *PLoS One* **2017,** *12* (7), e0180798.
98. Gutiérrez de la Rosa, S. Y.; Muñiz Diaz, R.; Villalobos Gutiérrez, P. T.; Patakfalvi, R.; Gutiérrez Coronado, Ó. Functionalized Platinum Nanoparticles with Biomedical Applications. *Int. J. Mol. Sci.* **2022,** *23* (16), 9404.
99. Devi, M. Synthesis and Characterization of Palladium Nanoparticles & Its Contribution in Photothermal Therapy of Cancer. *Int. J. Gen. Med. Pharm.* **2019,** *8* (5), 11–18.
100. Ma, Q.; Cheng, L.; Gong, F.; Dong, Z.; Liang, C.; Wang, M.; Feng, L.; Li, Y.; Liu, Z.; Li, C.; He, L. Platinum Nanoworms for Imaging-Guided Combined Cancer Therapy in the Second Near-Infrared Window. *J. Mater. Chem. B* **2018,** *6* (31), 5069–5079.
101. Brown, S. D.; Nativo, P.; Smith, J. A.; Stirling, D.; Edwards, P. R.; Venugopal, B.; Flint, D. J.; Plumb, J. A.; Graham, D.; Wheate, N. J. Gold Nanoparticles for the Improved Anticancer Drug Delivery of the Active Component of Oxaliplatin. *J. Am. Chem. Soc.* **2010,** *132* (13), 4678–4684.
102. Liu, Y.; Wang, D. D.; Zhao, L.; Lin, M.; Sun, H. Z.; Sun, H. C.; Yang, B. Polypyrrole-Coated Flower-Like Pd Nanoparticles (Pd NPs@ PPy) with Enhanced Stability and Heat Conversion Efficiency for Cancer Photothermal Therapy. *RSC Adv.* **2016,** *6* (19), 15854–15860.
103. Yun, Y. H.; Lee, B. K.; Park, K. Controlled Drug Delivery: Historical Perspective for the Next Generation. *J. Controlled Release* **2015,** *219*, 2–7.

104. Mubarak Ali, D.; Kim, H.; Venkatesh, P. S.; Kim, J. W.; Lee, S. Y. A Systemic Review on the Synthesis, Characterization, and Applications of Palladium Nanoparticles in Biomedicine. *Appl. Biochem. Biotechnol.* **2022,** , 1–20.
105. Mitchell, M. J.; Billingsley, M. M.; Haley, R. M.; Wechsler, M. E.; Peppas, N. A.; Langer, R. Engineering Precision Nanoparticles for Drug Delivery. *Nat. Rev. Drug Disc.* **2021,** *20* (2), 101–124.
106. Patra, J. K.; Das, G.; Fraceto, L. F.; Campos, E. V.; Rodriguez-Torres, M. D.; Acosta-Torres, L. S.; Diaz-Torres, L. A.; Grillo, R.; Swamy, M. K.; Sharma, S.; Habtemariam, S. Nano Based Drug Delivery Systems: Recent Developments and Future Prospects. *J. Nanobiotechnol.* **2018,** *16* (1), 1–33.
107. Chen, A.; Ostrom, C. Palladium-Based Nanomaterials: Synthesis and Electrochemical Applications. *Chem. Rev.* **2015,** *115* (21), 11999–12044.
108. Zhou, G.; Jiang, H.; Zhou, Y.; Liu, P.; Jia, Y.; Ye, C. Peptide-Coated Palladium Nanoparticle for Highly Sensitive Bioanalysis of Trypsin in Human Urine Samples. *Nanomater. Nanotechnol.* **2018,** *8*, 1847980418820391.
109. Shaili, E. Platinum Anticancer Drugs and Photochemotherapeutic Agents: Recent Advances and Future Developments. *Sci. Progress* **2014,** *97* (1), 20–40.
110. Kang, X.; Xiao, H. H.; Song, H. Q.; Jing, X. B.; Yan, L. S.; Qi, R. G. Advances in Drug Delivery System for Platinum Agents Based Combination Therapy. *Cancer Biol. Med.* **2015,** *12* (4), 362.
111. Abu-Surrah, A. S.; Kettunen, M. Platinum Group Antitumor Chemistry: Design and Development of New Anticancer Drugs Complementary to Cisplatin. *Curr. Med. Chem.* **2006,** *13* (11), 1337–1357.
112. Wheate, N. J.; Walker, S.; Craig, G. E.; Oun, R. The Status of Platinum Anticancer Drugs in the Clinic and in Clinical Trials. *Dalton Trans.* **2010,** *39* (35), 8113–8127.
113. Mukherjee, S.; Kotcherlakota, R.; Haque, S.; Bhattacharya, D.; Kumar, J. M.; Chakravarty, S.; Patra, C. R. Improved Delivery of Doxorubicin Using Rationally Designed PEGylated Platinum Nanoparticles for the Treatment of Melanoma. *Mater. Sci. Eng.: C* **2020,** *108*, 110375.
114. Ruiz, A. L.; Arribas, E. V.; McEnnis, K. Poly (Lactic-Co-Glycolic Acid) Encapsulated Platinum Nanoparticles for Cancer Treatment. *Mater. Adv.* **2022,** *3* (6), 2858–2870.
115. Kang, S.; Shin, W.; Kang, K.; Choi, M. H.; Kim, Y. J.; Kim, Y. K.; Min, D. H.; Jang, H. Revisiting of Pd Nanoparticles in Cancer Treatment: All-Round Excellence of Porous Pd Nanoplates in Gene-Thermo Combinational Therapy. *ACS Appl. Mater. Interfaces* **2018,** *10* (16), 13819–13828.
116. Shanthi, K.; Sreevani, V.; Vimala, K.; Kannan, S. Cytotoxic Effect of Palladium Nanoparticles Synthesized from Syzygium Aromaticum Aqueous Extracts and Induction of Apoptosis in Cervical Carcinoma. *Proc. Natl. Acad. Sci. India Sect. B: Biol. Sci.* **2017,** *87*, 1101–1112.
117. Gil, Y. G.; Kang, S.; Chae, A.; Kim, Y. K.; Min, D. H.; Jang, H. Synthesis of Porous Pd Nanoparticles by Therapeutic Chaga Extract for Highly Efficient Tri-Modal Cancer Treatment. *Nanoscale* 2018. *10* (42), 19810–19817.
118. Bagherzadeh, M.; Safarkhani, M.; Kiani, M.; Radmanesh, F.; Daneshgar, H.; Ghadiri, A. M.; Taghavimandi, F.; Fatahi, Y.; Safari-Alighiarloo, N.; Ahmadi, S.; Rabiee, N. MIL-125-Based Nanocarrier Decorated with Palladium Complex for Targeted Drug Delivery. *Sci. Rep.* **2022,** *12* (1), 1–5.

119. Nakata, S.; Arie, T.; Akita, S.; Takei, K. Wearable, Flexible, and Multifunctional Healthcare Device with an ISFET Chemical Sensor for Simultaneous Sweat pH and Skin Temperature Monitoring. *ACS Sensors* **2017,** *2* (3), 443–448.
120. Libanori, A.; Chen, G.; Zhao, X.; Zhou, Y.; Chen, J. Smart Textiles for Personalized Healthcare. *Nat. Electron.* **2022,** *5* (3), 142–156.
121. Deng, C.; Chen, J.; Nie, Z.; Si, S. A Sensitive and Stable Biosensor Based on the Direct Electrochemistry of Glucose Oxidase Assembled Layer-by-Layer at the multiwall carbon nanotube-modified electrode. Biosensors and Bioelectronics. 2010 Sep 15;26 (1), 213–219.
122. Kucherenko, I. S.; Soldatkin, O. O.; Kucherenko, D. Y.; Soldatkina, O. V.; Dzyadevych, S. V. Advances in Nanomaterial Application in Enzyme-Based Electrochemical Biosensors: A Review. *Nanosc. Adv.* **2019,** *1* (12), 4560–4577.
123. Li, Z.; Wang, X.; Wen, G.; Shuang, S.; Dong, C.; Paau, M. C.; Choi, M. M. Application of Hydrophobic Palladium Nanoparticles for the Development of Electrochemical Glucose Biosensor. *Biosens. Bioelectron.* **2011,** *26* (11), 4619–4623.
124. Sun, A.; Sheng, Q.; Zheng, J. A Hydrogen Peroxide Biosensor Based on Direct Electrochemistry of Hemoglobin in Palladium Nanoparticles/Graphene–Chitosan Nanocomposite Film. *Appl. Biochem. Biotechnol.* **2012,** *166*, 764–773.
125. Yan, T.; Zhu, L.; Ju, H.; Lei, J. DNA-Walker-Induced Allosteric Switch for Tandem Signal Amplification with Palladium Nanoparticles/Metal–Organic Framework Tags in Electrochemical Biosensing. *Anal. Chem.* **2018,** *90* (24), 14493–14499.
126. Qiu, J. D.; Shi, L.; Liang, R. P.; Wang, G. C.; Xia, X. H. Controllable Deposition of a Platinum Nanoparticle Ensemble on a Polyaniline/Graphene Hybrid as a Novel Electrode Material for Electrochemical Sensing. *Chem.—Eur. J.* **2012,** *18* (25), 7950–7959.
127. Harley-Trochimczyk, A.; Chang, J.; Zhou, Q.; Dong, J.; Pham, T.; Worsley, M. A.; Maboudian, R.; Zettl, A.; Mickelson, W. Catalytic Hydrogen Sensing Using Microheated Platinum Nanoparticle-Loaded Graphene Aerogel. *Sens. Actuators B: Chem.* **2015,** *206*, 399–406.
128. Singh, R.; Smitha, M. S.; Singh, S. P. The Role of Nanotechnology in Combating Multi-Drug Resistant Bacteria. *J. Nanosci. Nanotechnol.* **2014,** *14* (7), 4745–4756.
129. ur Rehman, K.; Khan, S. U.; Tahir, K.; Zaman, U.; Khan, D.; Nazir, S.; Khan, W. U.; Khan, M. I.; Ullah, K.; Anjum, S. I.; Bibi, R. Sustainable and Green Synthesis of Novel Acid Phosphatase Mediated Platinum Nanoparticles (ACP-PtNPs) and Investigation of Its In Vitro Antibacterial, Antioxidant, Hemolysis and Photocatalytic Activities. *J. Environ. Chem. Eng.* **2022,** *10* (3), 107623.
130. Tiri, R. N.; Gulbagca, F.; Aygun, A.; Cherif, A.; Sen, F. Biosynthesis of Ag–Pt Bimetallic Nanoparticles Using Propolis Extract: Antibacterial Effects and Catalytic Activity on NaBH4 Hydrolysis. *Environ. Res.* **2022,** *206*, 112622.
131. Hashimoto, M.; Yanagiuchi, H.; Kitagawa, H.; Honda, Y. Inhibitory Effect of Platinum Nanoparticles on Biofilm Formation of Oral Bacteria. *Nano Biomed.* **2017,** *9* (2), 77–82.
132. Adams, C. P.; Walker, K. A.; Obare, S. O.; Docherty, K. M. Size-Dependent Antimicrobial Effects of Novel Palladium Nanoparticles. *PloS One* **2014,** *9* (1), e85981.
133. Rajendran, S.; Prabha, S. S.; Rathish, R. J.; Singh, G.; Al-Hashem, A. Antibacterial Activity of Platinum Nanoparticles. In: *Nanotoxicity*; Elsevier, 2020; pp 275–281.
134. Sankarganesh, M.; Jose, P. A.; Raja, J. D.; Kesavan, M. P.; Vadivel, M.; Rajesh, J.; Jeyamurugan, R.; Kumar, R. S.; Karthikeyan, S. New Pyrimidine Based Ligand Capped Gold and Platinum Nano Particles: Synthesis, Characterization, Antimicrobial,

Antioxidant, DNA Interaction and In Vitro Anticancer Activities. *J. Photochem. Photobiol. B: Biol.* **2017,** *176*, 44–53.
135. Lopes, L. Q.; Ramos, A. P.; Copetti, P. M.; Acunha, T. V.; Iglesias, B. A.; Santos, R. C.; Machado, A. K.; Sagrillo, M. R. Antimicrobial Activity and Safety Applications of Meso-Tetra (4-Pyridyl) Platinum (II) Porphyrin. *Microb. Pathogen.* **2019,** *128*, 47–54.
136. Manikandan, V.; Velmurugan, P.; Park, J. H.; Lovanh, N.; Seo, S. K.; Jayanthi, P.; Park, Y. J.; Cho, M.; Oh, B. T. Synthesis and Antimicrobial Activity of Palladium Nanoparticles from Prunus× Yedoensis Leaf Extract. *Mater. Lett.* **2016,** *185*, 335–338.
137. Suleman, V. T.; Al-Hamdani, A. A.; Ahmed, S. D.; Jirjees, V. Y.; Khan, M. E.; Dib, A.; Al Zoubi, W.; Ko, Y. G. Phosphorus Schiff Base Ligand and Its Complexes: Experimental and Theoretical Investigations. *Appl. Organomet. Chem.* **2020,** *34* (4), e5546.
138. (a) Barbosa, H. F.; Attjioui, M.; Ferreira, A. P.; Moerschbacher, B. M.; Cavalheiro, É. T. New Series of Metal Complexes by Amphiphilic Biopolymeric Schiff Bases from Modified Chitosans: Preparation, Characterization and Effect of Molecular Weight on Its Biological Applications. *Int. J. Biol. Macromol.* **2020,** *145*, 417–428. (b) Hazarika, M.; Borah, D.; Bora, P.; Silva, A. R.; Das, P. Biogenic Synthesis of Palladium Nanoparticles and Their Applications as Catalyst and Antimicrobial Agent. *PLoS One* **2017,** *12* (9), e0184936.
139. Chen, X. M.; Lin, Z. J.; Chen, D. J.; Jia, T. T.; Cai, Z. M.; Wang, X. R.; Chen, X.; Chen, G. N.; Oyama, M. Nonenzymatic Amperometric Sensing of Glucose by Using Palladium Nanoparticles Supported on Functional Carbon Nanotubes. *Biosens. Bioelectron.* **2010,** *25* (7), 1803–1808.
140. Wang, L.; Jiang, K.; Shen, G. Wearable, Implantable, and Interventional Medical Devices Based on Smart Electronic Skins. *Adv. Mater. Technol.* **2021,** *6* (6), 2100107.
141. Medical Equipment Global Market Report, 2022. https://www.globenewswire.com/news-release/2022/05/13/2442731/0/en/Medical-Equipment-Global-Market-Report-2022.html
142. Kumar, P.; Dehiya, B. S.; Sindhu, A. Bioceramics for Hard Tissue Engineering Applications: A Review. *Int. J. Appl. Eng. Res.* **2018,** *13* (5), 2744–2752.
143. Świątkowska, I. Implant Metals and Their Potential Toxicity. In: *Biomarkers of Hip Implant Function*; Academic Press, 2023; pp 75–103.
144. Vishnu, J.; Manivasagam, G.; Mantovani, D.; Udduttula, A.; Coathup, M. J.; Popat, K. C.; Ren, P. G.; Prashanth, K. G. Balloon Expandable Coronary Stent Materials: A Systematic Review Focused on Clinical Success. *In Vitro Models* **2022,** *1* (2), 151–175.
145. Eid, K.; Eldesouky, A.; Fahmy, A.; Shahat, A.; Abd Elaal, R. Calcium Phosphate Scaffold Loaded with Platinum Nanoparticles for Bone Allograft. *Am. J. Biomed. Sci.* **2013,** *5* (4), 242–249.
146. Gautam, S.; Bhatnagar, D.; Bansal, D.; Batra, H.; Goyal, N. Recent Advancements in Nanomaterials for Biomedical Implants. *Biomed. Eng. Adv.* **2022,** , 100029.
147. Ferrero, M. E. Rationale for the Successful Management of EDTA Chelation Therapy in Human Burden by Toxic Metals. *BioMed Res. Int.* **2016,** *2016*.
148. Parasuraman, S. Toxicological Screening. *J. Pharm. Pharmacotherap.* **2011,** *2* (2), 74.
149. Briffa, J.; Sinagra, E.; Blundell, R. Heavy Metal Pollution in the Environment and Their Toxicological Effects on Humans. *Heliyon* **2020,** *6* (9), e04691.
150. Pati, R.; Das, I.; Mehta, R. K.; Sahu, R.; Sonawane, A. Zinc-Oxide Nanoparticles Exhibit Genotoxic, Clastogenic, Cytotoxic and Actin Depolymerization Effects by Inducing

Oxidative Stress Responses in Macrophages and Adult Mice. *Toxicol. Sci.* **2016,** *150* (2), 454–472.

151. Safranski, D. L.; Smith, K. E.; Gall, K. Mechanical Requirements of Shape-Memory Polymers in Biomedical Devices. *Polym. Rev.* **2013,** *53* (1), 76–91.
152. Cowley, A. A Healthy Future: Platinum in Medical Applications. *Platinum Metals Rev.* **2011,** *55* (2), 98–107.

CHAPTER 8

Stimuli-responsive Drug-delivery Carrier Using Metal–Organic Framework

RAJASEKHAR REDDY ALAVALA, PRIYAL SHAH, NACHIKET JOSHI, GSN KOTESWARA RAO, and MITAL PATEL

Shobhaben Pratapbhai Patel School of Pharmacy & Technology Management, SVKM's NMIMS, Vile Parle, Mumbai, Maharashtra, India

ABSTRACT

The multifunctional applications of framework materials are currently advancing and getting better every day. They were used in the field of the laboratory for land application due to the materials' excellent structural architectures and stabilities. For the scientific community in the relevant field, physiologically active metal–organic frameworks (MOFs) are greatly needed in this regard. With the careful selection of structural elements for the stimuli-responsive activity, MOFs can be created. MOFs were produced using a variety of metal ions and organic ligands, which resulted in unique constructions that are biocompatible, biodegradable, and suitable for medical use. The active pharmaceutical component can be released by the drug-delivery systems (DDSs) to carry out a requested therapeutic response. Recent years have seen substantial advancement in numerous new MOF and coordination polymer (CP) sections, which have gained favor over other distinctively defined systems due to their improved biocompatibility and adaptable loading capacities. These materials' porous features and high surface areas allowed the drug molecules to go to the target site more effectively. It has been thoroughly investigated how pharmaceuticals are loaded and released at the atomic level inside MOF pores when there are outside influences. This book chapter discusses the importance of several triggers in MOF-based targeted drug delivery. The stimuli-responsive MOF

Metals in Medicine, Volume 1: Metals for Tissue Engineering and Pharmaceutical Applications.
Sonali Sundram, Rishabha Malviya, and GSN Koteswara Rao

systems were classified according to the type of stimuli and explained with a suitable example. From a particular standpoint, further advances in stimulus-responsive smart MOFs and their applications are suggested.

8.1 INTRODUCTION

Nanomedicine can be defined as the use of nanomaterials for the diagnosis of illness, its monitoring, control, prophylaxis, and therapeutic strategies in a disease condition.[1] Nanomedicine involves the medicinal uses of materials, sensors, and devices at nano-level size, and prospective applications such as biological machines. Detection of the toxicity of the compounds is one of the current problems in nanomedicine.[2] Nanomaterials, such as biochemicals, can be valuable for both cell culture studies and animal experimentation. Thus far, nanomaterials in coherence with biomedical research have been useful in developing new diagnostic techniques and newly engineered. It makes use of unique properties of nanometric materials which are of size 10^{-9} m[3] Furthermore, this size is similar to the various bodily mechanisms, allowing nanoparticles to possibly cross membranes to gain access to the new sites of action, delivery, and interact with proteins or genetic material at various concentrations in the cell, blood, tissues, or within organs.[4]

It accounts for as many as 80 marketed preparations, in the fields of delivery, such as biomaterials, medical imaging, diagnostics, and therapy.[5] Nanomedicine offers the chance of early diagnosis and prevention, thereby, advancing therapeutic strategies and complementing the broad spectrum of diseases, majorly in cancer.[6,7] Overall, many nanomedicine preparations are currently in clinical trials, covering major diseases, such as neurological, cardiovascular, musculoskeletal, and inflammatory diseases.[8,9] Nanomedicines are used in the treatment of various diseases such as various forms of cancer, fungal infections, kidney disease, hypercholesterolemia, menopause conditions, chronic pain, multiple sclerosis, asthma, and emphysema.[10] Nanomedicines are present in different forms and have found applications in covid 19 vaccines for biomarker detection, in medical devices, magnetic resonance imagings (MRIs) for exact drug-delivery system (DDS), gene therapy, delicate surgeries, and in the treatment of diabetes.[11,12]

8.1.1 METAL–ORGANIC FRAMEWORKS (MOFs)

The metal–organic frameworks (MOFs) are crystal-like materials with highly porous structures and consists of a framework of organic compounds and metal atoms attached to them via coordinate bonds. Due to its adjustable porosity, chemical structure configuration, size, shape, and ease of derivatization or functionalization of surface, this is increasingly desirable for drug delivery.[13–15] MOFs have various biological applications for drug delivery and have gained prominence in recent years. When MOF materials are reduced to the nanoscale, they can operate as efficient nanocarriers for diagnostic imaging, chemotherapy, photothermal or photodynamic therapy.[16] Liposomes, micelles, dendrimers, microbubbles, and solid lipid nanoparticles have been explored as nanoparticle-based drug-delivery methods.[17]

Applications in Drug Delivery

Poor distribution is one of the main drawbacks of traditional chemotherapy, which is the requirement to utilize higher medication doses, frequently leads to dose-associated side or toxic effects. This necessitates finding new and effective DDSs.[18] A promising class of DDSs is MOFs, which can deliver antimicrobial agents, anticancer drugs, antiglaucoma medication, and hormones to the intended site of action. Recent scientific reports have demonstrated the use of MOF nanocarriers to attain organ or site-specific delivery of the drug, increased absorption rate, and controlled drug release.[19,20] Targeted delivery has so far been accomplished using three different methods: triggered delivery, direct delivery (such as folate, hyaluronic acid, and antibodies), and delivery due to the increased permeability and retention phenomena (e.g., temperature, pH, photoirradiation, and pressure). The pinocytosis is activated by clathrin and caveolin-mediated endocytosis, and sometimes independent endocytosis.[21,22]

Receptors are responsible for the cargo during clathrin-mediated endocytosis, which is tailed by the formation of clathrin-smeared vesicles that are typically in a size of 200 nm.[23] These clathrin vesicles develop into late endosomes after merging with early forms of the material. The resultant endosomes merge with lysosomes, which results into the DDS hydrolysis and the loaded drug molecules, subsequently reducing its therapeutic outcome.[24] On the contrary, endocytosis mediated by caveolin results in the development of indentations that are rich in lipid rafts.[25] Nanoparticles that have been ingested by a cell's caveolins can later be transported to other parts of the cell.[26] One of the biggest problems with various MOF-based DDS is premature drug release. Recent studies have demonstrated that several approaches, comprising the one-pot encapsulation of medicines into MOFs, the surface modification of the metal network, and activated drug release could be used to address this issue.[27,28] The combination of MOFs and various functional materials considerably increased the MOF performance which led to the development of novel functionality with real-world applications.[29] The MOF complexes of MOF-reduced graphene oxide (rGO), MOF-carbon nanotube (CNT), MOF-metal nanoparticles, and MOF-complexes are a few examples.[30,31] In this part, the current developments in MOF applications for the delivery of medicines in the biomedical field were discussed.

The pores of MOFs are typically stable throughout the removal of the guest molecules, which are frequently solvents and can be refilled with different substances. MOFs are, thus, attractive for storing gases such as carbon dioxide and hydrogen. Additional uses for MOFs include gas filtration, gas separation, water purification, catalysis, conducting solids, and supercapacitors.[32,33]

For intracellular delivery for cancer treatment, anticancer medications such as synthetic compounds such as cisplatin, and 5-fluorouracil and natural products such as doxorubicin, topotecan, and camptothecin have been integrated into MOFs.[19,34] For photothermal therapy, some organic dyes with near-infrared region (NIR) radiation have been utilized.[20] For photodynamic treatment, MOFs functionalized with photosensitizers were also prepared. Furthermore, the transport of many biomolecules using MOF nanocarriers has been researched recently. Organisms contain biological molecules, which are essential to biological operations.[35] They comprise tiny molecules such as amino acids and fatty acids as well as macromolecules including proteins, lipids, carbohydrates, and nucleic acids. A revolutionary method of treating diseases is to deliver these molecules with vital biological functions as biomolecular medicines.[36]

To reduce the problems caused by water contamination, researchers are focusing heavily on developing new techniques and enhancing and improving existing ones. Two of the most environmentally friendly processes used in water filtration are adsorption and photodegradation. Due to the affordable, and straightforward to operate designs required to treat wastewater, these technologies have many advantages. MOFs, as a new system of porous materials characterized by a crystal-like structure, are playing a critical role in these contexts.[37]

Due to the properties' alteration, MOFs are considered to be excellent candidates for application in the treatment of wastewater.[38] The objective of this chapter is to give a thorough overview of the most current studies that were described in the literature on the usage of MOFs for the adsorptive and photocatalytic abstraction of organic emerging pollutants from wastewater. This chapter will also briefly describe the MOF synthesis technologies. Moreover, the obstacles to producing MOF on a big scale in the future are finally acknowledged.

8.1.2 STIMULI-RESPONSIVE DRUG-DELIVERY SYSTEM

DDSs that respond to stimuli DDS seem to be a potential way to manage and target drug distribution. When the DDS is given, the release of the drug is initiated, regulated, and facilitated with the energy supplied externally by some action or external input.[39, 40] Agreeing to the type of stimuli or the kind of energy used that cause the release of the drug can be classified into three drug-delivery types (Fig. 8.1)[41,42]:

1. Physical stimuli such as thermal, ultrasound, osmotic pressure magnetic field, and electric field.
2. Chemical stimuli such as pH changes, ionic capacity, and presence of glucose.
3. Biological stimuli such as enzymes, receptors, and other macromolecules.

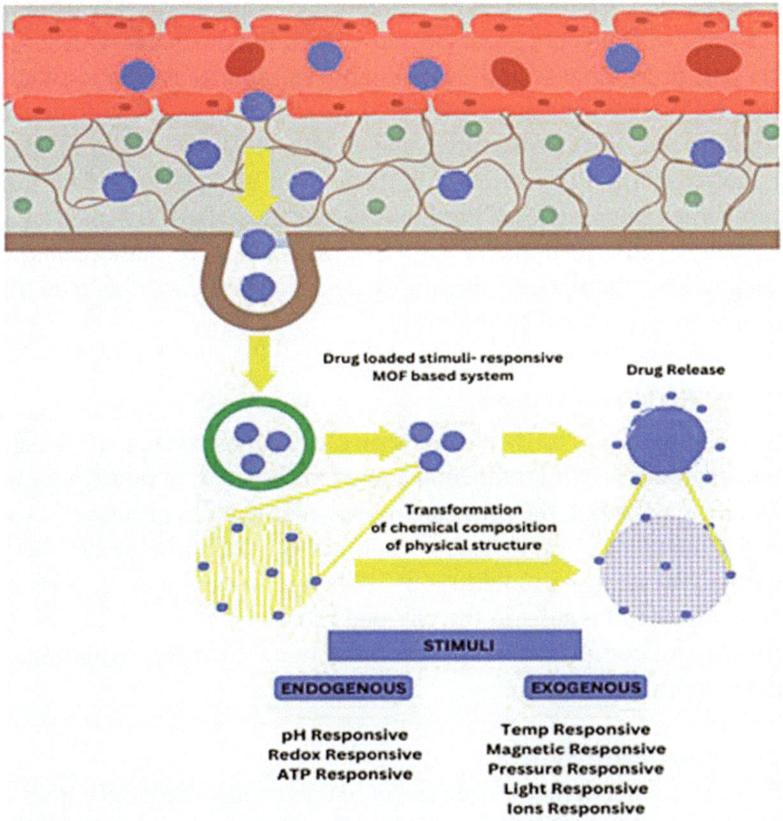

FIGURE 8.1 Drug-delivery types.

8.1.3 APPLICATIONS OF STIMULI-RESPONSIVE DRUG-DELIVERY SYSTEMS

It is possible to apply stimuli-responsive drug-delivery techniques by using an external element such as temperature, magnetic field, and electromagnetic field or ultrasonic waves. Exogenous or endogenous stimuli are intended to cause the desired release of a certain medication at predetermined sites throughout the body. This strategy has the advantage of directing a specific drug's administration to the intended spot and minimizing unwanted side effects. There are a variety of extrinsic physical stimuli that may be helpful in DDSs in addition to endogenous inputs, including light, magnetic fields, and temperature. Therapeutic effects of such DDSs are a function of reaction to the external stimuli, in contrast with smart DDSs that were known to be responsive to internal stimuli present in the tumor cells and hence, would only exhibit or display improved therapeutic properties under particular external physical stimuli applied to the tumor.[43–45]

Since cancer is a highly complex and predominant disease afflicting the 21st century, the current cancer treatment used in clinics has both severe side effects and only modest and individually variable therapeutic outcomes.[46] Various DDSs have been investigated in recent decades with the aim of cell-specific delivery of the drug and controlled release within the lesion with the expectation of overcoming those problems associated with present cancer therapy approaches.[47] Particularly, various DDSs activated by stimuli were successfully formulated with the assistance of nanotechnology to further increase therapeutic specificity, and their efficacy has recently been confirmed by preclinical animal trials.[48]

Internally Regulated systems

Often referred to as "self-regulated or closed-loop systems," these DDSs regulate the delivery of therapeutic agents in response to bodily stimuli such as pH, redox potential, the presence of enzymes such as proteases, or various other circumstances. A physical or chemical alteration in the architecture of the delivery system is brought on by a change in the biocomposition at the target location and results in the payload release. The physiological state of the illness site completely determines the release profile, which cannot be altered externally.[49]

Enzyme Responsive Systems

Proteases present as a major drug target in the management of tumors. Matrix metalloproteinases (MMPs), urokinase plasminogen activators (uPAs), and cathepsin are examples of cancer-associated proteases (CAPs) that are important in modifying tumor tissue as well as in the progression, invasion, and dissemination of illness.[50] MMPs are widely acknowledged to have a considerable part in the development and invasiveness of cancer due to evidence that they are overexpressed in many malignancies. In line to induce delivery once the substrate is broken down by the action of the enzyme inside the tumors, enzyme-receptive vectors are created using an enzyme-specific peptide.[51] The local distribution of chemotherapeutic medications using a protease-sensitive matrix is one use of these specifically created enzyme-stimulated vectors.[52] Cisplatin was further attached to the protease-cleavable peptide CGLDD.[53] The physiology of tumors depends heavily on proteases. MMPs, cathepsin, and uPAs, among others, are examples of CAPs that are essential for altering tumor tissue as well as for the invasion, spread, and progression of illness. It has been demonstrated that MMPs are overexpressed in most malignancies, and it was highly acknowledged that MMPs showed a substantial role in the progress and invasiveness of cancer.[54] Since the substrate is broken down by the action of enzymes inside the tumors, enzyme-stimulated vectors were created using an enzyme-specific peptide in line to initiate the delivery.[52] The adoption of a protease-sensitive base to deliver chemotherapeutic agents locally is one model of these specifically engineered enzyme-stimulated vectors. Furthermore, cisplatin was linked to the protease-cleavable peptide CGLDD.[53]

Externally Regulated system

Open-loop systems, also known as externally regulated systems, are vectors, whose ability to distribute drugs, which can be controlled by an external stimulus. The release pattern of the drug from these nano-vectors can be temporally and spatially adjusted to create an on-demand delivery of the drug at a specified dose because the length and intensity of the stimuli can be accurately regulated.[55] Here it is discussed that existing research carried out on thermal, photo, ultrasound, magnetic, and electrical stimuli. The stimuli-responsive DDS is nontoxic to cells, escaping the disadvantage drug leaking out of the membranes and its premature degradation as observed with conventional DDS, which leads to the inefficacy of the drug.[56,57] In contrast to the conventional DDS, smart stimuli-responsive DDS can be developed thanks to nanomaterial chemistry.

Stimuli-responsive DDS guarantees on-demand medication delivery to the intended target cancer cells in either a spatial or temporal manner. Inorganic compounds such as gold, zinc oxide, or metal oxides; and organic materials such as liposomes, micelles, peptides, synthetic polymers, or dendrimers are used to engineer the DDS.[58,59] These nanocarriers deliver the drug to specific cellular targets in reaction to both internal and exterior stimuli including thermal, photo, ultrasound, magnetic, and electrical stimuli, alteration in pH level, glutathione's (GSH's) redox ability, and enzymes.[60] In cancer therapy, DDS which can respond to more than one or two stimuli would hold more promise than a single stimulus-responsive DDS because it would significantly increase the drug delivery and accumulation in the cancer tissue, leading to improved tumor cell management.[61] A few multistimuli-responsive DDS are currently undergoing clinical trials to establish their safety and efficacy in this area.

8.2 STIMULI-RESPONSIVE MOFS FOR DRUG DELIVERY

Since it was first proposed, MOF, a type of organic–inorganic hybrid material, has received considerable interest. It has been used in many areas, including material storage, material separation, material purification, material catalysis, material sensing, material bioimaging, material energy storage, material medication delivery, and more. Relative to conventional materials, MOFs provide a variety of special features for use in DDSs. In addition to big pores, high porosity, and wide surface areas, other characteristics such as ease of functionalization, strong biocompatibility, water solubility, and biodegradability can also help to increase the loading efficiency of medications or guest molecules in the body. Also, by a variety of interactions, including hydrogen bonds, van der Waals forces, the "π–π" effect between aromatic rings, electrostatic contacts, coordination bonds, covalent bonds, and others, pharmaceuticals may be chemically conjugated or physically enclosed within the carriers. Smart materials will undergo molecular conformational changes, protonation, or hydrolytic cleavage under stimuli due to the introduction of stimuli-responsive groups or materials into MOF structure, such as imidazolyl (pH), disulfide bond (GSH), porphyrin (light), and others. This results in the release of guest molecules. Different types of stimuli-responsive MOFs are discussed in detail in the following sections (Fig. 8.2).

8.2.1 PH-RESPONSIVE MOFs

Numerous pH-responsive MOFs were prepared and proven for targeted drug delivery. To promote localized delivery of the interested drug to various

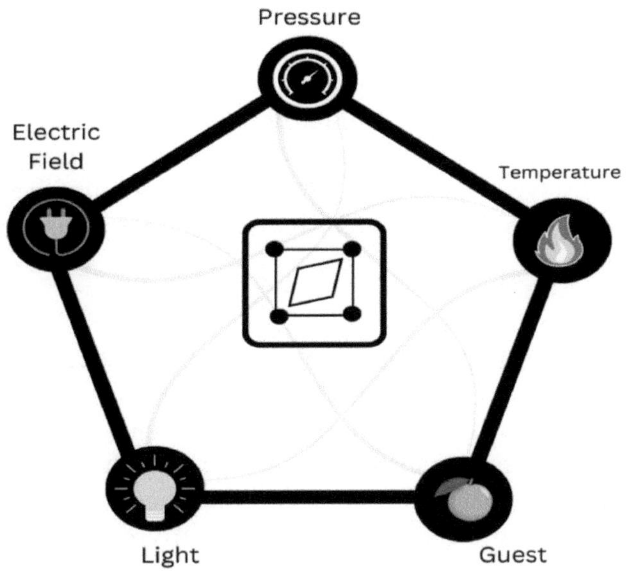

FIGURE 8.2 Different types of stimuli-responsive MOFs.

parts of the body, such as the tumor tissue, the gastrointestinal tract, or the cytoplasmic endosomal/lysosomal sections, pH-responsive devices use the changes in the pH.[62] Regardless of the oxygen content, cancerous tissue favors aerobic glycolysis as the main resource for energy. As a result, lactate builds up in the tumor's microenvironment, which lowers the extracellular matrix's pH.[63] This process is sometimes described as the "Warburg effect." This not only provides the increased energy requirement of the rapidly proliferating cancerous cells but also provides the crucial precursor molecules for the biosynthesis of other macromolecules.[64] pH-responsive vectors are characteristically constructed employing the polymers that comprise ionizable weak bases or acids. Metals that have been incorporated into these complex structures include Zinc and Zirconium. The rationale behind using zinc corresponds to it being the second-most abundant metal in the body after iron. Due to this, it is thought that the zinc-based MOFs would be biocompatible.

These MOFs have found infancy in applications in prosthetics for the heart, dressing of wounds, and bioimaging techniques, as well as in cancer diagnosis and therapeutics. MIL series of MOFs have also been studied and investigated for their biomedical applications owing to their biocompatibility, bioactivity, and good mechanical properties.[62] Recently, there was a study reported for the oxaliplatin in copper MOF with Magnetite nanoparticles and was evaluated for the simulated in vitro experiments for drug release at pH 1.2 and 7.4, which match with the gastric and intestinal conditions respectively. It reveals that 35% of the drug was released at gastric pH in 30 minutes, whereas 85% of the drug was released at intestinal pH in 9 hours. It was also observed that the drug loading is good at ambient conditions (20 mg/L in 10 min) and the MOF is following the Langmuir adsorption isotherm model.[63]

8.2.2 MAGNETICALLY RESPONSIVE METAL–ORGANIC FRAMEWORK

From the standpoint of chemical design, the harmonization of magnetism and absorbency presents a challenge because these two characteristics are antagonistic to each other. For example, while magnetic interactions call for proximity among the metal centers, which are typically the spin carriers, absorbency is usually promoted using lengthy linkers, which are commonly too lengthy for assembling the magnetism to occur at temperatures of absolute zero and above.[65,66] To create porous magnetic materials, various synthetic pathways may be designed, some of which are detailed as follows. Primarily, the utilization of shorter linkers in the creation of magnetic MOFs will be discussed, with specific instances employing cyanides, formates, diazines, and lactates. When combined with lengthy linkers, it can create wide pore spaces.[67] Second, a new synthetic approach—the metallo-ligand approach—that involves employing premade complexes to create magnetic MOFs. Finally, the demonstration of the radical ligands can be used to combine exchange coupling and porosity, and several examples of the usage of various radicals will be discussed. Using MOFs for selective adsorption is a successful technique for cleaning up hydrocarbon fuels. Given that the adsorption take place in liquid phases, MOFs magnetic properties should considerably ease the separation and recycling of adsorbents.[68,69]

The elimination of methylene blue (MB) was investigated using a novel, straightforward, and effective method for creating a magnetic MOF as an adsorbent to get rid of organic chemicals from fabricated water samples.[70] The innovative adsorbents combine the benefits of magnetic MOFs in nano-size to have a high capacity, less expensive, quick elimination, and simple solid-phase separation, creating them as an operative sorbent for treating wastewater. The resultant magnetic MOF complexes, often referred to as MFCs, exhibit substantial surface areas up to 79.52 m^2/g, outstanding magnetic capacity of 14.89 emu/g, substantial mesoporous volume (0.09 cm^3/g), and good chemical and mechanical stability.[1]

8.2.3 ION-RESPONSIVE METAL–ORGANIC FRAMEWORK

Ion-responsive MOFs have drawn a lot of attention from researchers because they provide a fresh method of drug delivery. Ionic interactions between ionic drug moieties and MOFs regulate the diffusion and release of pharmaceuticals in the DDS based on ion-responsive MOFs.[72] As a subclass of MOFs that contain uncoordinated ions in the porous voids, ionic metal–organic frameworks (iMOFs) are significant. Depending on how charged the framework is, iMOFs are additionally divided into anionic and cationic MOFs. Even though cationic MOFs possess inherent characteristics that make them good materials for anion reception, the synthetic methods required for target-specific applications are more difficult and have received less attention. Neutral N-donor bi-/multidentate ligands are typically utilized to create cationic MOFs which leave the anionic portion of the metal salt as the only component responsible for preserving the charge balance.[73,74]

Due to the necessity of a counter-cooperative ion's participation in both their creation and composition, cationic MOFs are an exceptional class of MOFs. These frameworks are typically made of neutral nitrogen-donating ligands, imposing a partial positive pore environment that is countered by residual counterions residing in the empty space. Despite this, cationic MOFs have demonstrated remarkable success in the sequestration of anions because the uncoordinated or weakly coordinated counter ions in the framework offer a superb platform for anion exchange. The majority of the earliest reports of anion-exchangers, and cationic MOFs are 1D or 2D coordination polymers (CPs) that date back to the early 2000s.[72]

It is desired for the MOF materials to have hydrolytic stability, quick anion adsorption kinetics, greater binding affinity, extreme anion adsorption capability, selectivity toward a specific anion binding, structure stability after the adsorption of counter ion, and most importantly reusability. Current research in this field has significantly improved the aforementioned qualities, opening the door for biological and environmental applications. Although the majority of the work on anion receptor chemistry still concentrates on soft materials, solution-phase molecular assemblies, and small molecules, using MOFs as an alternate approach has inherent advantages in the simplicity of achieving high-affinity anion binding. This is mostly due to the MOF's numerous metal ions, which can operate as direct anion coordination sites, supply anions with electrostatic interactions, or increase anion binding by polarizing the ligand in situations where an anion is binding to functional groups on the ligand.[72,73]

Additionally, compared to bulk water, the clustering of organic ligands within MOFs can offer a low-dielectric microenvironment to improve the anion binding. It is challenging to achieve selective binding toward a specific anion while employing MOFs as anion receptors. When designing small-molecule anion receptors, size and shape matching between the receptor and anion are often implemented to achieve anion selectivity. It is difficult to apply a similar idea to MOF-based anion receptors since doing so involves generating a well-preorganized anion-binding chamber.[72]

8.2.4 THERMAL RESPONSIVE METAL–ORGANIC FRAMEWORK

Polymers are incorporated by an in situ polymerization strategy with the help of regulated loads into the pores of the mesoporous MOFs. The MOF polymer comprises an unknown thermal activated water absorption and releases behavior initiating from the thermosensitive phase transition of polymer poly(*N*-isopropylacrylinamide), the results provided awareness on the expansion of stimuli-responsive porous absorbent constituents that are used for water purification as well as heat-transfer applications.[75] In comparatively mild-operating environments, thermal-responsive MOFs are flexible; the capacity to modify themselves when there are thermal stimuli while retaining a typical crystal structure is desirable for highly engineered mechanisms of some specialized actuators and sensors (Fig. 8.3). The thermal-responsive MOFs are designed according to electronic dispersion data supported by Density function theory, with materials which are isoreticular in nature such as MIL-53 (A1), MIL-53 (A1), FA(DUT-4), DUT-5, and MIL-53 out of which only MIL53 (Al) and MIL (53) have been studied to manage this change within realistic temperature ranges, thus being potentially feasible approaches.[76,77]

Unusual thermomechanical characteristics, such as "colossal" positive thermal expansion (PTE) and volumetric or uniaxial negative thermal expansion (NTE), have just lately been observed. These research studies have only concentrated on complex coordination networks with no voids that are open to visitors. There is currently no logical approach for the implementation and manipulation of such "extreme" thermomechanical properties in archetypal MOFs that are porous coordination networks.[75] The use of functionalized

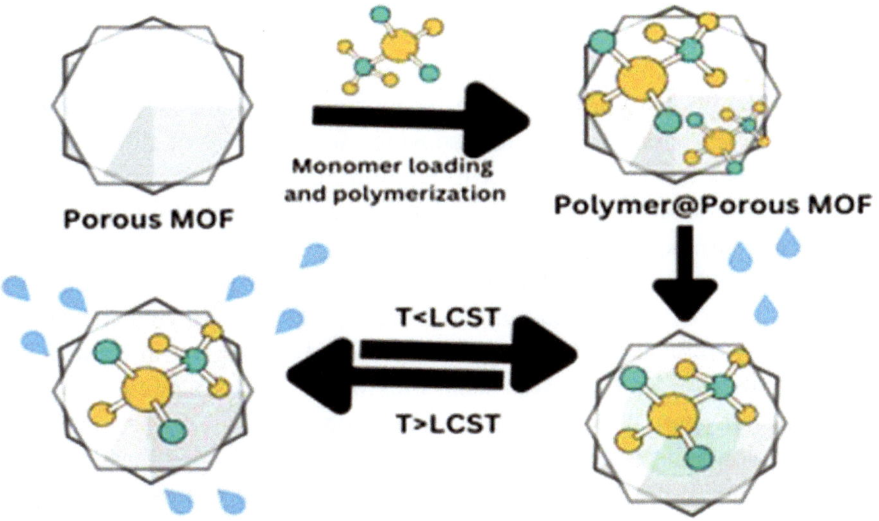

FIGURE 8.3 Thermal responsive MOFs.

linkers with pendant flexible substituents has allowed us to show how extreme thermomechanical features, such as huge framework expansion with uniaxial NTE and PTE, as well as temperature-responsive breathing, may be realized in MOFs. The unusual thermomechanical behavior is thought to result from the linear side chains' enhanced thermal movements (vibrations, rotations) as a function of temperature. The durable and structurally well-defined framework backbone interacts with the adaptable substituents to provide a surprising structural response in the hybrid solid/liquid materials that is temperature dependent. Crucially, according to the idea of mixed linker MOFs, the specific properties of each MOF are governed by the chain length and chemical makeup of the pendent side chains, allowing for a precise fine-tuning of the thermomechanical properties. The development of new functional hybrid materials for applications in sensing, heat storage/transfer, or for temperature switchable devices may be facilitated by our novel methodology using mixed fuels, which is theoretically transferable to a wide range of other MOF systems.[75,76]

8.2.5 PRESSURE-RESPONSIVE MOFs

These were synthesized and examined heavily in the recent past. Their novelty resides in possessing a high exterior area and their capability to withhold the additives to MOFs. Pressure-responsive MOFs focus on high-pressure crystallography measurements which are employed in examining the materials. It is feasible to approach pressures that are 4–6 times greater than ambient conditions. These pressure-responsive MOFs are used in molecular separation, gas storage, chemical sensing, and delivery of drug materials. Pressure-responsive MOFs work by exploiting the gate phenomenon. This opening and closing of the gate is dependent upon external pressure. This pressure is termed as gate opening pressure.[78,79]

In a recent publication a new (3,24)-connected MOF, porous coordination network (PCN)-69, maintains its mesoporosity following the removal of the guest molecules.[78] When O_2 was the adsorbate, an intriguing gate-opening sorption isotherm was seen. Flexible MOFs, which can achieve an expanded structure under pressurization, frequently exhibit abrupt increases in adsorption and decreases in pressure. It has been claimed that pressurization with supercritical gases can reveal the gate-opening pressure in flexible MOFs. Supercritical N_2, O_2, CH_4, and CO_2 high-pressure excess-adsorption isotherms were gathered in PCN-69.

All of the isotherms clearly showed a step, which is extremely uncommon in high-pressure gas-sorption isotherms and is a clear sign of the flexibility of the framework. The sequence of the gate-opening pressure, $N_2 > O_2 > CH_4 > CO_2$, is the reverse of the heat of adsorption and indicates the energy required to expand the framework. The gate-opening pressures in PCN-69 are higher than in previously published results, where the framework flexibility results from π–π stacking; this indicates a higher energy required to cause the curvature change. PCN-69 has solid network connectivity and a pressurized expandable scaffold. This flexibility results from the geodesic ligand adopted pressure-responsive curvature change, which is supported by model simulation, powder X-ray diffraction (PXRD), and gas–sorption experiments. This is the first instance of a flexible MOF caused by covalent-bond bending and curvature change that we are aware of.[78]

8.2.6 PHOTORESPONSIVE MOFs

Light response is a specific stressor, which can induce a conformational and most importantly a nondestructive change in the structure which can be used to release the contents inside the MFs. These are MOFs combined that respond to light stimuli and have shown uses in sensors, storage of gas, and phase separations besides the delivery of drugs. These MOFs undergo certain changes in pores in the presence of ultraviolet–visible (UV–visible) light. Photoresponsive MOFs absorb the incident energy and get converted from a basic singlet state to excited singlet state. This energy, upon relaxation back to the basic singlet state, if released as a fluorescent photon, the result will be fluorescence. This unique property can be used in bioimaging. The electrons of the excited singlet state can react with cancerous cells to give type-I and type-II reactions. Type-I reaction causes the formation of reactive oxygen species (ROS), while in type-II reactions, a reactive singlet oxygen species is formed, both thereby assisting in killing the cancerous cells. Photoresponsive MOFs can be divided into two types, either they have photoresponsive elements involved intrinsically or they have phototherapeutic agents involved nonintrinsically. Intrinsic ones are again divided into two types, namely, organic-doped MOF or metal-doped MOF. Metal-doped MOFs consist of copper, iron, and manganese-based MOFs. There are many strategies to formulate such MOFs. Primarily, it can be formulated by using light-switchable guest materials. An example of such a MOF is spiropyran MOF. The closed ring of spiropyran structure (SP) is composed of an indoline ring joined to a benzopyran structure in a spiro arrangement. The open ring conformation is formed upon substitutions when irradiated with UV light. Another strategy that can be used to formulate photoresponsive MOFs is to encapsulate a photoswitchable guest molecule into the MOF, such that upon irradiation of UV light, its physicochemical properties such as pore size, porosity, acidity, and basicity would change. Such MOFs are called MOF composites. Some semiconductors that have found applications exploit an empty d-orbital of inorganic material. An example of such a MOF is NH_2-UiO-66-based composites. Reversible photocycloaddition of the styryl pyrene groups connected to the MOFs produces effective gating capabilities and enables numerous cycles of charging and discharging of small molecules.[80] The photoresponsive MOFs can be employed by loading and unloading a hydrogenation catalyst called tetramethyl ethylenediamine (TEMED). The light-gated technique creates hydrogels of different sizes and forms by allowing control over the catalyst's release.[81]

8.2.7 MOISTURE-RESPONSIVE MOFs

Moisture-responsive MOFs are effective but they possess challenges such as sensitivity one of the greatest efficient ways to resolve this issue is to change the surface of MOFs from the hydrophilic to hydrophobic groups.[82] To dramatically increase the moisture or water resistance of MOF materials, we offer a general strategy to change lipophilic polydimethylsiloxane (PDMS) on their surface using a simple vapor deposition method. As exemplary susceptible MOFs, HKUST-1, ZnBT, and MOF-5 were effectively coated with PDMS; the coated samples successfully retained the crystalline and porosity features of the original materials. Surprisingly, the PDMS coating nearly completely preserved the surface areas of these MOFs. As a result of such a coating procedure, MOFs may be used in extensive sectors including gas sorption and catalysis where there is moisture or the presence of water. Due to their higher heats of regeneration, prolonged cycling durations, and high-molecular-weight components, indoor moisture management tools using conventional desiccating agents or adsorbents are even less competitive than VCAC.[83,84]

One study reported the use of a brand-new higher temperature chilling system that can regulate humidity using porous MOFs. The exterior of the condenser and evaporator are immediately coated with MOFs. Relative to a traditional VCAC, the system has no extra parts. Incoming air can have its sensible and latent loads concurrently removed by the evaporator without lowering the conditions under its dew point temperature. All of the leftover heat from the condenser is used to power the regeneration of wet MOFs. The amphiphilic MOFs employed in the study feature great hydrothermal stability, low-cost raw material synthesis, and high water uptake. They might therefore be scaled up for extensive air-cooling applications.[85]

8.2.8 REDOX-RESPONSIVE MOFs

As a promising platform for regulated drug administration, MOFs, a special family of hybrid porous materials made from metal ions and organic ligands, which have garnered a lot of attention lately. Coating of the stimuli-responsive agents inside the complex and modified MOFs or modification of their surfaces after the synthesis with sensitive agents are the existing techniques for creating MOF-based responsive DDS.[86] With iron, aluminum, or zirconium serving as the metal nodules and 4,4′-dithiobisbenzoic acid (DTBA) serving as the organic ligand, a novel intrinsic redox-responsive MOF carrier, known as MOF-M (DTBA) (where M can be Fe, Al or Zr) was discovered. Glutathione (GSH) is frequently overexpressed in cancer cells, and can break the disulfide link in DTBA (Fig. 8.4). The right size and characteristics for a medication were found in MOF-Zr based on DTBA synthesized at 40°C. Curcumin (CCM) was added to MOF-Zr (DTBA) to create nanoparticles of CCM@MOF-Zr (DTBA), which released their contents more quickly than free CCM and caused more cell death in cell line study. According to in vivo data, free CCM had much lower antitumor activity than CCM@ MOF-Zr (DTBA). The applicability of MOFs in theranostics, molecular imaging, and drug administration may be expanded by using this technique for building responsive MOFs-based nanocarriers. Another example of redox-responsive MOF is the combination of folic acid (FA) and anhydride bonds anchored onto the MOF structures to get effective release patterns of 5-fluorouracil. This was encapsulated inside UiO-66-NH_2 nanostructures along with a synergistically acting drug dichloroacetic acid. The additional concentration of GSH upon release reacts with the thiolate moiety and is oxidized, thereby achieving redox stimuli-responsive drugs release in MOFs. The microscopy confirmed that the addition of folic acid onto the surface of MOF can be proved to be beneficial in achieving targeted drug delivery for cancer therapy.[87–89]

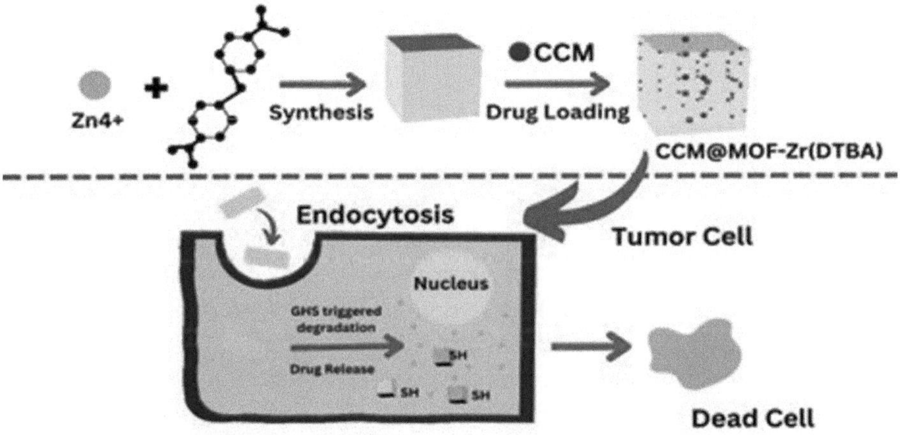

FIGURE 8.4 Breakdown of disulfide linkage in DTBA.

8.2.9 ATP-RESPONSIVE MOFs

These are nanoparticles that consist of MOF modified with nucleic acid binding sites. Here an example of the adenosine triphosphate (ATP)-sensitive zeolitic imidazole framework-90 (ZIF-90) is discussed as a versatile carrier for CRISPR/Cas9 genome editing and cytosolic protein delivery.[90] ZIF-90/ protein nanoparticles were created when imidazole-2-carbaldehyde, Zn^{2+}, self-assembled with the help of protein to effectively encapsulate it. It was discovered that the competition among the ATP and the Zn^{2+} of ZIF-90 caused the breakdown of ZIF-90 nanoparticles in the ATP presence, thus removing the protein part from the MOF. The ZIF-90/protein can transfer a wide range of therapeutic peptides inside the cellular assembly, irrespective of its mass and shape.[91] When RNase A which is toxic to the cells, is effectively delivered, tumor cell growth is inhibited, and when the genome-editing protein Cas9 is successfully delivered, HeLa cells' production of the green fluorescent protein (GFP) is knocked out with an efficiency of up to 35%. As ATP is increased in diseased cells, it was anticipated that the distribution of ATP-sensitive proteins would create new possibilities for enhanced protein or peptide delivery and editing of the CRISPR/Cas9 genome to treat specific diseases.[92] ATP was detected using a new technique of radiometric surface-enhanced Raman scattering (SERS) method built on stimuli-receptive DNA derivatized MOFs. As a result, ATP had a detection limit of 0.4 nM and a range of 1–200 nM. The ratiometric SERS biosensor technique gives a lower detection limit and more improved performance than the traditional SERS detection based on a single signal response, which may have the ability to detect different biomolecules or metal ions.[93]

8.2.10 COMPETITIVE BINDING AGENT'S RESPONSIVE STIMULI

This type of MOF is known for its easy functionalization, desirable host guests or desirable host–guest performance. Modification of nanomaterials with these agents can offer a new avenue for possible biological applications. β-cyclodextrin (β-CD) and supramolecular materials such as pillar arenes can change the surface structure of MOFs upon modifications and for the advancement of stimuli-responsive DDS. When there is a high affinity toward binding between competitive binding agents and a supramolecular material on a surface the release of drugs loaded in the MOF is triggered by the addition of a competitive binding agent.[94–96]

Based on the zinc-based MOF UMCM-1-NH_2, a monodispersed theranostic nanoplatform (102 nm) with dual stimuli-responsive (pH and competitive binding agent) drug release capacity was created. UMCM-1-NH2 was connected to positively charged "stalks" in this experiment. The negatively charged carboxylatopillar arene (CP5), a pillar arene-based supramolecular switch that serves as a gatekeeper, was then loaded with rhodamine 6G (Rh6G) or DOX and attached to the stalks with the aid of host-guest complexation.[97] By addition of methyl viologen salts, which will act as competitive binding agents competing with ATP, leading to trigger of the drug release due to increased binding affinity with CP5. CP5 is known for not having any charge in the intracellular acidic tumor cell, which can lessen the noncovalent binding energy among the π stalk and CP5, thus free drug is released. This theragnostic nano-platform had a high-level drug filling capability, drug release in responsive to stimulus, minimal cytotoxicity, excellent biodegradability, and great biocompatibility, and this can act as a new tool and can help in drug delivery for cancer treatment.[98,99]

β-CD@UiO-68-azo is an example of stimulus-responsive that was a mechanized MOF and comprised of a cyclodextrin (CD) ring providing a doorkeeper to monitor the release of its contents. This system shows the delivery of contents activated by the accumulation of competitive agents. Amantadine, hereby used as a competitive agent, had a superior binding affinity to CD and activated the dissociation of the CD nucleus from the azobenzene parts and therefore released the contents. Additionally, since CD possesses a superior binding affinity to the *trans*-form of azobenzene than to *cis*-form of azobenzene, exposure to ultraviolet (UV) light, which *trans*-forms azobenzene from *trans*-form to *cis*-form, also leads to its dissociation on the MOF surface. This MOF-based system may offer a unique platform for on-command drug delivery.[100,101]

8.3 MULTIPLE STIMULI-RESPONSIVE MOFs

To overcome challenges related to the human body and the complexities of the nature of cancer besides attempting to improve the therapeutic effectiveness, DDSs generally need multiple stimuli-responsive MOFs. Thus, MOFs based on multiple stimuli-responsive materials have been created to attain more specific cancer therapeutics that not only help in the controlled release of drugs but also have various biomedical applications as well.[102–104] For the surface functionalization of MOFs, a clever technique based on coordination chemistry has recently been reported. The stability of the nanocarrier is an issue when using the technology in vivo, though, as the conveyed cargoes are restricted to particular His-tagged and phosphate-modified proteins. The development of programmable MOFs for nanotherapeutic delivery calls for the immediate development of a universal technique that can change the surface of various MOFs. The development of effective delivery platforms will also enable the targeted distribution and stimuli-responsive release of a variety of medications for the treatment of cancer. For targeted cancer therapy, it is essential to prepare therapeutic MOFs with combinational therapies that can target and react to the tumor microenvironment. The development of a generic method for making stimuli-responsive, multifunctional MOF nanoparticles that can easily combine various functional molecular units with various MOFs and, preferably, have superior capabilities for effective therapeutic delivery, would be helpful.[103]

To create effective nanotherapeutics, polydopamine (PDA), undoubtedly the most adaptable coating material for surface treatment and a superior photothermal transduction material, is combined with MOF, a rapidly growing nanomotif with varied designability. These stimuli-responsive, multifunctional MOFs display the following characteristics: First, because of the special and practical conjugation properties of PDA, the PDA-modified MOFs preloaded with chemotherapy drugs have better solubility, and the outer surface of PDA can be easily linked with functional molecules of interest. For targeted medication administration, various MOF types, including ZIF-8, MIL101, and UiO-66 functionalized with PDA, were successfully coupled with targeting molecules including aptamer and FA. Second, the created nanocarriers for controlled cancer therapy are stimuli-responsive and stable under healthy settings but break down in an acidic environment or near tumor tissue. Last, but not the least, the PDA's capping layer is a multipurpose interface that functions as a therapeutic element with strong photothermal transduction efficiency. This interface enables the combination of chemotherapy and photothermal therapy in addition to offering a surface that is practical for the conjugation of targeted compounds. Overall, the produced stimuli-responsive multifunctional MOFs effectively and continuously deliver nanotherapeutics to cancer cells. The developed approach can be used to treat MOFs of various sorts using chemophoto-thermal combination therapy.[103]

8.4 CHALLENGES AND FUTURE PROSPECTS

Future prospects should mainly focus on the kinds of MOFs that can be extensively used in management of cancer which can help in trespassing existing concerns and shortcomings of the standard DDS. Certain other challenges faced are that the MOFs are difficult and complex in construction as well as with the understanding of how they work on human bodies.[105] Each model holds its own challenges, for example, the external stimuli-responsive model has more flexibility than the internal stimuli-responsive model, hence, more studies and extensive research should be done in the field of preparation of MOFs based on such model DDS. To overcome such challenges, proper optimization should be carried out for such systems preceding clinical purposes by creating organized studies on in-vivo experimentations and their stability.

8.5 CONCLUSION

It is well-established that MOFs are porous in nature and have higher drug loading capacities as well as help in easy functionalization in addition to being biocompatible in nature. However, more work and extensive research are required to uncover novel multifunctional MOFs. More research is deemed necessary to determine the potential toxicity profiles. Hence, MOFs based on certain modes of stimulus have low toxicity, the ability to degrade in the environment, and high therapeutic effectiveness are favorable research paths, but their clinical applications remain far in sight.

KEYWORDS

- **drug-delivery systems**
- **targeted drug delivery**
- **metal-organic frameworks**
- **stimuli-responsive**
- **surface modification**
- **cancer drug delivery**

REFERENCES

1. Sakaguchi, M. An Introduction to Nanotechnology. *Br. Biomed. Bull.* **2021,** *9* (2), 06.
2. Gu, N.; Sheng, J. Introduction to Nanomedicine. In: *Nanomedicine*; Springer Nature: Singapore, 2022; pp 1–14.
3. Al Sharabati, M.; Sabouni, R.; Husseini, G. A. Biomedical Applications of Metal–Organic Frameworks for Disease Diagnosis and Drug Delivery: A Review. *Nanomaterials* **2022,** *12* (2), 277.

4. Schlich, M.; Palomba, R.; Costabile, G.; Mizrahy, S.; Pannuzzo, M.; Peer, D.; Decuzzi, P. Cytosolic Delivery of Nucleic Acids: The Case of Ionizable Lipid Nanoparticles. *Bioeng. Transl. Med.* **2021,** *6* (2), e10213.
5. Abdel-Mageed, H. M.; AbuelEzz, N. Z.; Radwan, R. A.; Mohamed, S. A. Nanoparticles in Nanomedicine: A Comprehensive Updated Review on Current Status, Challenges and Emerging Opportunities. *J. Microencapsulation* **2021,** *38* (6), 414–436.
6. Li, L.; He, R.; Yan, H.; Leng, Z.; Zhu, S.; Gu, Z. Nanotechnology for the Diagnosis and Treatment of Alzheimer's Disease: A Bibliometric Analysis. *Nano Today* **2022,** *47*, 101654.
7. Bozzer, S.; Dal Bo, M.; Grimaldi, M. C.; Toffoli, G.; Macor, P. Nanocarriers as a Delivery Platform for Anticancer Treatment: Biological Limits and Perspectives in B-Cell Malignancies. *Pharmaceutics* **2022,** *14* (9), 1965.
8. Tuteja, J.; Sand, A. Role of Nanomedicine for Targeted Drug Delivery in Life-Threatening Diseases. In: *Nanobiotechnology for the Livestock Industry*–; Elsevier, 2023; pp 189–217.
9. Kumar, R.; Gulia, K. The Convergence of Nanotechnology-Stem Cell, Nanotopography-Mechanobiology, and Biotic-Abiotic Interfaces: Nanoscale Tools for Tackling the Top Killer, Arteriosclerosis, Strokes, and Heart Attacks. *Nano Select* **2021,** *2* (4), 655–687.
10. Shukla, R.; Thok, K.; Kakade, S.; Handa, M.; Beg, S. Clinical Translation Status of Nanoformulations. In: *Nanoformulation Strategies for Cancer Treatment*–; Elsevier, 2021; pp 303–338.
11. Singh, P.; Singh, D.; Sa, P.; Mohapatra, P.; Khuntia, A.; K Sahoo, S. Insights from Nanotechnology in COVID-19: Prevention, Detection, Therapy and Immunomodulation. *Nanomedicine* **2021,** *16* (14), 1219–1235.
12. Weiss, C.; Carriere, M.; Fusco, L.; Capua, I.; Regla-Nava, J. A.; Pasquali, M.; Scott, J. A.; Vitale, F.; Unal, M. A.; Mattevi, C.; Bedognetti, D. Toward Nanotechnology-Enabled Approaches Against the COVID-19 Pandemic. *ACS Nano* **2020,** *14* (6), 6383–6406.
13. Lee, Y. R.; Kim, J.; Ahn, W. S. Synthesis of Metal-Organic Frameworks: A Mini Review. *Korean J. Chem. Eng.* **2013,** *30*, 1667–1680.
14. Xiao, X.; Zou, L.; Pang, H.; Xu, Q. Synthesis of Micro/Nanoscaled Metal–Organic Frameworks and Their Direct Electrochemical Applications. *Chem. Soc. Rev.* **2020,** *49* (1), 301–331.
15. Seth, S.; Matzger, A. J. Metal–Organic Frameworks: Examples, Counterexamples, and an Actionable Definition. *Crystal Growth Design.* **2017,** *17* (8), 4043–4048.
16. Huang, Y.; He, S.; Cao, W.; Cai, K.; Liang, X. J. Biomedical Nanomaterials for Imaging-Guided Cancer Therapy. *Nanoscale* **2012,** *4* (20), 6135–6149.
17. Yao, Y.; Zhou, Y.; Liu, L.; Xu, Y.; Chen, Q.; Wang, Y.; Wu, S.; Deng, Y.; Zhang, J.; Shao, A. Nanoparticle-Based Drug Delivery in Cancer Therapy and Its Role in Overcoming Drug Resistance. *Front. Mol. Biosci.* **2020,** *7*, 193.
18. Deshantri, A. K.; Moreira, A. V.; Ecker, V.; Mandhane, S. N.; Schiffelers, R. M.; Buchner, M.; Fens, M. H. Nanomedicines for the Treatment of Hematological Malignancies. *J. Controlled Release.* **2018,** *287*, 194–215.
19. Sun, Y.; Zheng, L.; Yang, Y.; Qian, X.; Fu, T.; Li, X.; Yang, Z.; Yan, H.; Cui, C.; Tan, W. Metal–Organic Framework Nanocarriers for Drug Delivery in Biomedical Applications. *Nano-Micro Lett.* **2020,** *12*, 1–29.
20. Ma, X.; Lepoitevin, M.; Serre, C. Metal–Organic Frameworks Towards Bio-Medical Applications. *Mater. Chem. Front.* **2021,** *5* (15), 5573–5594.

21. Bilal, M.; Qindeel, M.; Raza, A.; Mehmood, S.; Rahdar, A. Stimuli-Responsive Nanoliposomes as Prospective Nanocarriers for Targeted Drug Delivery. *J. Drug Deliv. Sci. Technol.* **2021,** *66,* 102916.
22. Mura, S.; Nicolas, J.; Couvreur, P. Stimuli-Responsive Nanocarriers for Drug Delivery. *Nat. Mater.* **2013,** *12* (11), 991–1003.
23. Takei, K.; Haucke, V.; Slepnev, V.; Farsad, K.; Salazar, M.; Chen, H.; De Camilli, P. Generation of Coated Intermediates of Clathrin-Mediated Endocytosis on Protein-Free Liposomes. *Cell* **1998,** *94* (1), 131–141.
24. Yin, Q.; Shen, J.; Zhang, Z.; Yu, H.; Li, Y. Reversal of Multidrug Resistance by Stimuli-Responsive Drug Delivery Systems for Therapy of Tumor. *Adv. Drug Deliv. Rev.* **2013,** *65* (13–14), 1699–1715.
25. Filippini, A.; D'alessio, A. Caveolae and Lipid Rafts in Endothelium: Valuable Organelles for Multiple Functions. *Biomolecules* **2020,** *10* (9), 1218.
26. Fröhlich, E. Cellular Elimination of Nanoparticles. *Environ. Toxicol. Pharmacol.* **2016,** *46,* 90–94.
27. Hasan, M. N.; Bera, A.; Maji, T. K.; Pal, S. K. Sensitization of Nontoxic MOF for Their Potential Drug Delivery Application Against Microbial Infection. *Inorg. Chim. Acta* **2021,** *523,* 120381.
28. Wang, P.; Jin, Z.; Song, G.; Zhang, X. B. Recent Progress and Strategies for Precise Framework Structure-Enabled Drug Delivery Systems. *Mater. Today Sustain.* **2021,** *13,* 100065.
29. Freund, R.; Zaremba, O.; Arnauts, G.; Ameloot, R.; Skorupskii, G.; Dincă, M.; Bavykina, A.; Gascon, J.; Ejsmont, A.; Goscianska, J.; Kalmutzki, M. The Current Status of MOF and COF Applications. *Angew. Chem. Int. Ed.* **2021,** *60* (45), 23975–24001.
30. Gurusamy, L.; Anandan, S.; Wu, J. J. Nanomaterials Derived from Metal-Organic Frameworks for Energy Storage Supercapacitor Application. In: *Metal-Organic Frameworks for Chemical Reactions–*; Elsevier, 2021; pp 441–470.
31. Zeeshan, M.; Shahid, M. State of the Art Developments and Prospects of Metal–Organic Frameworks for Energy Applications. *Dalton Trans.* **2022,** *51* (5), 1675–1723.
32. Farha, O. K.; Hupp, J. T. Rational Design, Synthesis, Purification, and Activation of Metal–Organic Framework Materials. *Acc. Chem. Res.* **2010,** *43* (8), 1166–1175.
33. Meek, S. T.; Greathouse, J. A.; Allendorf, M. D. Metal-Organic Frameworks: A Rapidly Growing Class of Versatile Nanoporous Materials. *Adv. Mater.* **2011,** *23* (2), 249–267.
34. Attia, M. *Development of Metal-Organic Framework Based Magnetic Nanocomposites for Controlled Drug Delivery to Treat Glioblastoma*; Doctoral dissertation, The University of Texas at San Antonio.
35. Sargazi, S.; Fatima, I.; Kiani, M. H.; Mohammadzadeh, V.; Arshad, R.; Bilal, M.; Rahdar, A.; Díez-Pascual, A. M.; Behzadmehr, R. Fluorescent-Based Nanosensors for Selective Detection of a Wide Range of Biological Macromolecules: A Comprehensive Review. *Int. J. Biol. Macromol.* **2022,** *206,* 115–1147.
36. Sapsford, K. E.; Algar, W. R.; Berti, L.; Gemmill, K. B.; Casey, B. J.; Oh, E.; Stewart, M. H.; Medintz, I. L. Functionalizing Nanoparticles with Biological Molecules: Developing Chemistries That Facilitate Nanotechnology. *Chem. Rev.* **2013,** *113* (3), 1904–2074.
37. Nasrollahzadeh, M.; Sajjadi, M.; Iravani, S.; Varma, R. S. Starch, Cellulose, Pectin, Gum, Alginate, Chitin and Chitosan Derived (Nano) Materials for Sustainable Water Treatment: A Review. *Carbohydr. Polym.* **2021,** *251,* 116986.

38. Bazer-Bachi, D.; Assié, L.; Lecocq, V.; Harbuzaru, B.; Falk, V. Towards Industrial Use of Metal-Organic Framework: Impact of Shaping on the MOF Properties. *Powder Technol.* **2014,** *255*, 52–59.
39. Baek, S.; Singh, R. K.; Khanal, D.; Patel, K. D.; Lee, E. J.; Leong, K. W.; Chrzanowski, W.; Kim, H. W. Smart Multifunctional Drug Delivery Towards Anticancer Therapy Harmonized in Mesoporous Nanoparticles. *Nanoscale* **2015,** *7* (34), 14191–14216.
40. Arun, A.; Malrautu, P.; Laha, A.; Ramakrishna, S. Gelatin Nanofibers in Drug Delivery Systems and Tissue Engineering. *Eng. Sci.* **2021,** *16*, 71–81.
41. Lopes, J. R.; Santos, G.; Barata, P.; Oliveira, R.; Lopes, C. M. Physical and Chemical Stimuli-Responsive Drug Delivery Systems: Targeted Delivery and Main Routes of Administration. *Curr. Pharm. Design* **2013,** *19* (41), 7169–7184.
42. Delcea, M.; Möhwald, H.; Skirtach, A. G. Stimuli-Responsive LbL Capsules and Nanoshells for Drug Delivery. *Adv. Drug Deliv. Rev.* **2011,** *63* (9), 730–747.
43. Zhu, D.; Roy, S.; Liu, Z.; Weller, H.; Parak, W. J.; Feliu, N. Remotely Controlled Opening of Delivery Vehicles and Release of Cargo by External Triggers. *Adv. Drug Deliv. Rev.* **2019,** *138*, 117–132.
44. Armenia, I.; Ayllón, C. C.; Herrero, B. T.; Bussolari, F.; Alfranca, G.; Grazú, V.; de la Fuente, J. M. Photonic and Magnetic Materials for On-Demand Local Drug Delivery. *Adv. Drug Deliv. Rev.* **2022,** , 114584.
45. Gelmi, A.; Schutt, C. E. Stimuli-Responsive Biomaterials: Scaffolds for Stem Cell Control. *Adv. Healthcare Mater.* **2021,** *10* (1), 2001125.
46. Widmer, N.; Bardin, C.; Chatelut, E.; Paci, A.; Beijnen, J.; Levêque, D.; Veal, G.; Astier, A. Review of Therapeutic Drug Monitoring of Anticancer Drugs Part Two–Targeted Therapies. *Eur. J. Cancer.* **2014,** *50* (12), 2020–2036.
47. Liu, C. C.; Zhao, J. J.; Zhang, R.; Li, H.; Chen, B.; Zhang, L. L.; Yang, H. Multifunctionalization of Graphene and Graphene Oxide for Controlled Release and Targeted Delivery of Anticancer Drugs. *Am. J. Transl. Res.* **2017,** *9* (12), 5197.
48. Quader, S.; Kataoka, K. Nanomaterial-Enabled Cancer Therapy. *Mol. Therapy* **2017,** *25* (7), 1501–1513.
49. Mayegowda, S. B.; Sureshkumar, K.; Sahana, M.; Ramakrishnappa, T. 4 pH and Thermo-responsive Systems. *Polym. Biomater.: Fabric. Prop. App.* **2023**.
50. Zhang, X. X.; Eden, H. S.; Chen, X. Peptides in Cancer Nanomedicine: Drug Carriers, Targeting Ligands and Protease Substrates. *J. Controlled Release* **2012,** *159* (1), 2–13.
51. Shim, M. K.; Yang, S.; Sun, I. C.; Kim, K. Tumor-Activated Carrier-Free Prodrug Nanoparticles for Targeted Cancer Immunotherapy: Preclinical Evidence for Safe and Effective Drug Delivery. *Adv. Drug Deliv. Rev.* **2022,** , 114177.
52. Shahriari, M.; Zahiri, M.; Abnous, K.; Taghdisi, S. M.; Ramezani, M.; Alibolandi, M. Enzyme Responsive Drug Delivery Systems in Cancer Treatment. *J. Controlled Release* **2019,** *308*, 172–189.
53. Law, B.; Tung, C. H. Proteolysis: a biological process adapted in drug delivery, therapy, and imaging. Bioconjugate chemistry. 2009 Sep 16;20 (9), 1683–95.
54. Niland, S.; Riscanevo, A. X.; Eble, J. A. Matrix Metalloproteinases Shape the Tumor Microenvironment in Cancer Progression. *Int. J. Mol. Sci.* **2022,** *23* (1), 146.
55. Jia, R.; Teng, L.; Gao, L.; Su, T.; Fu, L.; Qiu, Z.; Bi, Y. Advances in Multiple Stimuli-Responsive Drug-Delivery Systems for Cancer Therapy. *Int. J. Nanomed.* **2021,** *16*, 1525.

56. Yadav, N.; Mudgal, D.; Anand, R.; Jindal, S.; Mishra, V. Recent Development in Nanoencapsulation and Delivery of Natural Bioactives Through Chitosan Scaffolds for Various Biological Applications. *Int. J. Biol. Macromol.* **2022.**
57. von Haartman, E. Design and Evaluation of Nanoparticle-Based Delivery Systems: Towards Cancer Theranostics.
58. El-Sawy, H. S.; Al-Abd, A. M.; Ahmed, T. A.; El-Say, K. M.; Torchilin, V. P. Stimuli-Responsive Nano-Architecture Drug-Delivery Systems to Solid Tumor Micromilieu: Past, Present, and Future Perspectives. *ACS Nano* **2018,** *12* (11), 10636–10664.
59. Armenia, I.; Ayllón, C. C.; Herrero, B. T.; Bussolari, F.; Alfranca, G.; Grazú, V.; de la Fuente, J. M. Photonic and Magnetic Materials for On-Demand Local Drug Delivery. *Adv. Drug Deliv. Rev.* **2022,** 114584.
60. Rana, A.; Adhikary, M.; Singh, P. K.; Das, B. C.; Bhatnagar, S. "Smart" Drug Delivery: A Window to Future of Translational Medicine. *Front. Chem.* **2023,** *10,* 1095598.
61. Liu, D.; Yang, F.; Xiong, F.; Gu, N. The Smart Drug Delivery System and Its Clinical Potential. *Theranostics* **2016,** *6* (9), 1306.
62. De, D.; Sahoo, P. The Impact of MOFs in pH-Dependent Drug Delivery Systems: Progress in the Last Decade. *Dalton Trans.* **2022,** *51* (26), 9950–9965.
63. Kohan Hoosh Nejad, A.; Ahmad Panahi, H.; Keshmirizadeh, E.; Torabi Fard, N. Fabrication of a pH-Responsive Drug Delivery System Based on the Super-Paramagnetic Metal-Organic Framework for Targeted Delivery of Oxaliplatin. *Int. J. Polym. Mater. Polym. Biomater.* **2022,** 1–0.
64. Schiliro, C.; Firestein, B. L. Mechanisms of Metabolic Reprogramming in Cancer Cells Supporting Enhanced Growth and Proliferation. *Cells* **2021,** *10* (5), 1056.
65. Lu, A. H.; Salabas, E. E.; Schüth, F. Magnetic Nanoparticles: Synthesis, Protection, Functionalization, and Application. *Angew. Chem. Int. Ed.* **2007,** *46* (8), 1222–1244.
66. Mancuso, J. L.; Mroz, A. M.; Le, K. N.; Hendon, C. H. Electronic Structure Modeling of Metal–Organic Frameworks. *Chem. Rev.* **2020,** *120* (16), 8641–8715.
67. Espallargas, G. M.; Coronado, E. Magnetic Functionalities in MOFs: From the Framework to the Pore. *Chem. Soc. Rev.* **2018,** *47* (2), 533–557.
68. Qiu, S.; Xue, M.; Zhu, G. Metal–Organic Framework Membranes: From Synthesis to Separation Application. *Chem. Soc. Rev.* **2014,** *43* (16), 6116–6140.
69. Ahmed, I.; Jhung, S. H. Adsorptive Desulfurization and Denitrogenation Using Metal-Organic Frameworks. *J. Hazard. Mater.* **2016,** *301,* 259–276.
70. Dong, X.; Lin, Y.; Ren, G.; Ma, Y.; Zhao, L. Catalytic Degradation of Methylene Blue by Fenton-Like Oxidation of Ce-Doped MOF. *Colloids Surfaces A: Physicochem. Eng. Aspects* **2021,** *608,* 125578.
71. Zhao, X.; Liu, S.; Tang, Z.; Niu, H.; Cai, Y.; Meng, W.; Wu, F.; Giesy, J. P. Synthesis of Magnetic Metal-Organic Framework (MOF) for Efficient Removal of Organic Dyes from Water. *Sci. Rep.* **2015,** *5* (1), 11849.
72. Wu, X.; Macreadie, L. K.; Gale, P. A. Anion Binding in Metal-Organic Frameworks. *Coord. Chem. Rev.* **2021,** *432,* 213708.
73. Desai, A. V.; Manna, B.; Karmakar, A.; Sahu, A.; Ghosh, S. K. A Water-Stable Cationic Metal–Organic Framework as a Dual Adsorbent of Oxoanion Pollutants. *Angew. Chem.* **2016,** *128* (27), 7942–7946.
74. Deng, S. Q.; Mo, X. J.; Zheng, S. R.; Jin, X.; Gao, Y.; Cai, S. L.; Fan, J.; Zhang, W. G. Hydrolytically Stable Nanotubular Cationic Metal–Organic Framework for Rapid and

Efficient Removal of Toxic Oxo-Anions and Dyes from Water. *Inorg. Chem.* **2019,** *58* (4), 2899–2909.

75. Henke, S.; Schneemann, A.; Fischer, R. A. Massive Anisotropic Thermal Expansion and Thermo-Responsive Breathing in Metal–Organic Frameworks Modulated by Linker Functionalization. *Adv. Funct. Mater.* **2013,** *23* (48), 5990–5996.
76. Liu, J.; Goetjen, T. A.; Wang, Q.; Knapp, J. G.; Wasson, M. C.; Yang, Y.; Syed, Z. H.; Delferro, M.; Notestein, J. M.; Farha, O. K.; Hupp, J. T. MOF-Enabled Confinement and Related Effects for Chemical Catalyst Presentation and Utilization. *Chem. Soc. Rev.* **2022,** *51* (3), 1045–1097.
77. Qian, Q.; Asinger, P. A.; Lee, M. J.; Han, G.; Mizrahi Rodriguez, K.; Lin, S.; Benedetti, F. M.; Wu, A. X.; Chi, W. S.; Smith, Z. P. MOF-Based Membranes for Gas Separations. *Chem. Rev.* **2020,** *120* (16), 8161–8266.
78. Ying, Y.; Zhang, Z.; Peh, S. B.; Karmakar, A.; Cheng, Y.; Zhang, J.; Xi, L.; Boothroyd, C.; Lam, Y. M.; Zhong, C.; Zhao, D. Pressure-Responsive Two-Dimensional Metal–Organic Framework Composite Membranes for CO_2 Separation. *Angew. Chem. Int. Ed.* **2021,** *60* (20), 11318–11325.
79. Yuan, D.; Zhao, D.; Zhou, H. C. Pressure-Responsive Curvature Change of a "Rigid" Geodesic Ligand in a (3, 24)-Connected Mesoporous Metal–Organic Framework. *Inorg. Chem.* **2011,** *50* (21), 10528–10530.
80. Ou, R.; Zhang, H.; Zhao, C.; Hegab, H. M.; Jiang, L.; Truong, V. X.; Wang, H. Photoresponsive Styrylpyrene-Modified MOFs for Gated Loading and Release of Cargo Molecules. *Chem. Mater.* **2020,** *32* (24), 10621–10627.
81. Butova, V. V.; Burachevskaya, O. A.; Podshibyakin, V. A.; Shepelenko, E. N.; Tereshchenko, A. A.; Shapovalova, S. O.; Il'in, O. I.; Bren, V. A.; Soldatov, A. V. Photo Switchable Zirconium MOF for Light-Driven Hydrogen Storage. *Polymers* **2021,** *13* (22), 4052.
82. Zhang, W.; Hu, Y.; Ge, J.; Jiang, H. L.; Yu, S. H. A Facile and General Coating Approach to Moisture/Water-Resistant Metal–Organic Frameworks with Intact Porosity. *J. Am. Chem. Soc.* **2014,** *136* (49), 16978–16981.
83. Ding, M.; Cai, X.; Jiang, H. L. Improving MOF Stability: Approaches and Applications. *Chem. Sci.* **2019,** *10* (44), 10209–10230.
84. Joseph, J.; Iftekhar, S.; Srivastava, V.; Fallah, Z.; Zare, E. N.; Sillanpää, M. Iron-Based Metal-Organic Framework: Synthesis, Structure and Current Technologies for Water Reclamation with Deep Insight into Framework Integrity. *Chemosphere* **2021,** *284*, 131171.
85. Jayaramulu, K.; Geyer, F.; Schneemann, A.; Kment, Š.; Otyepka, M.; Zboril, R.; Vollmer, D.; Fischer, R. A. Hydrophobic Metal–Organic Frameworks. *Adv. Mater.* **2019,** *31* (32), 1900820.
86. Ahmed, A.; McHugh, D.; Papatriantafyllopoulou, C. Synthesis and Biomedical Applications of Highly Porous Metal–Organic Frameworks. *Molecules* **2022,** *27* (19), 6585.
87. Saeb, M. R.; Rabiee, N.; Mozafari, M.; Mostafavi, E. Metal-Organic Frameworks (MOFs)-Based Nanomaterials for Drug Delivery. *Materials* **2021,** *14* (13), 3652.
88. Wang, C.; Liu, D.; Lin, W. Metal–Organic Frameworks as a Tunable Platform for Designing Functional Molecular Materials. *J. Am. Chem. Soc.* **2013,** *135* (36), 13222–13234.

89. Zhao, D.; Zhang, W.; Yu, S.; Xia, S. L.; Liu, Y. N.; Yang, G. J. Application of MOF-Based Nano Therapeutics in Light-Mediated Cancer Diagnosis and Therapy. *J. Nanobiotechnol.* **2022,** *20* (1), 1–28.
90. Wang, Y.; Shahi, P. K.; Xie, R.; Zhang, H.; Abdeen, A. A.; Yodsanit, N.; Ma, Z.; Saha, K.; Pattnaik, B. R.; Gong, S. A pH-Responsive Silica–Metal–Organic Framework Hybrid Nanoparticle for the Delivery of Hydrophilic Drugs, Nucleic Acids, and CRISPR-Cas9 Genome-Editing Machineries. *J. Controlled Release* **2020,** *324*, 194–203.
91. Yang, X.; Tang, Q.; Jiang, Y.; Zhang, M.; Wang, M.; Mao, L. Nanoscale ATP-Responsive Zeolitic Imidazole Framework-90 as a General Platform for Cytosolic Protein Delivery and Genome Editing. *J. Am. Chem. Soc.* **2019,** *141* (9), 3782–3786.
92. Deng, J.; Wang, K.; Wang, M.; Yu, P.; Mao, L. Mitochondria Targeted Nanoscale Zeolitic Imidazole Framework-90 for ATP Imaging in Live Cells. *J. Am. Chem. Soc.* **2017,** *139* (16), 5877–5882.
93. Xu, X.; Liu, C.; Wang, Y.; Koivisto, O.; Zhou, J.; Shu, Y.; Zhang, H. Nanotechnology-Based Delivery of CRISPR/Cas9 for Cancer Treatment. *Adv. Drug Deliv. Rev.* **2021,** *176*, 113891.
94. Cai, W.; Wang, J.; Chu, C.; Chen, W.; Wu, C.; Liu, G. Metal–Organic Framework-Based Stimuli-Responsive Systems for Drug Delivery. *Adv. Sci.* **2019,** *6* (1), 1801526.
95. Liu, Z.; Shi, J.; Han, R.; Wang, H.; Wang, Y.; Gan, Y. Competitive-Binding Activated Supramolecular Nanovalves Based on β-Cyclodextrin Complexes. *ChemistrySelect* **2017,** *2* (19), 5341–5347.
96. Zhang, H.; Liu, Z.; Shen, J. Cyclodextrins Modified/Coated Metal–Organic Frameworks. *Materials* **2020,** *13* (6), 1273.
97. He, L.; Liu, Y.; Lau, J.; Fan, W.; Li, Q.; Zhang, C.; Huang, P.; Chen, X. Recent Progress in Nanoscale Metal-Organic Frameworks for Drug Release and Cancer Therapy. *Nanomedicine* **2019,** *14* (10), 1343–1365.
98. Xing, K.; Fan, R.; Wang, F.; Nie, H.; Du, X.; Gai, S.; Wang, P.; Yang, Y. Dual-Stimulus-Triggered Programmable Drug Release and Luminescent Ratiometric pH Sensing from Chemically Stable Biocompatible Zinc Metal–Organic Framework. *ACS Appl. Mater. Interfaces* **2018,** *10* (26), 22746–22756.
99. Rahaman, S. J.; Samanta, A.; Mir, M. H.; Dutta, B. Metal-Organic Frameworks (MOFs), A Promising Candidate for Stimuli-Responsive Drug Delivery. *ES Mater. Manufac.* **2022,** *19*, 792.
100. Han, Y.; Liu, W.; Huang, J.; Qiu, S.; Zhong, H.; Liu, D.; Liu, J. Cyclodextrin-Based Metal-Organic Frameworks (CD-MOFs) in Pharmaceutics and Biomedicine. *Pharmaceutics* **2018,** *10* (4), 271.
101. Karmakar, A.; Samanta, P.; Desai, A. V.; Ghosh, S. K. Guest-Responsive Metal–Organic Frameworks as Scaffolds for Separation and Sensing Applications. *Acc. Chem Res.* **2017,** *50* (10), 2457–2469.
102. Maranescu, B.; Visa, A. Applications of Metal-Organic Frameworks as Drug Delivery Systems. *Int. J. Mol. Sci.* **2022,** *23* (8), 4458.
103. Feng, J.; Xu, Z.; Dong, P.; Yu, W.; Liu, F.; Jiang, Q.; Wang, F.; Liu, X. Stimuli-Responsive Multifunctional Metal–Organic Framework Nanoparticles for Enhanced Chemo-Photothermal Therapy. *J. Mater. Chem. B* **2019,** *7* (6), 994–1004.
104. Masoudifar, R.; Pouyanfar, N.; Liu, D.; Ahmadi, M.; Landi, B.; Akbari, M.; Moayeri-Jolandan, S.; Ghorbani-Bidkorpeh, F.; Asadian, E.; Shahbazi, M. A. Surface Engineered

Metal-Organic Frameworks as Active Targeting Nanomedicines for Mono-and Multi-Therapy. *Appl. Mater. Today*. **2022,** *29*, 101646.

105. Ibrahim, M.; Sabouni, R.; A Husseini, G. Anti-Cancer Drug Delivery Using Metal Organic Frameworks (MOFs). *Curr. Med. Chem*. **2017,** *24* (2), 193–214.

CHAPTER 9

Metallic Scaffold for Tissue Engineering

AJAYKUMAR CHITTIPOLU

Vision College of Pharmaceutical Sciences, JNTUH, Hyderabad, Telangana, India

ABSTRACT

The shape and mechanical properties of bone are characterized by viscoelasticity and anisotropy, which make it a complicated porous composite structure. High toughness, specific strength, and low stiffness are the defining characteristics of natural bone's exceptional mechanical capability. Because they offer a 3D framework for distributing reparative cells or regeneration factors in an organized manner to repair or regenerate damaged tissues, porous scaffolds are essential to hard tissue engineering (TE) procedures. Materials intended for mending or rebuilding hard tissues must be strong, resistant to deterioration, and have high biocompatibility since hard tissues are what maintain the body's mechanical stability. Successful bone TE scaffold creation demands a concurrent engineering strategy that integrates several research domains. Researchers have developed metallic scaffolds that are effective for a number of medical and dental applications over the past three decades. The application of TE requires the surface modification of metals that have already been shown to be biocompatible, since the metal surface must be regulated to promote cell adhesion, proliferation, and adsorption of vital biomolecules. This chapter summarizes the design and progress of the metallic scaffolds, with the intensive characterization of host tissues as well as the reported biocompatibility of each of these metallic structures that have been conceived to be used in the specific reconstruction of small or large bone defects.

Metals in Medicine, Volume 1: Metals for Tissue Engineering and Pharmaceutical Applications.
Sonali Sundram, Rishabha Malviya, and GSN Koteswara Rao

9.1 INTRODUCTION

Human skeletal tissues have intricated internal layouts and three-dimensional (3D) geometries, which make it difficult for cells kept in 2D to accurately mimic them. Natural bone has a special mechanical performance that is distinguished by its low stiffness, high specific strength, and high toughness, which offers a 3D framework for distributing regeneration factors to regenerate or repair damaged tissues. Since the body's hard tissues are what keep it mechanically stable, materials used to repair, replace, and/or restore them must be strong, resistant to degradation and corrosion, have good wear resistance, and have good biocompatibility.[1,2] Biomaterials are synthetic or natural substances that are used to build implants or other structures that restore the shape and function of biological tissue that has been lost or damaged.[3,4] As a result, biomaterials help prolong human life and improve quality of life. To meet the needs of an aging population, the field of study of biomaterials has undergone significant expansion. The heart, blood vessels, shoulders, knees, hips, elbows, ears, and orthodontic structures are just a few of the body parts that use biomaterials as replacement implants.[4] A metal must be biocompatible to function as a biomaterial, which means that it must not have a negative effect on living things.[5] It also requires excellent wear resistance, strong osseointegration, and great corrosion resistance. To put it another way, the materials used to make implants should be completely non-toxic and shouldn't cause any allergic or inflammatory reactions in people.[6]

Because of this, the material used to replace the bone should have mechanical properties that are similar to those of bone. Since then, it has been recommended that new tissues be made by planting cells on scaffolds made of biomaterials that are compatible with living things.[7] The ideal bone scaffold should possess both osteoconductive and osteoinductive qualities. Bone's component phases and hierarchical structural structure provide its mechanical qualities.[8] Compressive, bending, and fracture toughness strengths are used to characterize these characteristics.[9] The major elements of bone are collagen and hydroxyl-carbonate apatite, with a porosity of 10–30% in the cortical bone's outer layer and 30–90% in the cancellous bone's inner layer. While some bones, like the talus, are heavily compressed, certain bones, like the ribs, are more exposed to tensile stress. Successful bone tissue engineering (TE) scaffold creation demands a concurrent engineering strategy that integrates several research domains.[10,11] Because the metal surface needs to be regulated to promote cell adhesion and proliferation as well as the adsorption of vital biomolecules, surface modification of metals that have already been demonstrated to be biocompatible is a crucial need for their application in TE.[12] A thorough evaluation of the host tissue's characteristics is logically the first step in designing a hard tissue-engineered scaffold.

In the field of bioengineering, nanotechnology is being used to change traditional treatments, which often do not work and do not give patients long-term comfort.[13] The nanoscale hierarchical structure of human tissues shows how important it is to study the "tiny" to solve the bigger problems. Nanomaterials are helpful because they can mimic the nanoenvironment of tissue and change biological reactions in a big way.[14,15] According to reports, nanomaterials can act as nanostructured vehicles for effective drug delivery devices that can pass through biological barriers.[15] Materials such as growth factors, medicines, contrast agents, and targeting ligands, can be added to nanoparticles with higher surface area to volume ratios to create multifunctional materials.[16] Theranostic agents are those nanocomposites that may be used for both treatment and diagnostics. Such nanoparticles assist in transporting medications selectively to the target region, reducing the negative consequences of accumulation and toxicity.[17,18] Recently, multifunctional scaffolds for TE purposes have been made using nanoparticles. Strategies based on nanotechnology have been developed to treat bone-related disorders as a consequence of extensive study into the manufacture of improved biomaterials with desirable surface qualities, mechanical strength, and durability.[19,20]

Because their structural, mechanical, and occasionally chemical qualities closely mimic those of genuine biological tissues, biomaterials made using nanoengineering and nanofabrication techniques provide intriguing biomimetic methods.[20,21] Porosity, complexity, chemical composition, and spatial geometry of nanoscaffolds may be used to regulate the adhesion and proliferation of cells with desired capabilities. Unique scaffolds for orthopedic TE, including bone, tendons, ligaments, and cartilage, may be created using nanostructures with unusual forms such as hollow tubes, sheets, fibers, spheres, and nets.[22,23]

This paper discusses in detail about how metallic nanoparticle-based nanoscaffolds can be used to help bone tissue grow back. A number of nanoscale metals, including copper, platinum, silver, titanium (Ti), iron oxide, zinc, strontium, gold, and palladium, as well as their oxides, are explored in relation to their potential function in bone tissue regeneration. Additionally, methods to improve mechanical qualities, bioactive properties, and biocompatibility are provided.

9.1.1 TISSUE ENGINEERING'S IMPORTANCE

The creation of biosubstitutes to restore, preserve, or enhance the function of tissue or organs uses biological sciences and engineering concepts, which is an interdisciplinary discipline with a wide variety of application fields. To obtain practical applications, TE is a multidisciplinary research effort that combines clinical medicine, biochemistry, biology, and materials science. Regenerative medicine, also known as tissue engineering, has recently emerged as a viable method for mending damaged tissues and avoiding the problems that occur with traditional organ donation procedures. Due to the rising need for organ transplants in clinical medicine, TE has emerged as a substitute.

To fulfill the requirements of regeneration and repair, the cellular material must be capable of effectively colonizing the host cell and integrating the scaffolds with diverse cell types that can enhance the osteogenic lineage's ability to generate tissues in vivo or release certain soluble chemicals for the lineage. Before being implanted into the target region, these cells may be selectively grown ex vivo. Depending on elements such as the severity of the damage, patient age, anatomical location, and other pathological variables, these scaffold qualities should be tailored for a particular application. The mechanical properties of the scaffold, such as its strength, must be less protective against physiological stress.[24] In cell regeneration, the scaffold contains several cell types taken from a donor or a patient. Extended cells come from adult stem cells such as blood cells, teeth, fatty tissue, embryonic stem cells, bone marrow, induced pluripotent stem cells, genetically engineered cells, and peripheral blood-derived stem cells, whereas bone marrow aspirate-derived platelet-rich plasma cells are the main source for non-expended cells.[25,26] Because these cells may take many different shapes when generated by verbal or chemical substances, a scaffold with certain qualities is crucial.

Even though many discoveries have been made in TE, the commercialization of these newly found functions has grown a lot because they could be used to treat diseases. Therefore, it is crucial to combine certain clinical, mechanical, and biological features that are not just theoretical but may also play a role in actual execution to increase the adoption of clinical applications of such technologies.[25] The basic needs for host integration, proliferation, cell development, and vascularization must be met by an adequate scaffold, and materials must naturally decay during or after the healing process.

9.1.2 CHARACTERISTICS OF SCAFFOLD

The biocompatibility and nontoxicity characteristics of scaffolds are among their biological characteristics. To create a new matrix, cells growing on scaffolds must be allowed to divide and differentiate unhindered and freely.[27,28] Therefore, a scaffold is deemed to be a suitable scaffold for TE applications if it can accurately and fully match the features of the tissues.[28] However, as was already indicated, factors including the chosen cell line, the underlying substance, the surface qualities, and the scaffolding structure affect how the supporting cell performs.

Biocompatibility allows for the simultaneous development of new tissue and matrix breakdown. For the system to dispose of the matrix without upsetting other members, it should not be hazardous. Because they have an impact on how scaffolds interact with tissues and organs, a scaffold's biological characteristics are a crucial modifying concern.[29] Additionally, the structure must prevent host immune reactions. The notion of immune-inert biomaterials has recently been put into practice, and their immune-modulatory properties control the immune system (i.e., reduced NK cell activity and T and B cell-mediated immunity).

9.1.3 CHARACTERISTICS OF THE STRUCTURE

Tissue is very complicated in all 3D and has complicated mechanical properties related to how it moves mass. To reach this key goal of TE,[26] biological scaffolds that provide cells, proteins, and genes for tissue reconstruction must be used. This will make the structures and functions less complicated. There is no doubt that biological materials and structures cannot be used to make complex tissue environments. These environments are made up of a wide range of cell types that interact with various cytokines to create extracellular matrices within cells that have hierarchical features and a mechanical function that is highly nonlinear and two-phase.[30] The ultimate physical properties of the scaffold are influenced by the material selection (Fig. 9.1). It is generally preferred that the scaffold be more porous to increase its mechanical capacity and promote cell growth.[31] The proper pore size in a scaffold also encourages high-mass oxygen transfer throughout the scaffold, improves cell motility, and increases water absorption.

Recently, it has been suggested that bioactive composite materials could be used to combine the benefits of two or more different materials, such as metals, ceramics, and polymers. For applications in TE, composite materials improve the scaffold's properties and allow controlled breakdown.[32] Polymer-ceramic composites have good mechanical properties and are osteoconductive, which makes them good materials for engineering bone tissue. For investigations on bone healing, composites of the three primary natural bones hydroxyapatite (HA), calcium phosphate (CP), and tricalcium phosphate (TCP)-with collagen, chitosan, gelatin, and poly (L-lactic acid) have been extensively employed as scaffolding materials.[33] The introduction of structures that mimic and match bone characteristics as well as matrices for bone mineralization and cell differentiation has been made possible by the reinforcement of high-density polyethylene (HDPE) and poly (L-lactide-co-glycolide acid) (PLGA) with HA. Composites made of CP and polymers combine bioactivity and mechanical strength. Nanocomposites made of collagen and bioglass have improved ALP expression and early mineralization. For orthopedic applications, a straightforward calcium phosphate coating process on glasses, metals, organic polymers, silk fibers, inorganic ceramics, and collagens, can increase biocompatibility or boost bioreactivity. These composite scaffolds' mechanical reinforcement has not yet been able to keep up with the demands of living bone tissue. Human mesenchymal stem cells have been proven to proliferate and differentiate at a greater rate on Fe foam covered with calcium phosphate than on untreated samples. Even while the coating boosts bioactivity, it prevents Fe foams from degrading.[34] The compressive yield is increased with the addition of phosphorus and is equivalent to that of normal bone. In vitro testing has revealed that Fe alloys degrade quicker than the pure form.[34,35] The mechanical and degradation characteristics of the construct, cell regeneration, and degradation product movement are all impacted by the creation of porous structures using all biodegradable metals.[2] In animal tests, metallic scaffolds with carbon and Ta deposits on their grids demonstrated good biocompatibility.

9.2 MATERIALS AND LIMITATIONS OF CURRENTLY USED METALLIC SCAFFOLDS

Several different materials are often used as implants in dentistry and orthopedic surgery to replace lost bone, help bones heal, or treat bone problems.[1] The biggest problem with metallic biomaterials is that they cannot be recognized by living things. Surface modification offers a technique to get around this limitation by maintaining the mechanical capabilities of well-known biocompatible metals while enhancing their surface biocompatibility.[37,38]

To enhance communication between cells and facilitate their organization within the porous scaffold, it was also desirable to put cell-recognizable ligands and signaling growth factors on the surface of the scaffolds.[39,40] In reality, the scaffold design and manufacturing can contain biofactors that affect cell proliferation, differentiation, migration, morphologies, and gene expression to speed up cell growth and control cell activities.[41] The potential release of poisonous metallic ions and/or particles through corrosion or wear is another drawback of the present metallic biomaterials.[42] These particles can trigger allergic responses and inflammatory cascades, which decrease biocompatibility and result in tissue loss. To prevent this issue and establish a direct bond with the tissue, the material surface may benefit from the correct treatment.[42,43] On the contrary, some metallic materials, depending on the material's qualities, are too weak to be ordered into the necessary architecture with a regulated porosity structure, while some metals, depending on the design, are too stiff and would shatter. The processing needs for each metallic substance vary, as does the degree to which each metal may be processed to create a scaffold.[44]

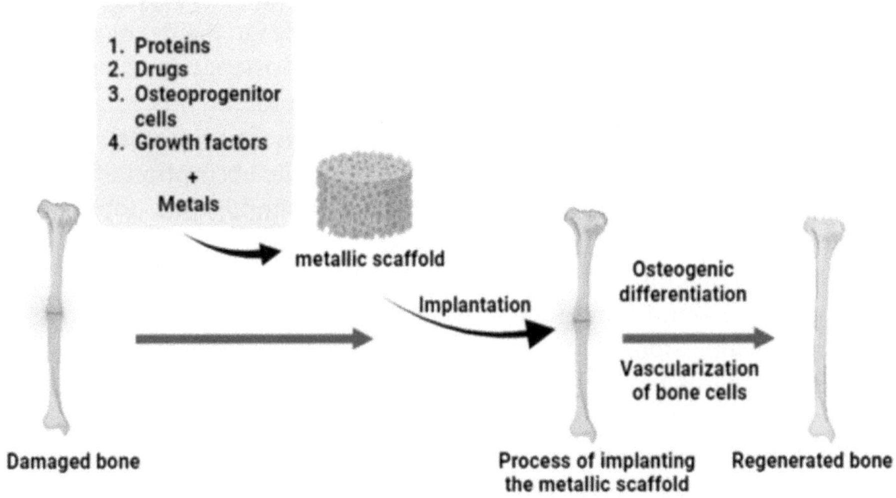

FIGURE 9.1 Regeneration of defected bone through implantation of metallic scaffolds.

9.2.1 TANTALUM

A biomaterial with a distinctive set of physical and mechanical qualities is porous tantalum. It contains totally linked pores and a high volume of porosity (>80%), which enables quick and secure bone ingrowth.[45] Additionally, it possesses a bone-like elasticity modulus, which reduces stress shielding. High levels of bone development on the scaffold itself, as well as significant cortical bone growth between the trabecular networks, have both been shown in studies.[46,47] The trabecular metals own initial stability is also greater than that of common materials such as cobalt chrome.[48] Additionally, compared to current biological fixation methods, this novel material provides greater osteoconduction. The initial clinical results and preclinical investigations suggest the use of porous tantalum as an alternative to conventional orthopedic implant materials, even though this technology is still in its infancy.[1,49].

Ta porous scaffold exhibits a high friction coefficient. Rahbek, O. et al.[50] Implantation of porous Ta components in the knee joints of dogs for 8 weeks. Weekly polyethylene (PE) particle injection into the knees was done to determine the resistance to migration of PE particles. Porous Ta exhibited superior bone ingrowth, more bone marrow, less fibrous tissue, and less PE particle migration compared with glass bead-blasted Ti. Porous Ta showed resistance to the migration of PE particles and superior bone formation. According to research by Gao et al.,[49] applying NaOH to porous Ta scaffold surfaces may effectively encourage the development of apatite, increasing the bioactivity and capacity of osteogenesis and vascularization. Furthermore, Wang et al. found that protein was substantially more abundant on a Ta_2O_5 surface than on porous Ta scaffolds' untreated surfaces, suggesting that the Ta_2O_5 layer aids in the absorption of proteins by Ta. Porous Ta implants removed from rat femoral bone defects were histologically examined by Wauthle et al.[52] They reported that new bone was growing quickly within implant pores, and the porous Ta scaffolds had a good connection to the tissues around them. Other studies of porous Ta produced conclusions that were relatively positive. After four, eight, and sixteen weeks of healing, Hacking et al.[53] removed dorsal subcutaneous porous Ta implants from dogs and examined their histological sections under transmission light microscopy. The porous Ta scaffold included highly vascularized connective tissue after 16 weeks of implantation. Vascularity was visible at the porous Ta implants' interface in a soft-tissue peel test. To create porous Ta scaffolds with high mechanical strength and an appropriate elastic modulus, the biomechanical parameters of porous Ta should be optimized. The clinical stability and long-term survival of the implant rely on this optimization.

9.2.2 MAGNESIUM

Particularly intriguing is the use of magnesium and related alloys in surgical procedures; these alloys have a lot of potential since they are completely bioresorbable, have characteristics aligned with bone,[54] do not cause an inflammatory or systemic response, promote bone formation, and play a part in cell attachment.[55] Additionally, the second operation for the removal of the scaffold can be avoided due to the biodegradability of the scaffold.

All of these factors imply that magnesium has a lot of potential as a load-bearing biomaterial in biomedical applications, such as coronary stents.[54,56] Researchers have focused on the use of magnesium–rare-earth alloys with new elemental contributions of praseodymium, neodymium, and cerium, for bone fixation devices for osteo applications.[57] Mg–Ca alloys have recently been created and tested as biodegradable biomaterials for orthopedic applications in vitro and in vivo.[58]

Although expressions about the toxicity of dissolved magnesium, demonstrated that it was effectively eliminated from the body through urine.[59,60] Even though several potential methods for reducing corrosion have been suggested, including coating it with ceramic material, Ti, or by using Mg alloys such as WE43, LAE442, AZ31, AZ91, and Mg–Mn–Zn alloys,[61–63] concern still exists regarding the use of pure magnesium due to the material's rapid dissolution rate under physiological conditions, which could result in hypermagnesia. For porous scaffolds of magnesium or its alloys, there aren't many long-term survival statistics available, but the material appears to show potential for applications involving bone ingrowth, including trabecular bone regeneration.[64,65] For instance, activating the canonical Wnt signaling pathway causes Mg^{2+} to first have an osteogenic impact in the marrow cavity before encouraging BMSC development into osteoblasts.[66]

9.2.3 TITANIUM AND TITANIUM ALLOYS

Ti has been discovered to be highly tolerated and essentially inert in the environment of the human body. Ti may osseointegrate with bone under ideal conditions. Ti also offers great biocompatibility and develops a highly stable passive layer of TiO_2 on its surface.[67,68] The passive layer is quickly recreated, even if it is destroyed. The physicochemical characteristics of the oxide coating, such as crystallinity and impurity segregation, have been shown to be particularly significant in the case of Ti because they protect the metal substrate against corrosion.[69] Comparing Ti alloys to stainless steels and Cr–Co alloys, they exhibit higher biocompatibility. Total joint implants employ Ti–aluminum–vanadium alloys more frequently than commercially pure Ti because they have greater mechanical qualities.[59,70]

However, as metals such as vanadium are poisonous in their elemental form, concerns have been raised concerning the existence of long-term Ti-6Al-4V implants.[63] The creation of novel beta Ti alloys with non-toxic alloying components such as Ta, Nb, and Zr is the result of these worries.[71] These new Ti alloys are still in the research and development stages and do not appear to have reached the market yet. In general, Ti alloys and porous Ti show strong biocompatibility.[72] For the past 20 years, spine fusion surgery has been successfully performed using bioactive Ti meshes. For more than 15 years, anterior lumbar interbody fusion (ALIF) has been performed successfully using a Ti mesh cage that has been molded into a cylindrical shape. Additionally, Ti mesh cages containing autografts were employed for bone grafting during spinal fusion. Complications and second-site morbidity are only a couple of the variables that limit this.[73,74]

Zaharin et al.[74] examined several Ti-6A-l4V porous scaffolds Their findings showed that scaffolds built on cube and gyroid unit cells with hole sizes of 300 mm had characteristics similar to those of bone. Additionally, they concluded that increases in porosity reduced the scaffolds' yield strength and elastic modulus. In a previous study, Bobyn et al.[75] looked at how variations in the pore size of cobalt-base alloy implants affected the pace of bone development. For this, powder-coated, cast cobalt-base alloy implants were inserted into canine femurs for some time. The findings showed that the highest bone ingrowth and fixing strength were achieved at pore diameters between 50 and 400 m.

Use hydroxyapatite to give the Ti mesh cage with a porous network the bioactivity it needs to allow osteoconduction. Ti and its alloys are not ferro-magnetic and do not affect patients in magnetic resonance imaging (MRI) machines. Ti osseointegration may be helped by adding certain growth factors to the scaffold.[76–78]

Increased bone regeneration has frequently been achieved using TGF- and BMP-2 distribution via Ti scaffolds in situations where there are existing gaps, such as craniofacial restoration or augmentation of bone or peri-implant deficiencies.[79,80] The later growth factors have the ability to trigger particular cellular reactions that hasten the development of new tissue. To promote the development of mineralized extracellular matrix (ECM) onto the cells/scaffold constructions, stem cells have also been grown in vitro onto Ti scaffolds.[81]

9.2.4 *NICKEL–TITANIUM ALLOY (NITINOL)*

The superplasticity, shape memory effect, improved biocompatibility, and high damping qualities that nitinol exhibits, even in a porous form, have a variety of uses. Because of its high biocompatibility and near resemblance to the bone in terms of compressive strength and elastic modulus, porous Ni–Ti has been utilized for the treatment of scoliosis.[82] According to extensive in vivo research and preclinical experience, nitinol is extremely biocompatible. Furthermore, Ni–Ti with changed surfaces has been shown to have high biocompatibility.[83,84] Nitinol is biocompatible, and this alloy may provide significant improvements in the orthopedic industry based on its physical characteristics and SME (85). These improvements in developing scaffolds that adapt to the human body's temperature after implantation were made possible by nitinol's SME.[86] The discharge of Ni ions does cause allergy and toxicity issues for Ni–Ti alloys. The usage of Ni–Ti alloys has been limited in Europe and the USA due to worries about Ni toxicity and probable carcinogenicity.[87] The oxidation of Ni–Ti and its alloy surfaces to obtain Ni-free surfaces. Several alternative Ni-free shapes are being developed, and their biological performances will need to be evaluated in the future.[88]

The impact of porosity on the osseointegration of porous Ni–Ti implants in the rat femur was investigated by Kujala et al.[89] The porosity and mean pore size of three distinct specimens were used. Higher porosity creates more surface area, which may promote more bone fusion. When resorbable implants are subjected to deep bone ingrowth, interconnecting pores are necessary to create room for vascular ingrowth, which is necessary for ongoing bone remodeling.[90] At the interface between the implants, no fibrous tissue was discovered. This was understood to indicate a direct bond between the implant and bone.

9.3 CONCLUSION

Since TE has many uses, both old and new ways of making scaffolds have been used to move the field forward. The TE approach is a cutting-edge method for creating scaffolds to be employed in tissue and organ structure, according to prior research. The continuous development of technology and the synthesis of materials will also aid in the development of new techniques. Additionally, 3D printing, one of the prototyping methods, will be crucial in major applications pertaining to the scaffold-based area. Future directions of research in this field will probably focus on the efficient combinations of osteoinductive materials, osteoinductive growth factors, and cell-based tissue regeneration approaches using composite constructs as carriers to reconstruct and repair hard tissues. The goal is to obtain a functional replacement of the injured hard tissue in a procedure that avoids the step of bone harvesting. Therefore, a perfectly controlled hybrid scaffold still remains to be developed.

KEYWORDS

- **metallic scaffolds**
- **tissue repair**
- **bone regeneration**
- **bone tissue**
- **tissue engineering**

REFERENCES

1. Zhang, L.; Yang, G.; Johnson, B. N.; Jia, X. Three-Dimensional (3D) Printed Scaffold and Material Selection for Bone Repair. *Acta Biomaterialia* **2019,** *84*, 16–33.
2. Gao, G.; Kim, B. S.; Jang, J.; Cho, D. W. Recent Strategies in Extrusion-Based Three-Dimensional Cell Printing Toward Organ Biofabrication. *ACS Biomater. Sci. Eng.* **2019,** *5* (3), 1150–1169.
3. Collins, M. N.; Ren, G.; Young, K.; Pina, S.; Reis, R. L.; Oliveira, J. M. Scaffold Fabrication Technologies and Structure/Function Properties in Bone Tissue Engineering. *Adv. Funct. Mater.* **2021,** *31* (21), 2010609.
4. Raghavendra, G. M.; Varaprasad, K.; Jayaramudu, T. Biomaterials: Design, Development and Biomedical Applications. In: *Nanotechnology Applications for Tissue* Engineering; William Andrew Publishing, 2015; pp 21–44.
5. Schmalz, G.; Galler, K. M. Biocompatibility of Biomaterials–Lessons Learned and Considerations for the Design of Novel Materials. *Dental Mater.* **2017,** *33* (4), 382–393.
6. Vasvani, S.; Kulkarni, P.; Rawtani, D. Hyaluronic Acid: A Review on Its Biology, Aspects of Drug Delivery, Route of Administrations and a Special Emphasis on Its Approved Marketed Products and Recent Clinical Studies. *Int. J. Biol. Macromol.* **2020,** *151*, 1012–1029.
7. Tahmasebi, E.; Alam, M.; Yazdanian, M.; Tebyanian, H.; Yazdanian, A.; Seifalian, A.; Mosaddad, S. A. Current Biocompatible Materials in Oral Regeneration: A

Comprehensive Overview of Composite Materials. *J. Mater. Res. Technol.* **2020,** *9* (5), 11731–11755.
8. Hu, C.; Ashok, D.; Nisbet, D. R.; Gautam, V. Bioinspired Surface Modification of Orthopedic Implants for Bone Tissue Engineering. *Biomaterials* **2019,** *219*, 119366.
9. Feng, G.; Kang, Y.; Meng, T.; Hu, Y. Q.; Li, X. H. The Influence of Temperature on Mode I Fracture Toughness and Fracture Characteristics of Sandstone. *Rock Mech. Rock Eng.* **2017,** *50*, 2007–2019.
10. Niu, X.; Li, N.; Du, Z.; Li, X. Integrated Gradient Tissue-Engineered Osteochondral Scaffolds: Challenges, Current Efforts and Future Perspectives. *Bioactive Mater.* **2023,** *20*, 574–597.
11. Collins, M. N.; Ren, G.; Young, K.; Pina, S.; Reis, R. L.; Oliveira, J. M. Scaffold Fabrication Technologies and Structure/Function Properties in Bone Tissue Engineering. *Adv. Funct. Mater.* **2021,** *31* (21), 2010609.
12. Cai, S.; Wu, C.; Yang, W.; Liang, W.; Yu, H.; Liu, L. Recent Advance in Surface Modification for Regulating Cell Adhesion and Behaviors. *Nanotechnol. Rev.* **2020,** *9* (1), 971–989.
13. Mantha, S.; Pillai, S.; Khayambashi, P.; Upadhyay, A.; Zhang, Y.; Tao, O.; Pham, H. M.; Tran, S. D. Smart Hydrogels in Tissue Engineering and Regenerative Medicine. *Materials* **2019,** *12* (20), 3323.
14. Hosseini, F. S.; Laurencin, C. T. Advanced Electrospun Nanofibrous Stem Cell Niche for Bone Regenerative Engineering. *Regen. Eng. Transl. Med.* **2022,** 1–6.
15. Joseph, M. M.; Narayanan, N.; Nair, J. B.; Karunakaran, V.; Ramya, A. N.; Sujai, P. T.; Saranya, G.; Arya, J. S.; Vijayan, V. M.; Maiti, K. K. Exploring the Margins of SERS in Practical Domain: An Emerging Diagnostic Modality for Modern Biomedical Applications. *Biomaterials.* **2018,** *181*, 140–181.
16. Farzin, A.; Etesami, S. A.; Quint, J.; Memic, A.; Tamayol, A. Magnetic Nanoparticles in Cancer Therapy and Diagnosis. *Adv. Healthcare Mater.* **2020,** *9* (9), 1901058.
17. Jin, Y.; Wang, H.; Yi, K.; Lv, S.; Hu, H.; Li, M.; Tao, Y. Applications of Nanobiomaterials in the Therapy and Imaging of Acute Liver Failure. *Nano-Micro Lett.* **2021,** *13*, 1–36.
18. Barani, M.; Rahdar, A.; Mukhtar, M.; Razzaq, S.; Qindeel, M.; Olam, S. A.; Paiva-Santos, A. C.; Ajalli, N.; Sargazi, S.; Balakrishnan, D.; Gupta, A. K. Recent Application of Cobalt Ferrite Nanoparticles as a Theranostic Agent. *Mater. Today Chem.* **2022,** *26*, 101131.
19. Liao, J.; Han, R.; Wu, Y.; Qian, Z. Review of a New Bone Tumor Therapy Strategy Based on Bifunctional Biomaterials. *Bone Res.* **2021,** *9* (1), 18.
20. Hajiali, H.; Ouyang, L.; Llopis-Hernandez, V.; Dobre, O.; Rose, F. R. Review of Emerging Nanotechnology in Bone Regeneration: Progress, Challenges, and Perspectives. *Nanoscale* **2021,** *13* (23), 10266–10280.
21. Mostafavi, E.; Soltantabar, P.; Webster, T. J. Nanotechnology and Picotechnology: A New Arena for Translational Medicine. In: *Biomaterials in Translational Medicine*; Academic Press, 2019; pp 191–212.
22. Lei, T.; Zhang, T.; Ju, W.; Chen, X.; Heng, B. C.; Shen, W.; Yin, Z. Biomimetic Strategies for Tendon/Ligament-to-Bone Interface Regeneration. *Bioactive Mater.* **2021,** *6* (8), 2491–2510.
23. Anjum, S.; Rahman, F.; Pandey, P.; Arya, D. K.; Alam, M.; Rajinikanth, P. S.; Ao, Q. Electrospun Biomimetic Nanofibrous Scaffolds: A Promising Prospect for Bone Tissue Engineering and Regenerative Medicine. *Int. J. Mol. Sci.* **2022,** *23* (16), 9206.

24. Kopp, A.; Derra, T.; Müther, M.; Jauer, L.; Schleifenbaum, J. H.; Voshage, M.; Jung, O.; Smeets, R.; Kröger, N. Influence of Design and Post-Processing Parameters on the Degradation Behavior and Mechanical Properties of Additively Manufactured Magnesium Scaffolds. *Acta Biomaterialia* **2019,** *98*, 23–35.
25. Bohr, A.; Memarzadeh, K. The Rise of Artificial Intelligence in Healthcare Applications. In: *Artificial Intelligence in Healthcare*; Academic Press, 2020; pp 25–60.
26. Eltom, A.; Zhong, G.; Muhammad, A. Scaffold Techniques and Designs in Tissue Engineering Functions and Purposes: A Review. *Adv. Mater. Sci. Eng.* **2019,** *2019*.
27. Żylińska, B.; Silmanowicz, P.; Sobczyńska-Rak, A.; Jarosz, Ł.; Szponder, T. Treatment of Articular Cartilage Defects: Focus on Tissue Engineering. *In Vivo* **2018,** *32* (6), 1289–1300.
28. Hanemann, B. *Perfused Tumor-Tissue Model for Invasion Analysis*; Doctoral dissertation, Worcester Polytechnic Institute.
29. Boumiza, M. Study of End-Use Properties of Polylactic Acid Fiber-Závěrečná práce projektu ERASMUS+.
30. Morgan, E. F.; Gerstenfeld, L. C. The Bone Organ System: Form and Function. In: *Marcus and Feldman's Osteoporosis*; Academic Press, 2021; pp 15–35.
31. Freedman, B. R.; Mooney, D. J. Biomaterials to Mimic and Heal Connective Tissues. *Adv. Mater.* **2019,** *31* (19), 1806695.
32. Mondal, S.; Pal, U. 3D Hydroxyapatite Scaffold for Bone Regeneration and Local Drug Delivery Applications. *J. Drug Deliv. Sci. Technol.* **2019,** *53*, 101131.
33. Qu, H.; Fu, H.; Han, Z.; Sun, Y. Biomaterials for Bone Tissue Engineering Scaffolds: A Review. *RSC Adv.* **2019,** *9* (45), 26252–26262.
34. Ho, W. F.; Lee, M. H.; Thomas, J. L.; Li, J. A.; Wu, S. C.; Hsu, H. C.; Lin, H. Y. Porous Biphasic Calcium Phosphate Granules from Oyster Shell Promote the Differentiation of Induced Pluripotent Stem Cells. *Int. J. Mol. Sci.* **2021,** *22* (17), 9444.
35. Meskinfam, M.; Bertoldi, S.; Albanese, N.; Cerri, A.; Tanzi, M. C.; Imani, R.; Baheiraei, N.; Farokhi, M.; Fare, S. Polyurethane Foam/Nano Hydroxyapatite Composite as a Suitable Scaffold for Bone Tissue Regeneration. *Mater. Sci. Eng.: C* **2018,** *82*, 130–140.
36. Zhou, J.; Zhang, Z.; Joseph, J.; Zhang, X.; Ferdows, B. E.; Patel, D. N.; Chen, W.; Banfi, G.; Molinaro, R.; Cosco, D.; Kong, N. Biomaterials and Nanomedicine for Bone Regeneration: Progress and Future Prospects. *Exploration* **2021,** *1* (2), 20210011.
37. Florea, D. A.; Albuleț, D.; Grumezescu, A. M.; Andronescu, E. Surface Modification—A Step Forward to Overcome the Current Challenges in Orthopedic Industry and to Obtain an Improved Osseointegration and Antimicrobial Properties. *Mater. Chem. Phys.* **2020,** *243*, 122579.
38. Pałka, K.; Pokrowiecki, R. Porous Titanium Implants: A Review. *Adv. Eng. Mater.* **2018,** *20* (5), 1700648.
39. Nemati, S.; Kim, S. J.; Shin, Y. M.; Shin, H. Current Progress in Application of Polymeric Nanofibers to Tissue Engineering. *Nano Convergence* **2019,** *6* (1), 1–6.
40. Bahraminasab, M.; Janmohammadi, M.; Arab, S.; Talebi, A.; Nooshabadi, V. T.; Koohsarian, P.; Nourbakhsh, M. S. Bone Scaffolds: An Incorporation of Biomaterials, Cells, and Biofactors. *ACS Biomater. Sci. Eng.* **2021,** *7* (12), 5397–5431.
41. Toosi, S.; Behravan, J. Osteogenesis and Bone Remodeling: A Focus on Growth Factors and Bioactive Peptides. *Biofactors* **2020,** *46* (3), 326–340.
42. Krajewska, B. Urease-Aided Calcium Carbonate Mineralization for Engineering Applications: A Review. *J. Adv. Res.* **2018,** *13*, 59–67.

43. Qin, W.; Wang, C. Y.; Ma, Y. X.; Shen, M. J.; Li, J.; Jiao, K.; Tay, F. R.; Niu, L. N. Microbe-Mediated Extracellular and Intracellular Mineralization: Environmental, Industrial, and Biotechnological Applications. *Adv. Mater.* **2020,** *32* (22), 1907833.
44. Ying, H.; Han, W. Q. Metallic Sn-Based Anode Materials: Application in High-Performance Lithium-Ion and Sodium-Ion Batteries. *Adv. Sci.* **2017,** *4* (11), 1700298.
45. Han, Q.; Wang, C.; Chen, H.; Zhao, X.; Wang, J. Porous Tantalum and Titanium in Orthopedics: A Review. *ACS Biomater. Sci. Eng.* **2019,** *5* (11), 5798–5824.
46. Davoodi, E.; Montazerian, H.; Mirhakimi, A. S.; Zhianmanesh, M.; Ibhadode, O.; Shahabad, S. I.; Esmaeilizadeh, R.; Sarikhani, E.; Toorandaz, S.; Sarabi, S. A.; Nasiri, R. Additively Manufactured Metallic Biomaterials. *Bioactive Mater.* **2021.**
47. Mani, G.; Porter, D.; Grove, K.; Collins, S.; Ornberg, A.; Shulfer, R. A Comprehensive Review of Biological and Materials Properties of Tantalum and Its Alloys. *J. Biomed. Mater. Res. Part A* **2022,** *110* (6), 1291–1306.
48. Pałka, K.; Pokrowiecki, R. Porous Titanium Implants: A Review. *Adv. Eng. Mater.* **2018,** *20* (5), 1700648.
49. Gao, H.; Yang, J.; Jin, X.; Qu, X.; Zhang, F.; Zhang, D.; Chen, H.; Wei, H.; Zhang, S.; Jia, W.; Yue, B. Porous Tantalum Scaffolds: Fabrication, Structure, Properties, and Orthopedic Applications. *Mater. Design* **2021,** *210*, 110095.
50. Rahbek, O.; Kold, S.; Zippor, B.; Overgaard, S.; Søballe, K. Particle Migration and Gap Healing Around Trabecular Metal Implants. *Int. Orthopaedics* **2005,** *29*, 368–374.
51. Wang, Y.; Chai, W.; Wang, Z. G.; Zhou, Y. G.; Zhang, G. Q.; Chen, J. Y. Superelastic Cage Implantation: A New Technique for Treating Osteonecrosis of the Femoral Head with Mid-Term Follow-Ups. *J. Arthroplasty* **2009,** *24* (7), 1006–1014.
52. Wauthle, R.; Van Der Stok, J.; Yavari, S. A.; Van Humbeeck, J.; Kruth, J. P.; Zadpoor, A. A.; Weinans, H.; Mulier, M.; Schrooten, J. Additively Manufactured Porous Tantalum Implants. *Acta Biomaterialia* **2015,** *14*, 217–225.
53. Hacking, S. A.; Bobyn, J. D.; Toh, K. K.; Tanzer, M.; Krygier, J. J. Fibrous tissue ingrowth and attachment to porous tantalum. *J. Biomed. Mater. Res.* **2000,** *52* (4), 631–638.
54. Rider, P.; Kačarević ŽP, Elad, A.; Tadic, D.; Rothamel, D.; Sauer, G.; Bornert, F.; Windisch, P.; Hangyási, D. B.; Molnar, B.; Bortel, E. Biodegradable Magnesium Barrier Membrane Used for Guided Bone Regeneration in Dental Surgery. *Bioactive Mater.* **2022,** *14*, 152–168.
55. Thanigaivel, S.; Priya, A. K.; Balakrishnan, D.; Dutta, K.; Rajendran, S.; Soto-Moscoso, M. Insight on Recent Development in Metallic Biomaterials: Strategies Involving Synthesis, Types and Surface Modification for Advanced Therapeutic and Biomedical Applications. *Biochem. Eng. J.* **2022,** 108522.
56. Zhang, Z.; Jia, B.; Yang, H.; Han, Y.; Wu, Q.; Dai, K.; Zheng, Y. Zn0.8Li0.1Sr—A Biodegradable Metal with High Mechanical Strength Comparable to Pure Ti for the Treatment of Osteoporotic Bone Fractures: In Vitro and In Vivo Studies. *Biomaterials* **2021,** *275*, 120905.
57. Alvarez, K.; Nakajima, H. Metallic Scaffolds for Bone Regeneration. *Materials* **2009,** *2* (3), 790–832.
58. Miao, H.; Zhang, D.; Chen, C.; Zhang, L.; Pei, J.; Su, Y.; Huang, H.; Wang, Z.; Kang, B.; Ding, W.; Zeng, H. Research on Biodegradable Mg–Zn–Gd alloys for Potential Orthopedic Implants: In Vitro and in Vivo Evaluations. *ACS Biomater. Sci. Eng.* **2019,** *5* (3), 1623–1634.

59. De Baaij, J. H.; Hoenderop, J. G.; Bindels, R. J. Magnesium in Man: Implications for Health and Disease. *Physiol. Rev.* **2015**.
60. Volarevic, V.; Djokovic, B.; Jankovic, M. G.; Harrell, C. R.; Fellabaum, C.; Djonov, V.; Arsenijevic, N. Molecular Mechanisms of Cisplatin-Induced Nephrotoxicity: A Balance on the Knife Edge Between Renoprotection and Tumor Toxicity. *J. Biomed. Sci.* **2019,** *26* (1), 1–4.
61. Li, L.; Zhang, M.; Li, Y.; Zhao, J.; Qin, L.; Lai, Y. Corrosion and Biocompatibility Improvement of Magnesium-Based Alloys as Bone Implant Materials: A Review. *Regen. Biomater.* **2017,** *4* (2), 129–137.
62. Liu, C.; Ren, Z.; Xu, Y.; Pang, S.; Zhao, X.; Zhao, Y. Biodegradable Magnesium Alloys Developed as Bone Repair Materials: A Review. *Scanning* **2018,** *2018*.
63. Chen, Q.; Thouas, G. A. Metallic Implant Biomaterials. *Mater. Sci. Eng.: R: Rep.* **2015,** *87*, 1–57.
64. Zhou, H.; Liang, B.; Jiang, H.; Deng, Z.; Yu, K. Magnesium-Based Biomaterials as Emerging Agents for Bone Repair and Regeneration: From Mechanism to Application. *J. Magnesium Alloys* **2021,** *9* (3), 779–804.
65. Liu, Y.; Zheng, Y.; Chen, X. H.; Yang, J. A.; Pan, H.; Chen, D.; Wang, L.; Zhang, J.; Zhu, D.; Wu, S.; Yeung, K. W. Fundamental Theory of Biodegradable Metals—Definition, Criteria, and Design. *Adv. Funct. Mater.* **2019,** *29* (18), 1805402.
66. Hung, C. C.; Chaya, A.; Liu, K.; Verdelis, K.; Sfeir, C. The Role of Magnesium Ions in Bone Regeneration Involves the Canonical WNT Signaling Pathway. *Acta Biomaterialia* **2019,** *98*, 246–255.
67. Zhang, L. C.; Chen, L. Y. A Review on Biomedical Titanium Alloys: Recent Progress and Prospect. *Adv. Eng. Mater.* **2019,** *21* (4), 1801215.
68. Kaur, M.; Singh, K. Review on Titanium and Titanium Based Alloys as Biomaterials for Orthopaedic Applications. *Mater. Sci. Eng.: C* **2019,** *102*, 844–862.
69. Luo, Y. H.; Wei, H. X.; Tang, L. B.; Wang, Z. Y.; He, Z. J.; Yan, C.; Mao, J.; Dai, K.; Zheng, J. C. Nickel-Rich and Cobalt-Free Layered Oxide Cathode Materials for Lithium Ion Batteries. *Energy Storage Mater.* **2022**.
70. Mehta, N.; Hall, D. J.; Pourzal, R.; Garrigues, G. E. The Biomaterials of Total Shoulder Arthroplasty: Their Features, Function, and Effect on Outcomes. *JBJS Rev.* **2020,** *8* (9), e19.
71. Mohammad, N. F.; Ahmad, R. N.; Rosli, N. M.; Manan, M. A.; Marzuki, M.; Wahi, A. Sol Gel Deposited Hydroxyapatite-Based Coating Technique on Porous Titanium Niobium for Biomedical Applications: A Mini Review. *Mater. Today: Proc.* **2021,** *41*, 127–135.
72. Kopova, I.; Stráský, J.; Harcuba, P.; Landa, M.; Janeček, M.; Bačákova, L. Newly developed Ti–Nb–Zr–Ta–Si–Fe Biomedical Beta Titanium Alloys with Increased Strength and Enhanced Biocompatibility. *Mater. Sci. Eng.: C* **2016,** *60*, 230–238.
73. (a) Hee, H. T.; Majd, M. E.; Holt, R. T.; Pienkowski, D. Better Treatment of Vertebral Osteomyelitis Using Posterior Stabilization and Titanium Mesh Cages. *Clin. Spine Surg.* **2002,** *15* (2), 149–156. (b) Kersten, R. F. M. R.; van Gaalen, S. M.; de Gast, A.; Öner, F. C. Polyetheretherketone (PEEK) Cages in Cervical Applications: A Systematic Review. *Spine J.* **2015,** *15* (6), 1446–1460.
74. Zaharin, H. A.; Abdul Rani, A. M.; Azam, F. I.; Ginta, T. L.; Sallih, N.; Ahmad, A.; Yunus, N. A.; Zulkifli, T. Z. Effect of Unit Cell Type and Pore Size on Porosity and

Mechanical Behavior of Additively Manufactured Ti6Al4V Scaffolds. *Materials* **2018,** *11* (12), 2402.
75. Bobyn, J. D.; Pilliar, R. M.; Cameron, H. U.; Weatherly, G. C. The Optimum Pore Size for the Fixation of Porous-Surfaced Metal Implants by the Ingrowth of Bone. *Clin. Orthopaedics Relat. Res.®* **1980,** *150*, 263–270.
76. Wang, X.; Xu, S.; Zhou, S.; Xu, W.; Leary, M.; Choong, P.; Qian, M.; Brandt, M.; Xie, Y. M. Topological Design and Additive Manufacturing of Porous Metals for Bone Scaffolds and Orthopaedic Implants: A Review. *Biomaterials* **2016,** *83*, 127–141.
77. Wang, Z.; Wang, Y.; Yan, J.; Zhang, K.; Lin, F.; Xiang, L.; Deng, L.; Guan, Z.; Cui, W.; Zhang, H. Pharmaceutical Electrospinning and 3D Printing Scaffold Design for Bone Regeneration. *Adv. Drug Deliv. Rev.* **2021,** *174*, 504–534.
78. Park, S. Y.; Kim, K. H.; Kim, S.; Lee, Y. M.; Seol, Y. J. BMP-2 Gene Delivery-Based Bone Regeneration in Dentistry. *Pharmaceutics* **2019,** *11* (8), 393.
79. von Wilmowsky, C.; Moest, T.; Nkenke, E.; Stelzle, F.; Schlegel, K. A. Implants in Bone: Part, I. A Current Overview About Tissue Response, Surface Modifications and Future Perspectives. *Oral Maxillofacial Surg.* **2014,** *18*, 243–257.
80. Mahon, O. R.; Browe, D. C.; Diaz-Payno, P. J.; Pitacco, P.; Cunningham, K. T.; Mills, K. H.; Dunne, A.; Kelly, D. J. Extracellular Matrix Scaffolds Derived from Different Musculoskeletal Tissues Drive Distinct Macrophage Phenotypes and Direct Tissue-Specific Cellular Differentiation. *J. Immunol. Regen. Med.* **2021,** *12*, 100041.
81. Ramezannejad, A.; Xu, W.; Xiao, W. L.; Fox, K.; Liang, D.; Qian, M. New Insights into Nickel-Free Superelastic Titanium Alloys for Biomedical Applications. *Curr. Opin. Solid State Mater. Sci.* **2019,** *23* (6), 100783.
82. Jafary-Zadeh, M.; Praveen Kumar, G.; Branicio, P. S.; Seifi, M.; Lewandowski, J. J.; Cui, F. A Critical Review on Metallic Glasses as Structural Materials for Cardiovascular Stent Applications. *J. Funct. Biomater.* **2018,** *9* (1), 19.
83. Razavi, M. Metallic Scaffolds. *Biomater. Tissue Eng.* **2017,** *4*, 170–194.
84. Bandyopadhyay, A.; Mitra, I.; Goodman, S. B.; Kumar, M.; Bose, S. Improving Biocompatibility for Next Generation of Metallic Implants. *Progress Mater. Sci.* **2022,** 101053.
85. Choudhary, N.; Kaur, D. Shape Memory Alloy Thin Films and Heterostructures for MEMS Applications: A Review. *Sens. Actuators A: Phys.* **2016,** *242*, 162–181.
86. Sharma, N.; Kumar, K.; Kumar, V. Post-processing of NiTi Alloys: Issues and Challenges. *Powder Metall. Metal Ceram.* **2018,** *56* (9–10), 599–609.
87. Močnik, P.; Kosec, T. A Critical Appraisal of the Use and Properties of Nickel–Titanium Dental Alloys. *Materials* **2021,** *14* (24), 7859.
88. Mishnaevsky Jr., L.; Levashov, E.; Valiev, R. Z.; Segurado, J.; Sabirov, I.; Enikeev, N.; Prokoshkin, S.; Solov'yov, A. V.; Korotitskiy, A.; Gutmanas, E.; Gotman, I. Nanostructured Titanium-Based Materials for Medical Implants: Modeling and Development. *Mater. Sci. Eng: R: Rep.* **2014,** *81*, 1–9.
89. Kujala, S.; Ryhänen, J.; Danilov, A.; Tuukkanen, J. Effect of Porosity on the Osteointegration and Bone Ingrowth of a Weight-Bearing Nickel–Titanium Bone Graft Substitute. *Biomaterials* **2003,** *24* (25), 4691–4697.
90. Zhu, S. L.; Yang, X. J.; Chen, M. F.; Li, C. Y.; Cui, Z. D. Effect of Porous NiTi Alloy on Bone Formation: A Comparative Investigation with Bulk NiTi Alloy for 15 Weeks In Vivo. *Mater. Sci. Eng: C* **2008,** *28* (8), 1271–1275.

Index